S0-AZA-244

Cellular Mechanisms of Sensory Processing

The Somatosensory System

NATO ASI Series

Advanced Science Institutes Series

A series presenting the results of activities sponsored by the NATO Science Committee, which aims at the dissemination of advanced scientific and technological knowledge, with a view to strengthening links between scientific communities.

The Series is published by an international board of publishers in conjunction with the NATO Scientific Affairs Division

A Life Sciences	Plenum Publishing Corporation
B Physics	London and New York
C Mathematical and Physical Sciences	Kluwer Academic Publishers Dordrecht, Boston and London
D Behavioural and Social Sciences	
E Applied Sciences	
F Computer and Systems Sciences	Springer-Verlag Berlin Heidelberg New York
G Ecological Sciences	London Paris Tokyo Hong Kong
H Cell Biology	Barcelona Budapest
I Global Environmental Change	

NATO-PCO DATABASE

The electronic index to the NATO ASI Series provides full bibliographical references (with keywords and/or abstracts) to more than 30000 contributions from international scientists published in all sections of the NATO ASI Series. Access to the NATO-PCO DATABASE compiled by the NATO Publication Coordination Office is possible in two ways:

- via online FILE 128 (NATO-PCO DATABASE) hosted by ESRIN, Via Galileo Galilei, I-00044 Frascati, Italy.

- via CD-ROM "NATO Science & Technology Disk" with user-friendly retrieval software in English, French and German (© WTV GmbH and DATAWARE Technologies Inc. 1992).

The CD-ROM can be ordered through any member of the Board of Publishers or through NATO-PCO, Overijse, Belgium.

Series H: Cell Biology, Vol. 79

Cellular Mechanisms of Sensory Processing

The Somatosensory System

Edited by

Laszlo Urban

Sandoz Institute for Medical Research
5 Gower Place
London WC1E 6BN, U.K.

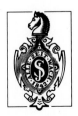

Springer-Verlag
Berlin Heidelberg New York London Paris Tokyo
Hong Kong Barcelona Budapest
Published in cooperation with NATO Scientific Affairs Division

Proceedings of the NATO Advanced Research Workshop on Cellular Mechanisms of Sensory Processing, held at Wye, Kent, U.K., April 1–3, 1993

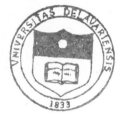

ISBN 3-540-57625-8 Springer-Verlag Berlin Heidelberg New York
ISBN 0-387-57625-8 Springer-Verlag New York Berlin Heidelberg

Library of Congress Cataloging-in-Publication Data.
NATO Advanced Research Workshop on Cellular Mechanisms of Sensory Processing (1993: Wye, England) Cellular mechanisms of sensory processing: the somatosensory system / edited by Laszlo Urban. p. cm. – (NATO ASI series. Series H. Cell biology; vol. 79)
"Proceedings of the NATO Advanced Research Workshop on Cellular Mechanisms of Sensory Processing, held at Wye, Kent, U.K., April 1-3, 1993" – T.p. verso.
Includes bibliographical references and index. ISBN 0-387-57625-8 (acid-free paper: New York). – ISBN 3-540-57625-8 (acid-free paper: Berlin). 1. Skin–Innervation–Congresses. 2. Sensory receptors–Congresses. 3. Ganglia, Sensory–Congresses. 4. Afferent pathways–Congresses. I. Urban, Laszlo, 1951- . II. Title. III. Series. QP369.N36 1993 599'.0182–dc20 93-46741

This work is subject to copyright. All rights are reserved, whether the whole or part of the material is concerned, specifically the rights of translation, reprinting, reuse of illustrations, recitation, broadcasting, reproduction on microfilm or in any other way, and storage in data banks. Duplication of this publication or parts thereof is permitted only under the provisions of the German Copyright Law of September 9, 1965, in its current version, and permission for use must always be obtained from Springer-Verlag. Violations are liable for prosecution under the German Copyright Law.

© Springer-Verlag Berlin Heidelberg 1994
Printed in Germany

Typesetting: Camera ready by authors
31/3145 - 5 4 3 2 1 0 - Printed on acid-free paper

PREFACE

The research field of somatosensory processing in mammals has experienced revolutionary changes in recent years. Accumulation of basic and clinical data has greatly accelerated, and new phenomena have emerged. With the aid of new, refined methods, molecular and cellular changes have been described, underlying the signal transduction-transmission between the internal/external environment and the central nervous system have been described. The discovery of the interaction between the nervous and the immune system has, for example changed our view on the development of inflammatory diseases, while the cloning of genes encoding different trophic factors has boosted studies revealing profound changes in the regeneration of neurons, and induction of changes in phenotype. The study of the pre- and postsynaptic modulation of transmitter release, and the examination of the combined effects of amino acid and peptide transmitters has become recently possible by using cultured cell lines and in vitro techniques. Although it is in embryonic state, computational properties of single DRG cells under normal and pathological conditions are being investigated. Results soon or later will have a great impact on pain research and consequently ultimately in clinical pain management.

This brief introduction indicates how our knowledge of the somatosensory system has increased dramatically recently. However, many investigators cultivate only a very specific field in the growing area of somatosensory research and find it difficult to integrate a more universal knowledge of their work. To process the large body of information requires interaction between scientists investigating different aspects of the same system or phenomen. On the other hand some aspects in somatosensory research are neglected because of technical difficulties (e.g. signal transduction in peripheral receptors). In this case results derived from studies in non-neural systems or in lower vertebrates may fill the gap and provide information for further studies.

Given this background, we organised a symposium, to provide the opportunity for integration of expertise in studying the function of the somatosensory system at the cellular level. The content of this book is based on the presentations at this NATO Advanced Research Workshop with the title *The Cellular Mechanisms of Sensory Processing*, held in Wye College (United Kingdom) from 31th March to 3rd April 1993.

As almost all speakers contributed to the book, the sequence of the presentations is reflected in the organisation of the chapters. Authors were deliberately given freedom to decide on the material which they wanted to present and discuss, and so some chapters provide more results and speculative discussion while others incorporate less data and focus on reviewing recent development. In order to give some structure to the book, chapters wich give a review of a certain area will preceed others which present more original findings. We believe that this format is particularly important in this book, because of the diversity of topics discussed.

I regret that even though the primary afferents and the spinal cord are a "fragment" of the sensory nervous system they are far more complicated than all of the aspects of present research concerning this area could be properly discussed within a workshop and presented in a coveringing book. Even as the meeting and the publication concentrate solely on cellular mechanisms, there remain many gaps which could be filled. Unfortunately we could not invite all colleagues working in this field therefore the book may represent debatable views, but I hope that it gives the reader a general view on the recent development and hot topics in the research field of the somatosensory system.

The chapters of his book were reviewed by the chairmen of each session which made inevitable delays, but the organising committee thought it necessary for the benefit of the publication. We encouraged the contributors to discuss controversial issues and allowed the presentation of unpublished original, even controversial, observations. Therefore some chapters contain data which are open to criticism with the view that they may trigger further experimental work and debate.

The workshop was sponsored by the Scientific Affairs Division of NATO. We would like to express our appreciation to NATO for the finantial support and help. We are most grateful to the Wellcome Trust to fund the attendance of young British scientists and to Sandoz Institute for Medical Research, Ily Lilly, Amersham and Pfizer for finantial support.

I am most grateful to Dr Andy Dray, Prof. Srdija Jeftinija, Prof. Peter W Reeh and Prof. Clifford J. Woolf who helped to organise the meeting as members of the organising committee. I was fortunate to have some enthusiastic colleagues, Dr Alyson J. Fox, Dr Istvan Nagy and Dr Stephen W.N. Thompson, who gave their best professional skills to run the meeting, and Miss Amanda Noble who helped me with the secretarial work. I wish to offer my thanks to all of the contributors and to everyone who helped with this project.

L. A. Urban

I wish to dedicate this book to Prof. Patrick D. Wall whose contribution made a major impact on our present understanding of the spinal sensory processing.

AUTHOR INDEX

Abbadie, C., 449

Baranauskas, G., 255
Belmonte, C., 87
Ben-Ari, Y., 161
Besson, J.-M., 449
Bond, A., 173
Bregestovski, P., 161

Dolphin, A.C., 47
Dray, A., 273, 379

Felipe, C., 297
French, A.S., 19

Gallar, J., 87
Gebhart, G.F., 401

Henry, J.L., 231
Holzer, P., 133
Honore, P., 449
Hunt, S.P., 297

Iadarola, M.J., 313

Jeftinija, S., 185
Jeftinija, K., 185
Jenkins, R., 297

Lecci, A., 217
Lev-Tov, A., 151
Liu, F., 185
Lodge, D., 173
Lopez-Briones, L.G. 87
Lücke, T., 195

Maggi, C.A., 217
Medina, I., 161
Meller, S.T., 401
Mendell, L.M., 3
Menon-Johansson, A., 47
Messersmith, D.J., 313

Nagy, I., 379
Neugebauer, V., 195

Nistri, A. 255

Pinco, M., 151
Pozo, M.A., 87

Radhakrishnan, V., 231
Reeh, P.W., 119

Schaible, H.-G., 195, 289
Schäfer, K.-H., 337
Schmidt, R.F., 289
Stoney, S.D. Jr., 63
Surprenant, A., 35
Sweeney, M.I., 47

Thompson, S.W.N., 379

Urban, L., 379

Weihe, E., 337
Wiesenfeld-Hallin, Zs., 361
Willis, W.D. Jr., 421
Xu, X.-J., 361
Woolf, C.J., 473

CHARACTERIZATION OF THE PRIMARY AFFERENT

DIVERSITY OF SOMATIC SPIKES IN DORSAL ROOT GANGLION
CELLS: IMPLICATIONS FOR DEVELOPMENT, FUNCTION AND
PLASTICITY
Lorne M. Mendell..3

ION CHANNELS UNDERLYING TRANSDUCTION AND ADAPTATION
IN MECHANORECEPTORS
Andrew S. French...19

SIGNAL TRANSDUCTION PROCESSES IN SENSORIMOTOR
NEURONES OF THE ENTERIC NERVOUS SYSTEM
Annmarie Surprenant 35

MODULATION OF VOLTAGE DEPENDENT CALCIUM CHANNELS
BY GABA$_B$ RECEPTORS AND G PROTEINS IN CULTURED RAT
DORSAL ROOT GANGLION NEURONS: RELEVANCE
TO TRANSMITTER RELEASE AND ITS MODULATION
Annette C. Dolphin, Anatole Menon-Johansson, Veronica Campbell,
Nick Berrow and Marva I. Sweeney 47

SIGNAL INTEGRATION IN THE AXON TREE DUE TO BRANCH
POINT FILTERING ACTION
S. David Stoney, Jr...63

POLYMODALITY IN NOCICEPTIVE NEURONS: EXPERIMENTAL
MODELS OF CHEMOTRANSDUCTION
Carlos Belmonte, Juana Gallar, Laura G. Lopez-Briones
and Miguel A. Pozo 87

CHEMICAL EXCITATION AND SENSITIZATION OF NOCICEPTORS
Peter W. Reeh...119

LOCAL EFFECTOR FUNCTIONS OF PRIMARY AFFERENT
NERVE FIBERS
Peter Holzer...133

TRANSMITTERS IN THE SOMATOSENSORY SYSTEM
(SYNAPTOLOGY OF THE SPINAL CORD)

EXITATORY AMINO ACID RECEPTORS IN THE IN VITRO
MAMMALIAN SPINAL CORD
Aharon Lev-Tov and M. Pinco 151

MODULATION OF NMDA CURRENTS IN HIPPOCAMPAL NEURONS
Pìotr Bregestovski, Igor Medina and Yezekiel Ben-Ari...................................161

EXCITATORY AMINO ACID RECEPTORS IN THE SPINAL CORD
David Lodge and Ann Bond...173

EXCITATORY AMINO ACID RELEASE IN DORSAL ROOT GANGLION
CULTURES
Fang Liu, Ksenija Jeftinija and Srdija Jeftinija 185

THE INVOLVEMENT OF EXCITATORY AMINO ACIDS AND THEIR
RECEPTORS IN THE SPINAL PROCESSING OF NOCICEPTIVE
INPUT FROM THE NORMAL AND INFLAMED KNEE
JOINT IN THE RAT
Hans-Georg Schaible, Volker Neugebauer, Thomas Lücke...........................195

TACHYKININ RECEPTORS AND THEIR ANTAGONISTS
Carlo Alberto Maggi and Alessandro Lecci 217

SYNAPTIC ACTIVATION BY THE RELEASE OF PEPTIDES
J.L. Henry and V. Radhakrishnan...231

TRH AND SUBSTANCE P INCREASE RAT MOTONEURONE
EXCITABILITY THROUGH A BLOCK OF A NOVEL K+ CONDUCTANCE
A. Nistri, N.D. Fisher And G. Baranauskas...255

DYNAMIC CHANGES IN THE SENSORY SYSTEM

INFLUENCES OF THE CHEMICAL ENVIRONMENT ON PERIPHERAL
AFFERENT NEURONS
Andy Dray..273

SILENT PRIMARY AFFERENTS
Robert F. Schmidt and H.-G. Schaible 289

SENSORY NEURONS AND PLASTICITY: THE ROLE OF IMMEDIATE
EARLY GENES
Carmen De Felipe, Robert Jenkins and Stephen P. Hunt 297

MOLECULAR BIOLOGY OF DYNORPHIN GENE EXPRESSION IN
RELATIONSHIP TO SPINAL CORD PROCESSING OF PAIN
Michael J.Iadarola and Donna J. Messerschmith...313

REGULATION OF CELLULAR PHENOTYPE IN THE NOCICEPTIVE
PATHWAY
Eberhard Weihe and Martin K.-H. Schafer 337

ALTERED FUNCTIONS OF NEUROPEPTIDES AND NITRIC OXIDE
IN SOMATOSENSORY AFFERENTS AND SPINAL CORD AFTER
PERIPHERAL NERVE LESIONS IN THE RAT
Zsuzsanna Wiesenfeld-Hallin and Xiao-Jun Xu...361

HYPEREXCITABILTY IN THE SPINAL DORSAL HORN:
COOPERATION OF NEUROPEPTIDES AND EXCITATORY
AMINO ACIDS
Laszlo Urban, Stephen W. N. Thompson, Istvan Nagy and Andy Dray 379

THE ROLE OF NITRIC OXIDE IN HYPERALGESIA
Stephen T. Meller and G.F. Gebhart 401

DYNAMIC CHANGES IN DORSAL HORN NEURONS
William D. Willis, Jr. 421

POSTSYNAPTIC CHANGES DURING SUSTAINED PRIMARY
AFFERENT FIBER STIMULATION AS REVEALED BY C-FOS
IMMUNOHISTOCHEMISTRY IN THE RAT SPINAL CORD
Catherine Abbadie, Prisca Honoré and Jean-Marie Besson 449

STRUCTURAL PLASTICITY OF PRIMARY AFFERENT TERMINALS
IN THE ADULT DORSAL HORN - REGENERATIVE SPROUTING
INDUCED BY PERIPHERAL NERVE INJURY
Clifford J. Woolf 473

SUBJECT INDEX 499

CHARACTERIZATION OF THE PRIMARY AFFERENT

DIVERSITY OF SOMATIC SPIKES IN DORSAL ROOT GANGLION CELLS: IMPLICATIONS FOR DEVELOPMENT, FUNCTION AND PLASTICITY

Lorne M. Mendell
Department of Neurobiology and Behavior
State University of New York at Stony Brook
Stony Brook, NY 11794
USA

INTRODUCTION

Dorsal root ganglion cells are superficially similar in that they all innervate a target in the periphery and project into the spinal cord. However, it has been appreciated for many decades that these neurons are in fact quite heterogeneous in their projections, both peripherally and centrally (for review see Willis and Coggeshall[55]). In the periphery individual cells can innervate receptors in skin, muscles, joints or viscera, and their laminar targets in the spinal cord are also quite diverse. It is important to appreciate that peripheral and central innervation is highly correlated so that, for example, neurons innervating muscle spindles project principally to laminae VI, VII and IX whereas C-fiber nociceptors project primarily into lamina II. These periphero- central correlations have been extremely important in determining the sensory channels through which individual modalities project in the spinal cord (for review see Willis and Coggeshall[55]).

In the last 2 decades it has become evident that individual dorsal root ganglion cells have intrinsic differences beyond their targets, both peripheral and central (see review: Koerber and Mendell[32]). These physiological differences extend well beyond axonal conduction velocity which has long been known to vary widely and to a certain extent systematically among dorsal root ganglion cells of different functional types. Recording from dorsal root ganglion cells *in vitro* has demonstrated that these neurons fall into 3 categories according to the configuration and properties

NATO ASI Series, Vol. H 79
Cellular Mechanisms of Sensory Processing
Edited by Laszlo Urban
© Springer-Verlag Berlin Heidelberg 1994

of their spikes.[58] At one extreme is spikes with relatively small amplitude, fast peak rate of rise and brief AHP (Figure 1, top). This spike is blocked by application of TTX. At the other extreme is a TTX-insensitive spike of relatively large amplitude with a slow peak rate of rise and a long AHP (Figure 1, bottom). This spike differs from the fast spike described above in having a characteristic hump on the falling limb. A third group of spikes is relatively long in duration, TTX-insensitive and has a long AHP; however, it exhibits no hump on the falling phase.

IONIC CURRENTS DETERMINING SPIKE CONFIGURATION

It is now clear that the differences in spike properties among DRG neurons are associated with differences in their ionic currents. The most definitive evidence for this is the division of these neurons into those whose somatic spikes are resistant or sensitive to TTX (see reviews: Koerber and Mendell[32], Nowycky[43]). Since the TTX-insensitive Na^+ current tends to have slower activation and inactivation time constants than the TTX-sensitive Na^+ current,[35] this factor could play an important role in the differences in peak rate of rise that have been reported[22,30] (but see[32]). Voltage clamp studies reveal that virtually all neurons have a mixture of TTX-sensitive and TTX-resistant Na^+ channels[35], and that the degree of Na^+ inward current surviving TTX administration reflects the relative proportions of these two types. Axons of cells with TTX-sensitive and TTX-resistant somatic spikes are sensitive to TTX.[47]

Most workers have attributed the hump seen on the descending limb of the spike to a Ca^{++} current.[10,16,46,58] These experiments were done in chick or in rodent and involved the use either of Ca^{++}-free solutions or Ca^{++} channel blockers. However, in recent experiments in bullfrog DRG neurons the TTX-resistant broad spikes were found to be totally abolished in Na^+-free solutions suggesting that in some cases the entire current is carried by Na^+ ions.[41]

Several different K^+ currents have been reported in mammalian DRG cells, including the delayed rectifier, the fast transient K^+ current (I_A), the inward rectifier (I_R) and the Ca^{++}-activated K^+ current (I_{Ca}) (see rev.[43]). The inward rectifying K^+ current has been reported to be larger in cells with myelinated axons than in those with unmyelinated axons.[17,18] Consistent with this is the finding that the inward rectifier is much weaker in cells with broad spikes (which includes all those with unmyelinated axons: see later) than in those with narrow spikes[30] (all of which have myelinated axons: see later). I_{Ca} has also been suggested to be vary among DRG neurons, being largest among the small cells that tend to generate larger AHPs (see rev.[43]). The observed variations in both these K^+ currents would tend to reduce the magnitude and duration of the after-hyperpolarization in the soma of myelinated afferents with narrow spikes.

Recent work by Campbell[4] in frog DRG neurons has demonstrated heterogeneity in Na^+ and K^+ channels among cells of different sizes. These studies were carried out under conditions known to minimise the Ca^{++} current. The very largest cells had only TTX-sensitive Na^+ channels although a minority of small cells also exhibited TTX-sensitive Na^+ channels only. Cells with a mix of TTX-sensitive and TTX-insensitive channels tended to be smaller in size. Large cells expressing only TTX-sensitive Na^+ channels tended to have K^+ channels with rapid activation time (similar to I_A - see review by Nowycky[43]). Conversely small cells with significant amounts of TTX-insensitive Na^+ channels had K^+ channels with longer activation time constants (similar to the delayed rectifier). A second group of small cells exhibited TTX-sensitive Na^+ channels and slowly activating K^+ channels. These data suggest that the largest DRG cells are homogeneous in having TTX-sensitive Na^+ channels and K^+ channels with rapid kinetics. The smallest cells are heterogeneous in their properties. Thus these channel properties are consonant with the action potential width measurements from these cells, with narrow spikes tending to have TTX-sensitive Na^+ and rapid K^+ channels whereas those with broad spikes have some TTX-insensitive Na^+ channels and the slow K^+ channels (Figure 1). A third group of cells, small in size, with TTX-sensitive Na^+ channels and slowly activating K^+ channels, would be expected to have somatic spikes intermediate in duration.

Ca^{++} channels are also reported to be differentially distributed among small and large DRG neurons[50,51,52]. Ca^{++} currents in the soma of sensory neurons have recently been shown to be divisible into (at least) 3 physiologically and pharmacologically distinct components[14], the N-, L- and T-channels. Small neurons in both frog and rat express both the L- and N- channel components whereas Ca^{++} current in large DRG cells of the frog is carried almost entirely by N-channels. Quantitative data in the rat[52] indicate that the L-channel carries a much larger fraction of the whole cell Ca^{++} current in small cells (20-27 µm) than in large cells (45-51 µM) whereas the fraction carried by N-channels is about the same across the entire size spectrum. T-channels have been found to be maximally expressed in medium-sized (33-38 µm) and small cells but not in large ones. These data suggest that L-type channels are confined to small cells which tend to be those with broad spikes (Figure 1; see Discussion).

CORRELATIONS OF SPIKE TYPE AND SENSORY RECEPTORS

The correlations just discussed have involved DRG cell size and it has been noted that particularly among small cells there is considerable heterogeneity in channel properties. Cell size is a relatively easy parameter to quantify, particularly in in vitro preparations, but it is well established that it is not strongly related to cell function (see review[55]). The lack of correlation between cell size and function is particularly marked for small cells where the smallest cells with unmyelinated axons, C-fibers, can innervate nociceptors or low threshold mechanoreceptors. The same is true of the smallest myelinated afferents, those with A-delta axons, which can innervate either low or high threshold receptors in the periphery.

AXON TYPE	SPIKE SHAPE	MECHANICAL THRESHOLD	g_{Na}	g_K	g_{Ca}	TRANS-MITTER
Aβ ---------- Aδ	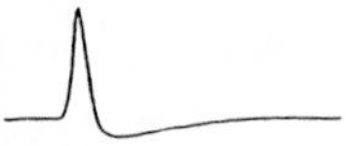	Low	TTX+	Rapidly-Activating -------------------- Slowly-Activating	N	Amino Acid
Aβ Aδ C	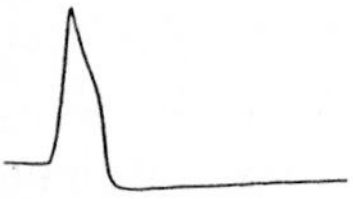	High	TTX+ TTX-	Slowly-Activating	N,L	Amino Acid, Peptide

Fig. 1. Correlation of properties in DRG cells with narrow and broad spikes. Cells with narrow spikes have A-beta or A- delta axons, and the spikes are TTX-sensitive. Cells with broad spikes can have A-beta, A-delta or C-fiber axons, and their spikes are resistant to TTX because of the presence of a relatively large proportion of TTX-insensitive Na+ channels. From studies of K+ and Ca++ channels as a function of cell size, it is speculated that large somata with narrow spikes have rapidly activating K+ channels as well as N-type Ca++ channels. As discussed in the text there is a population of small neurons with TTX-sensitive Na+ channels and slowly activating K+ channels which might correspond to low threshold A-delta afferents (D-Hairs). It is further speculated that these N channels are expressed in the synaptic terminals and that they are responsible for release of amino acids from these cells. In contrast somata with broad spikes have have slowly activating K+ channels and both N- and L-type Ca++ channels. The role of T-channels in this scheme is not considered, mainly because of their less certain role in transmitter release. However, since they are expressed mainly in small- and medium-sized cells, probably in cells with broad spikes. It is speculated that the additional L-channels in these cells are responsible for the release of peptides.

Experiments correlating electrophysiological properties of the soma with functional properties of the axon have been carried out largely *in vivo*. Membrane properties have been measured in terms of spike properties rather than the underlying ionic channel properties. One of the major concerns has been to determine whether it is cell size or receptor type innervated that is best correlated with the electrophysiological properties of the soma.

Cells in the nodose ganglion innervate 2 types of sensory receptors: baroreceptors and chemoreceptors. Belmonte and Gallego[3] demonstrated that baroreceptors have narrow spikes, resembling those described above as Type F whereas cells innervating chemoreceptors generated broad spikes with humps on the descending limb characteristic of Type H-neurons. Chemoreceptors have conduction velocities which are generally lower than those of these baroreceptors and so this system is not diagnostic for the question whether cell spike properties are associated with cell size or peripheral innervation. However, there is a population of baroreceptors with a low axonal conduction velocity; their spikes are broad like those of the chemoreceptors. Therefore, in this case the spike type appears to be more correlated with axonal conduction velocity than with receptor type.

Studies of neurons of the dorsal root ganglion have revealed that neurons with broad spikes innervate a special group of sensory receptors, the nociceptors (Figure 1). Among myelinated afferents (A-beta and A-delta afferents), these differences between nociceptors and non nociceptors are observed over the entire fiber size distribution.[12,30,47,49] Using either axonal conduction velocity or soma input resistance as a measure of cell size it is clear that in this portion of the axonal fiber spectrum receptor type rather than axonal conduction velocity is the major correlate of spike type. Among low threshold myelinated afferents with TTX-sensitive spikes, those with A-delta axons have broader spikes than those with A-beta axons[47], in agreement with the distribution of slowly and rapidly activating K^+ channels in small and large cells with TTX-sensitive Na channels[4] (Figure 1).

Among neurons with unmyelinated afferents (C-fibers) the situation is somewhat different. All these neurons have very broad spikes regardless of whether they innervate low or high threshold mechanoreceptors.[54] Thus in these neurons the spike appears to be determined by axonal conduction velocity rather than by receptor type.

DEVELOPMENTAL CORRELATIONS

Studies in neonatal animals have revealed that spike shape changes considerably over the neonatal period[15]. At birth virtually all cells have broad spikes with humps on their descending limb, but by the time the animal is 2 weeks of age, the spikes have become heterogeneous with respect to their shape with some being broad and others being narrow. Despite the similarity of spike shape at birth TTX sensitivity indicates some differentiation of membrane properties since some neurons (presumptive C neurons) have TTX-resistant spikes whereas others (presumptive A neurons) are only partially TTX-resistant. In addition presumptive A-neurons have lower thresholds to spike initiation by intracellular depolarization than C neurons. Thus C neurons exhibit very little change in spike and membrane properties during this 2 week postnatal period, whereas A neuron spikes become narrower and more sensitive to TTX. However, as pointed out above, even at 2 weeks the properties of A neurons are heterogeneous with some spikes having no inflection on the descending limb of the spike whereas others have such a component.

The changes in spike properties in development, i.e., the narrowing of the spike, has been studied most completely in Rohon Beard cells and spinal neurons.[1,44] Studies of populations at different stages of development have led to the conclusion that inward and outward currents change. Initially, inward current is carried largely by Ca^{++} although Na^+ current is also present in these neurons. As the cell matures the Ca^{++}/Na^+ current ratio tends to decrease overall, although the heterogeneity in spike shape seen in adults suggests a broad spectrum in these changes. In addition, an increase in the delayed rectifier as well as in Ca^{++}-dependent K^+ current has been reported which presumably would contribute to the narrowing of the spike.[44]

One of the implications of these observations is that myelinated nociceptors with broad spikes express properties of immature neurons even in the adult. This may be of importance in making inferences concerning the potential targets in the DRG for certain neurotrophins (see below).

TARGET FOR TROPHIC FACTORS

It is known from a wide variety of studies that cells of the dorsal root ganglion are targets for the action of Nerve Growth Factor (NGF). In very young animals NGF acts as a survival factor: in its absence many sensory neurons, particularly the small, peptidergic ones, fail to survive (see review[2]). However, high- affinity NGF receptors are expressed on neurons well beyond the period during which they are crucial for survival, i.e., beyond postnatal day 2.[38] One can ask whether it is only cells, which are immature as indicated by their spike shape, that are susceptible to NGF excess or deprivation beyond the survival period.

Physiological studies of the effects of administration of the antibody to NGF (anti-NGF) or excess NGF have revealed highly selective effects directed towards sensory neurons that signal nociception. Administration of NGF or anti-NGF in the immediate postnatal period has small but consistent effects on spike properties in afferents with myelinated axons, NGF tending to broaden the spike and anti-NGF tending to narrow it.[47] These effects are directed towards the subpopulation of cells with broad spikes that innervate HTMRs (high-threshold mechanoreceptors). At present the specific conductances regulated by NGF are not known although the fact that peak rate of rise is not affected whereas the duration of the falling phase is would tend to suggest the involvement of one of the K^+ or Ca^{++} conductances. It is tempting to speculate that the factor making these cells sensitive to regulation by NGF is the presence of the broad spike (and the metabolic and ionic processes implied by such a spike). However, it is important to recall that during the period of sensitivity, i.e., the postnatal period, most cells have broad spikes (see above), and so it is difficult to be certain that this property per se is the determining factor.

The effects of NGF and anti-NGF have also been studied on neurons maintained in organotypic culture.[6] It is interesting that under these conditions the effects of NGF and anti-NGF on spike properties are opposite to what has been reported in vivo, i.e., NGF narrows the spike and anti-NGF broadens it. It is difficult to reconcile these observations at present except to point out that the in vitro experiments have been carried out on neurons which are at a very different developmental stage. Furthermore these neurons are axotomized, and thus may have very different trophic support than neurons studied in vivo. The selectivity of NGF for nociceptive afferents has several additional manifestations. For example, administration of anti-NGF over a postnatal critical period results in a depletion of A-delta HTMRs in the absence of cell death.[38,48] The evidence from analysis of the adequate stimulus for single afferents in these preparations is that HTMRs are converted to a low threshold mechanoreceptor, the D-Hair. Since the spike properties of these 2 types of afferent are so different (the D-hair afferent has a narrow spike whereas the HTMR has a broad spike with a hump on the descending limb), one can investigate whether the membrane properties of these converted or respecified afferents are also changed. This appears to be the case based on finding no sensory fibers innervating D-hairs with HTMR-like broad spikes in anti-NGF treated animals[47]. In addition, NGF and anti-NGF administered in the neonatal period decrease[39] and increase,[38] respectively, the mechanical threshold of HTMRs. It is not clear at present whether these changes are in any way related to the presumptive ionic channel changes underlying the alterations in somatic spike properties.

AXOTOMY AND REGENERATION OF PRIMARY AFFERENTS

When the peripheral axon of a primary afferent is cut the properties of the spike are largely unaffected.[8,20] When axons regenerate into the periphery, they reinnervate sensory receptors which generally exhibit properties similar to those seen in intact animals (see review by Johnson and Munson[28]). An interesting question concerns the match between peripheral receptor type and dorsal root ganglion spike type and whether this is completely restored. Present evidence (Koerber and Mendell, in preparation) indicates that the match between spike width and receptor type seen in intact animals is largely although not completely restored. However, it cannot be decided at present whether this represents selective reinnervation or adaptation following random reinnervation.

When a transected muscle nerve is redirected to reinnervate the hairy skin, individual large diameter muscle afferents innervating hairs are found to have slow adaptation properties in response to natural stimulation of their cutaneous receptors[28,42]. Similar conclusions were reached by Lewin and MacMahon[37] and Koerber et al.[33]. The significance of this finding is that afferents innervating hairs normally adapt rapidly, i.e., there is no maintained discharge in response to maintained deflection of the hair. However, when these hairs are reinnervated by a muscle nerve, whose receptors are normally virtually all slowly adapting, most of the afferents now exhibit a discharge in response to maintained deflection of the hair. Similarly skin afferents forced to reinnervate muscle tend to be more rapidly adapting than those in normal muscle. Thus the results of these cross unions are reciprocal and both suggest that adaptation rate is a property of the nerve fiber rather than the receptor. Although this is likely to be a membrane property of the sensory fiber, spike properties do not segregate among slowly adapting and rapidly adapting fibers. For example, it is difficult to detect consistent differences between spikes of slowly adapting SA1 afferents and rapidly adapting hair afferents.[30] It is interesting that rapidly- and slowly-adapting afferents also differ consistently in their central actions, specifically in their ability to evoke responses of maintained amplitude during repetitive stimulation.[31,34] Thus peripheral and central adaptation appear to be correlated, but it is presently difficult to attribute these properties to a membrane specialization in the sensory ganglion cell.

The upshot of these experiments is the indication that the intrinsic properties of the sensory neuron play an important role in its encoding process. However, the somatic spike may not be the parameter that correlates with these properties.

WHAT IS THE FUNCTIONAL CONSEQUENCE OF THE DIFFERENCES IN SPIKE PROPERTIES?

A number of investigators have questioned the significance of these different spikes given the fact that the soma is not directly in the path between the periphery and the spinal cord. The possibility that the somal membrane acts as an element in a low pass filter has been discounted.[17,26,53] Although cells with broad spikes do exhibit blockade during high frequency stimulation, the failure appears to occur at the T-junction so that blockade of the orthodromically travelling spike into both the soma and the dorsal root occurs. The major determining factor appears to be not the spike shape but rather the degree of myelination of the axon branches in the vicinity of the T-shaped junction.[23]

Numerous authors have suggested that the somal membrane properties are indicative of properties of synaptic membrane and of the sensory ending. Thus they have explored to what extent synaptic properties or sensory transducer properties correspond with the somal membrane properties. In the periphery there has been a report that the adaptation rate of mechanoreceptors is correlated with the ability of the neuron to maintain a steady discharge in response to steady depolarization of the soma.[21] Kirchhoff et al.[29] have demonstrated that TTX sensitivity of sensory endings varies and matches that measured at the soma. However, Belmonte and Gallego[3] reported that steady depolarization of the somata of chemoreceptors evoked only a single spike in contrast to the steady discharge elicited by the adequate stimulus applied to their peripheral receptors.

Correlations have been found between properties of the soma and those of the synaptic terminals. Jia and Nelson[27] demonstrated that the depression of synaptic currents during repetitive stimulation of sensory or spinal neurons of adult mouse in culture corresponds to the amount of depression of somatic Ca^{++} currents during similar stimulation. Dunlap and Fischbach,[13] in noting that exogenous GABA shortens the somatic spike, have speculated that the action of axo-axonic synapses in causing pre-synaptic inhibition occurs via blockade of Ca^{++} channels (probably N-channels[19]) in the terminals.

DISCUSSION

The degree of differentiation of dorsal root ganglia somata is striking in view of their apparently minor role in transmitting impulses from the periphery to the spinal cord. The membrane differences in the soma implied by these differences in spike parameters do not predict the functional differences in sensory receptor or synaptic terminals in these different classes of cells. Correspondence of sensory or synaptic properties to the somal membrane will require investigation of the membrane properties of these somata in greater detail than is possible by inference from spike properties.

The recording of spike properties has revealed one very robust dividing line between cells, namely those that generate spikes with broad spikes having a hump on the descending limb and those having narrow spikes. Cells with broad spikes would be expected to accumulate a greater amount of Ca^{++} than cells with narrow spikes in response to activity. This accumulation would depend on which Ca^{++} channels are available and their conductance, which is subject to modulation[13] (see discussion in[51,52]). This Ca^{++} might initiate a sequence of biochemical changes that would be important for their function. In considering the possibilities one can begin by asking how changes in activity levels affect cells with broad spikes in a manner that is different from those with narrow spikes.

Recently, it has been reported that A-delta and C nociceptive neurons, which would be anticipated to have broad spikes, are the most prone of sensory neurons to undergo collateral sprouting in the skin in response to partial denervation of a neighbouring target[11]. It is interesting that impulse activity in these nociceptors has been found to accelerate this process[9] suggesting that activity- dependent Ca^{++} influx into these neurons could trigger the metabolic changes resulting in collateral sprouting of their terminals.

Dorsal root ganglion cells with broad spikes that innervate mechanoreceptors are nociceptors (disregarding for the moment that some unmyelinated afferents are low threshold mechanoreceptors). In the periphery these cells exhibit the property of sensitization by which they generate more activity in response to successive adequate stimuli, generally nociceptive ones.[5,7] Corresponding differences have been reported for the central effects exerted by these afferents in the spinal cord. One of the earliest such findings was a form of central sensitization referred to as "windup", whereby spinal neurons responded with increasing discharges to successive volleys at rates of at least 0.25 Hz in C fibers.[40] More recently,[31] the first of a pair of stimuli delivered to a single afferent fiber with a broad somatic spike has been shown to facilitate the response to a test stimulus delivered 50 ms later. For afferents with narrow spikes the conditioning effect is either to depress the test response or to facilitate it only slightly. Although it is tempting to attribute these effects directly to the channels underlying the broad somatic spike, i.e., to the enhanced Ca^{++} entry, this seems very unlikely to be the entire explanation given the relatively short duration of enhanced intracellular Ca^{++}. It seems more likely that the sensitization, both peripheral and central, is the consequence of the release of peptides known to be present in these cells and not in large diameter, low threshold afferents which do not elicit such effects.[55] In the periphery release of peptides such as substance P are responsible for initiating the inflammatory response which in turn leads to sensitization of nociceptors (see review by Campbell et al.[5]). In the spinal cord windup has been attributed to long lasting responses evoked by peptide release (see review by Woolf[56]). It has also been suggested that bursts of impulses confined to small diameter afferents, particularly C-fibers, initiate heterosynaptic facilitation of a flexor reflex that can last for many minutes to hours as a result of peptide release from the C- fibers.[57] The role of low threshold mechanoreceptors with unmyelinated axons and broad spikes is uncertain in this connection. These neurons terminate mostly in the inner layer of lamina II of the spinal cord,[45] where the terminals react positively for fluoride-resistant acid phosphatase (FRAP) but not for the peptides typically associated with small diameter afferents (see review by Hunt et al.[25]). They presumably have a different function than large diameter, low threshold mechanoreceptors, but this is not presently known.

One speculation is that the release of peptides requires large or long lasting Ca^{++} currents that would not be available in cells generating narrow spikes (Figure 1). This line of reasoning is based on the assumption that ion channels in the soma are replicated in the terminals (see Discussion[52]). Dunlap and her colleagues[24] have demonstrated that depolarization-induced release of substance P from chick sensory neurons in culture, as well as the broad somatic spike, are co-regulated by

Ca^{++}-channel activity, most clearly L-channels but perhaps also N-channels (see also,[36] for T-channels see legend to Figure 1). More recently, N-channels have been shown to be associated with glutamate release from sensory axons responsible for fast EPSPs.[19] The data of Scroggs and Fox[50,51,52] suggest that small sensory neurons with broad spikes, releasing both amino acids and peptides, have both N and L channels whereas large cells with narrow spikes, releasing amino acids, have only N-type Ca^{++} channels. Altogether, then, there appears to be an association between the broad spike, L-channels and peptide release, and between narrow spikes, N-channels and amino acid release (Figure 1). The place of low threshold C-fiber afferents with broad spikes in this scheme is unknown. They may release peptides that are different from those for which markers are currently available.

These considerations are highly speculative, as they rely on many assumptions concerning the role of Ca^{++} channels, but they emphasise that the ionic channels associated with the broad spikes of nociceptive sensory neurons may play an important role in determining at least some activity-dependent plasticity in their actions.

ACKNOWLEDGEMENT: The experiments in the author's laboratory were supported by NIH: R01-NS16996 (Javits Neuroscience Award) and NS P01- 14899.

REFERENCES

1. BACCAGLINI, P.I. AND SPITZER, N.C. (1977) Developmental changes in the inward current of the action potential of Rohon-Beard neurones. *J. Physiol.* **271**, 93-117.
2. BARDE, Y. (1989) Trophic factors and neuronal survival. *Neuron* **2**, 1525-1534.
3. BELMONTE, C. AND GALLEGO, R. (1983) Membrane properties of cat sensory neurones with chemoreceptor and baroreceptor endings. *J. Physiol.* **342**, 603-614.
4. CAMPBELL, D.T. (1992) Large and small vertebrate sensory neurons express different Na and K channel subtypes. *Proc. Nat. Acad. Sci.* **89**, 9569-9573.
5. CAMPBELL, J.N., RAJA, S.N., COHEN, R.H., MANNING, A.A.K AND MEYER, R.A. (1989) Peripheral neural mechanisms of nociception. In: *Textbook of Pain*. eds. P. D. Wall and R. Melzack. Churchill Livingston, Edinburgh.
6. CHALAZONITIS, A., PETERSON, E.R. AND CRAIN S.M. (1987) Nerve growth

factor regulates the action potential duration of mature sensory neurons. *Proc. Natl. Acad. Sci.* **84**, 289-293.

7. COHEN, R.H. AND PERL, E.R. (1990) Contributions of arachidonic derivatives and substance P to the sensitization of cutaneous nociceptors. *J. Neurophysiol.* **64**, 457- 464.

8. CZEH, G., KUDO, N. AND KUNO, M. (1977) Membrane properties and conduction velocity in sensory neurons following sensory or peripheral axotomy. *J. Physiol.* **270**, 165- 180.

9. DIAMOND, J., HOLMES, M. AND COUGHLIN, M. (1992) Endogenous NGF and nerve impulses regulate the collateral sprouting of sensory axons in the skin of the adult rat. *J Neurosci* **12**, 1454-1466

10. DICHTER, M.A. AND FISCHBACH, G.D. (1977) The action potential of chick dorsal root ganglion neurones maintained in cell culture. *J. Physiol.* **267**, 281-298.

11. DOUCETTE, R. AND DIAMOND, J. (1987) Normal and precocious sprouting of heat nociceptors in the skin of adult rats. *J. Comp. Neurol.* **261**, 592- 603.

12. DUDA, P. AND STRAUSS, P. (1981) Action potentials of dorsal root ganglion cells activated by nonpainful and painful stimuli in cats. *Pain* 11 Suppl 1, 206.

13. DUNLAP, K. AND FISCHBACH, G.D. (1981) Neurotransmitters decrease the calcium conductance activated by depolarization of embryonic chick sensory neurones. *J. Physiol.* **317**, 519-535.

14. FOX, A.P., NOWYCKY, M.C. AND TSIEN, R.W. (1987) Kinetic and pharmacological properties distinguishing three types of calcium currents in chick sensory neurones. *J. Physiol.* **394**, 149- 172.

15. FULTON, B.P. (1987) Postnatal changes in conduction velocity and soma action potential parameters of rat dorsal root ganglion neurones. *Neurosci. Lett.* **73**, 125-130.

16. GALLEGO, R. (1983) The ionic basis of action potentials in petrosal ganglion cells of the cat. *J. Physiol.* 342, 591-602.

17. GALLEGO, R. AND EYZAGUIRRE, C. (1978) Membrane and action potential characteristics of A- and C nodose ganglion cells studied in whole ganglia and in tissue slices. *J. Neurophysiol.* **41**, 1217-1232.

18. GORKE, K. AND PIERAU, F.-K. (1980) Spike potentials and membrane properties of dorsal root ganglion cells in pigeons. *Pflugers Arch.* **386**, 21-28.

19. GRUNER, W., SILVA L.R. AND DUNLAP, K. (1992) ω-conotoxin- sensitive

calcium current mediates presynaptic inhibition at the sensory neuron-spinal cord synapse. *Neurosci. Abstr.* **18**, 247.

20. GURTU, S. AND SMITH, P.A. (1988) Electrophysiological characteristics of hamster dorsal root ganglion cells and their response to axotomy. *J. Neurophysiol.* **59**, 408- 423.

21. HARPER, A.A. (1986) Soma-sensory receptor relationships in rat dorsal root ganglion (DRG) neurones. *J. Physiol.* **380**, 15P.

22. HARPER, A.A. AND LAWSON, S.N. (1985) Electrical properties of rat dorsal root ganglion neurones with different peripheral nerve conduction velocities. J. *Physiol.* **359**, 47-63.

23. HOHEISEL, U. AND MENSE, S. (1987) Observations on the morphology of axons and somata of slowly conducting dorsal root ganglion cells in the cat. *Brain Res.* **423**, 269-278.

24. HOLZ, G.G., IV, DUNLAP, K. AND KREAM, R.M. (1988) Characterization of the electrically evoked release of substance P from dorsal root ganglion neurons: methods and dihydropyridine sensitivity. *J. Neurosci.* **8**, 463-471.

25. HUNT, S.P., MANTYH, P.W. AND PRIESTLY, J.V. (1992) The organization of biochemically characterized sensory neurons. In: *Sensory Neurons: Diversity, Development and Plasticity.* ed. S.A. Scott. Oxford University Press, New York

26. ITO, M. AND SAIGA, M. (1959) The mode of impulse conduction through the spinal ganglion. Jap. *J. Physiol.* **9**, 33-42.

27. JIA M. AND NELSON P.G. (1986) Calcium currents and transmitter output in cultured spinal cord and dorsal root ganglion neurons. J. Neurophysiol. **56**, 1257-1267.

28. JOHNSON, R.D. AND MUNSON, J.B. (1992) Specificity of regenerating sensory neurons in adult mammals. In: *Sensory Neurons: Diversity, Development and Plasticity.* ed. S.A. Scott, Oxford University Press, New York

29. KIRCHHOFF, C.G., REEH, P.W. AND WADDELL, P.J. (1989) Sensory endings of C- and A-fibres are differentially sensitive to tetrodotoxin in rat skin in vitro. *J. Physiol.* **418,** 116P.

30. KOERBER, H.R., DRUZINSKY, R.E. AND MENDELL, L.M. (1988) Properties of somata of spinal dorsal root ganglion cells differ according to peripheral receptor innervated. *J. Neurophysiol.* 60, 1584-1596.

31. KOERBER, H.R. AND MENDELL, L.M. (1988) Functional specialization of central projections from identified primary afferent fibers. *J. Neurophysiol.* **60**, 1597-1614.

32. KOERBER, H.R. AND MENDELL, L.M. (1992) Functional heterogeneity of dorsal root ganglion cells. In: *Sensory Neurons: Diversity, Development and Plasticity.* ed. S.A. Scott. Oxford University Press, New York.

33. KOERBER, H.R., SEYMOUR, A.W. AND MENDELL, L.M. (1990) Specificity of regeneration and effects on central function following peripheral axotomy. *Neurosci. Abstr.* **16**, 561.

34. KOERBER, H.R., SEYMOUR, A.W. AND MENDELL, L.M. (1991) Tuning of spinal networks to frequency components of individual afferent spike trains. *J. Neurosci.* **11**, 3178-3187.

35. KOSTYUK, P.G., VESELOVSKY, N.S. AND TSYDRENKO, A.Y. (1981) Ionic currents in somatic membrane of rat dorsal root ganglion neurons-I: Sodium currents. *Neuroscience* **6**, 2423-2430.

36. LEMOS, J. AND NOWYCKY, M.C. (1989) Two types of calcium channels coexist in peptide- releasing vertebrate nerve terminals. *Neuron* **2**, 1419- 1426.

37. LEWIN G.R. AND MCMAHON S.B. (1991) Physiological properties of primary sensory neurons appropriately and inappropriately innervating skin in adult rats. J. Neurophysiol. **66,** 1205-1217.

38. LEWIN, G.R., RITTER, A.M. AND MENDELL, L.M. (1992) On the role of nerve growth factor in the development of myelinated nociceptors. *J. Neurosci.* **12**, 1896-1905.

39. LEWIN, G.R., RITTER, A.M. AND MENDELL, L.M. (In Press) Nerve growth factor induced hyperalgesia in the neonatal and adult rat. *J. Neurosci.*

40. MENDELL, L.M. (1966) Physiological properties of unmyelinated fibre projection to the spinal cord. *Exp. Neurol.* **16**, 316-332.

41. MORITA, K. AND KATAYAMA, Y. (1989) Bullfrog dorsal root ganglion cells having tetrodotoxin-resistant spikes are endowed with nicotinic receptors. *J. Neurophysiol.* **62,** 657-664.

42. NISHIMURA, H., JOHNSON, R.D. AND MUNSON, J.B. (1990) Properties of muscle afferents cross- innervating skin in cats. *Neurosci. Abstr.* **16**, 561.

43. NOWYCKY, M.C. (1992) Voltage-gated channels in dorsal root ganglion neurons. In: *Sensory Neurons: Diversity, Development and Plasticity.* ed. S.A. Scott, Oxford University Press, New York.

44. O'DOWD, D.K., RIBERA, A.B. AND SPITZER, N.C. (1988) Development of voltage-sensitive calcium, sodium and potassium currents in Xenopus spinal neurons. *J. Neurosci.* **8**, 792-805.

45. PERL, E.R. (1984) Pain and Nociception. In: *Handbook of Physiology Section I: The Nervous System Vol. III. Sensory Processes, Part 2* ed I. Darian-Smith. American Physiological Society, Bethesda, MD.

46. RANSOM, B.R. AND HOLZ, R.W. (1977) Ionic determinents of excitability in cultured mouse dorsal root ganglion and spinal cord cells. *Brain Res.* **136**, 445-453.

47. RITTER, A.M. AND MENDELL, L.M. (1992) The somal membrane properties of physiologically identified sensory neurons in the rat: effects of nerve growth factor. *J. Neurophysiol.* **68**, 2033-2041.

48. RITTER, A.M., LEWIN, G.R., KREMER, N.E. AND MENDELL, L.M. (1991) Requirement for nerve growth factor in the development of myelinated nociceptors in vivo. *Nature* **350**, 500-502.

49. ROSE, R.D., KOERBER, H.R., SEDIVEC, M.J. AND MENDELL, L.M. (1986) Somal action potential duration differs in identified primary afferents. *Neurosci. Lett.* **63**, 259-264.

50. SCROGGS, R.S. AND FOX, A.P. (1991) Distribution of dihydropyridine and w-conotoxin- sensitive calcium currents in acutely isolated rat and frog sensory neuron somata: diameter- dependent L channel expression in frog. *J. Neurosci.* **11**, 1334-1346.

51. SCROGGS R.S. AND FOX, A.P. (1992) Multiple Ca^{2+} currents elicited by action potential waveforms in acutely isolated adult rat dorsal root ganglion cells. *J. Neurosci.* **12**, 1789- 1801.

52. SCROGGS, R.S. AND FOX, A.P. (1992) Calcium current variation between acutely isolated adult rat dorsal root ganglion neurons of different size. *J. Physiol.* **445**, 639- 658.

53. STONEY, S.D., JR. (1990) Limitations on impulse conduction at the branch point of afferent axons in frog dorsal root ganglion. *Exp. Brain Res.* **80**, 512-524.

54. TRAUB, R.J. AND MENDELL, L.M. (1988) The spinal projection of individual identified A-delta - and C-fibers. *J. Neurophysiol.* **59**, 41-55.

55. WILLIS, W.D. AND COGGESHALL, R.E. (1991) Sensory Mechanisms of the Spinal Cord, 2nd edition, Plenum Press, New York and London.

56. WOOLF, C.J. (1991) Central mechanisms of acute pain. In: *Proceedings of the VIth World Congress on Pain* ed. M.R. Bond, J.E. Charlton and C.J. Woolf. Elsevier.

57. WOOLF, C.J. AND WALL, P.D. (1986) Relative effectiveness of C primary afferent fibers of different origins in evoking a prolonged facilitation of the flexor reflex in the rat. *J. Neurosci.* 6, 1433-1442.

58. YOSHIDA, S., MATSUDA, Y. AND SAMEJIMA, A. (1978) Tetrodotoxin-resistant sodium and calcium components of action potentials in dorsal root ganglion cells of the adult mouse. *J. Neurophysiol.* **41**, 1096-1106.

ION CHANNELS UNDERLYING TRANSDUCTION AND ADAPTATION IN MECHANORECEPTORS

Andrew S. French
Department of Physiology
University of Alberta
Edmonton, Alberta T6G 2H7
Canada

INTRODUCTION

The earliest events in the processing of sensory information happen in the periphery at the sensory receptors themselves. Some important features of this processing are sensitivity, response dynamics, and non-linear behavior. Here, we will deal with the events between a mechanical stimulus arriving at a receptor and the resulting train of action potentials entering the central nervous system. Similar processing is likely to occur in other senses.

The term "mechanotransduction" is often used loosely to describe the entire operation of a mechanoreceptor cell, or even to include some further processing. Here, it will be treated as a three-stage process comprising (1) mechanical coupling of the primary stimulus to the sensory cell membrane, (2) transduction of the membrane movement into a receptor current, that produces a receptor potential, and (3) encoding of the membrane potential into a train of action potentials.[8,31] The first of these stages, mechanical coupling, or transformation, usually involves the mechanical properties of the materials surrounding the sensory ending, which can be elaborate. The remaining two stages are now believed to be crucially dependent on the properties of various groups of ion channels in the membranes of sensory cells.

NATO ASI Series, Vol. H 79
Cellular Mechanisms of Sensory Processing
Edited by Laszlo Urban
© Springer-Verlag Berlin Heidelberg 1994

MECHANICAL COUPLING

Perhaps the best known example of mechanical coupling is in the Pacinian corpuscle, where the viscoelastic properties of the layers of membranous lamellae surrounding the sensory ending produce a rapidly adapting receptor current[33]. The detailed mechanical behavior of the lamellae is still poorly understood, and has recently been studied by imaging techniques.[37] Mechanical coupling has also been investigated in a range of other vertebrate sensory systems, including muscle spindles[32] and frog touch receptors.[3,50]

In invertebrates, viscoelastic behavior has been found in the crayfish stretch receptor[39] and in the campaniform sensilla of the cockroach.[5] Insects also provide interesting examples of internal mechanical structures which probably contribute to mechanical coupling. A variety of insect cuticular receptors contain highly organised microtubule arrangements which could provide a cytoskeleton to enhance the force created on the membrane by external displacement.[14] More elaborate theories suggested that such microtubule structures could provide essential links between membrane displacement and the ion channels responsible for the receptor current. However, other evidence indicated that they are neither crucial for mechanotransduction, nor involved in viscoelastic behavior, although they may contribute to receptor sensitivity.[14,30]

The major demonstrated effects of mechanical coupling on the processing of sensory information are attenuation and adaptation. Most mechanical structures, such as the hairs of mammals or insects, or the lamellae of the Pacinian corpuscle, reduce the amplitude of the displacement that appears at the sensory cell membrane, although they may increase its force through lever action. Few estimates are available of the displacement that actually occurs at the cell membrane, although several calculations from arthropods suggest a value of 1-10nm.[14] The viscous properties of some coupling systems cause rapidly changing stimuli to be conducted to the membrane more effectively than steady movements. However, the importance of this function is not understood in most sensory systems. Even in the Pacinian corpuscle, where viscosity has a role, there may be more powerful dynamic effects exerted by the ion channels associated with encoding.[33]

Mechanically-activated ion channels

Up to about 10 years ago, the mechanisms responsible for converting a mechanical deformation of the cell membrane to a receptor current were a matter of speculation. For example, it was still considered possible that stretching of a suitably located cell membrane could lead directly to some increase in membrane conductance through disturbance of the lipid bilayer. Then, reports began to appear of ion channels which were activated directly by membrane deformation.[2,22] In many respects these channels were similar to those that had already been discovered in a variety of tissues, providing sensitivity to membrane potential, chemical transmitters, and internal cellular messengers. However, these new channels were selectively activated by changing the pressure on the patch pipette, which was assumed to cause deformation of the membrane patch containing the channel.

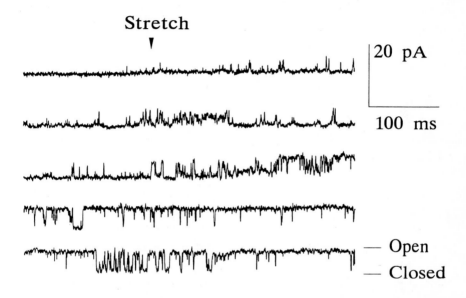

Figure 1. Patch clamp recording of a single mechanically-activated channel in a cell from a cockroach chordotonal organ. Suction, to produce membrane stretch, was applied at the time indicated by the arrow. Brief openings appeared immediately, but full opening of the channel required more than 1 s.

Figure 1 shows an example of a mechanically-activated ion channel observed in the membrane of a tissue-cultured mechanoreceptor cell from a cockroach antennal chordotonal organ.[44] This recording demonstrates the characteristics found in many recordings of mechanically-activated channels. They display the normal kinetic properties seen in other types of channels, with rapid transitions between completely open and completely closed states. The major difference is that they respond with great sensitivity to membrane stretch, but are usually insensitive to voltage or chemical agents. In contrast, voltage- and chemically-activated ion channels are insensitive to membrane deformation.

The effect of the mechanical stimulus on the channels is not to change their conductance, but to change their probability of being open. This is shown clearly in Figure 1, where the applied suction causes the channel to shift from being mainly closed to being mainly open, but does not affect the open channel current. This shows that the channel protein can not be modelled as a pore that is stretched to a wider diameter by the membrane tension, but must be similar to other ion channels, with relatively separate controls of channel conductance and the probability of being open[24]. Mechanically-activated channels with a range of different cation conductances have now been found (Figure 2), just as for the voltage- and chemically-activated ion channels.

Another interesting feature of the recording in Figure 1 is the delay in onset of the channel activity after the stimulus. Very little is known about the time-dependent responses of these channels, and it is possible that they could contribute to mechanoreceptor dynamics. Adaptation of channel activity to a maintained stimulus has been reported in several cases.[23,43]

The properties of mechanically-activated ion channels, their distribution and possible functions, have been the subject of several reviews.[17,34,40] Figure 2 summarises the distributions of ionic selectivity and single channel conductances for most of the channels discovered so far in eukaryotic cells. Mechanically-activated channels have also been found in bacteria and plants, where large conductances and some anion conductances have been found, but in most other cases, the channels are permeable to potassium, monovalent cations, or both monovalent and divalent cations. Some channels are sensitive to voltage in addition to mechanical sensitivity, and others seem to be inactivated, instead of activated, by membrane stretch. However, the general picture is of moderate conductance cation channels, primarily sensitive to membrane stretch.

The physical connection between membrane stretch and channel activation is still unknown. A series of studies have produced models of channel kinetics with one or more closed states selectively sensitive to stretch, but the actual connection remains elusive. There is evidence suggesting that cytoskeletal components provide an important mechanical link to the channels, while other work indicates that deformation of the lipid bilayer alone may be adequate to change channel activity. Some of this work was reviewed recently.[17] One case in which a putative mechanical link has been deduced experimentally and visualised with scanning electron

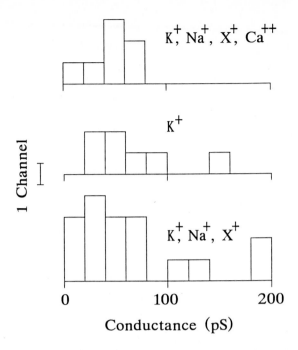

Figure 2. Distributions of mechanically-activated channels based on single channel conductance and cation permeation. Each entry in the histograms represents a separate type of channel.

microscopy is in auditory hair cells.[27,28] Here, the evidence suggests that a single mechanically-activated channel is present in each stereocilium, and that mechanical links connect each channel to the neighboring cilium, so that bending of the bundle applies tension to the links and opens the channels.

A central problem is that most examples of mechanically-activated channels have not been found in cells whose primary function is mechanoreception. Instead, they have been observed in a wide variety of cell types, including muscle, fibroblasts, epithelia, and endothelia. Possible functions of the channels in these cells include volume regulation, control of movement, and detection of external stress.[17] Therefore, it seems possible that all, or most cells have mechanically-activated channels, and it is difficult to correlate them directly with sensory transduction. Two types of mechanically-activated channels were found in crayfish stretch receptor neurons[7], and one type was seen in cockroach chordotonal neurons.[44] However, in both these cases, it was difficult to know if the channels were from areas of the membrane that are involved in transduction. The nature of the channels in auditory hair cells is also unclear. Discrete single-channel recordings of a 50 pS channel have been reported,[36] but careful noise analysis has suggested a much smaller conductance for the channels carrying the receptor current.[26]

Most mechanically-activated channels are selectively permeable to cations. Some mechanoreceptor currents are dependent on sodium ions[17] and some receptors are surrounded by a high concentration of sodium[21,42] or potassium[45]. The most parsimonious model of mechanotransduction is that sodium or potassium ions pass through mechanically-activated ion channels similar to those already known, and create the receptor current. However, we still lack a clear demonstration of this model.

ENCODING AND RAPID SENSORY ADAPTATION

In most cases, the receptor potential created by the mechanically-activated channels is encoded into action potentials by processes similar to those described by Hodgkin and Huxley.[25] While the basic Hodgkin-Huxley model predicts that action potentials can be produced continuously by a steady membrane current, many neurons actually slow their rate of discharge to a constant stimulus, or even cease firing completely. In receptor cells this effect causes adaptation of the response to a maintained stimulus. The Pacinian corpuscle has this kind of adaptation. When most of the lamellae surrounding the sensory ending were removed, the adaptation in the receptor current was reduced but the action potential discharge still adapted rapidly.[33]

A number of mechanisms could lead to adaptation of action potential discharge, including calcium-activated potassium channels, electrogenic sodium pumps, external ion accumulation or slow activation or inactivation of voltage-activated ion channels.[17,29] Most sensory neurons are too small to penetrate with electrodes using present technology, so that experiments to test hypotheses of adaptation are often difficult. We have used the single sensory neuron in the cockroach femoral tactile spine as a model of rapid sensory adaptation. The tactile spine has been a useful general mechanoreceptor preparation because it can be easily stimulated mechanically or electrically, and the resulting afferent action potentials can also be easily detected.[4,9,18,38]

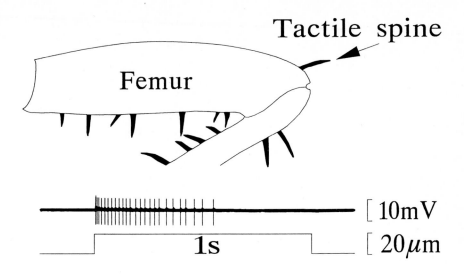

Figure 3. The cockroach tactile spine, a rapidly adapting insect mechanoreceptor. The spine is located on the dorsal surface of the femur, close to the femoro-tibial joint (upper). Step movements of the spine inwards along its long axis cause bursts of action potentials which adapt to silence after a few seconds or less (lower).

As shown in Figure 3, a step mechanical deflection of the tactile spine causes a burst of action potentials in the afferent axon which adapts rapidly and completely to silence. The cause of this adaptation was initially thought to be linked to the dense arrangement of microtubules in the sensory ending, but experiments with microtubule-dissociating drugs showed that although the sensitivity of the receptor neuron was reduced, the time course of its dynamic response persisted in the absence of microtubules.[30] Similar findings were made in another insect cuticular mechanoreceptor.[6]

Measurement of the receptor potential in the neuron by decremental conduction along the axon failed to find any evidence of adaptation during the mechanical coupling or transduction stages, indicating that rapid adaptation occurs later, during the encoding of action potentials.[10] This was confirmed by experiments with direct electrical stimulation of the neuron, where rapid adaptation was demonstrated without any mechanical stimulus, and the frequency response of the neuron was similar with either mechanical or electrical stimulation.[9]

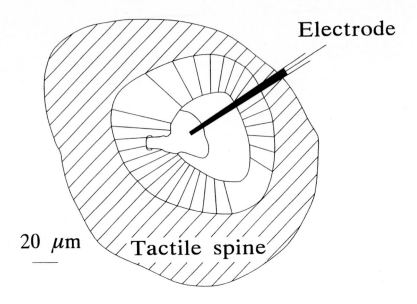

Figure 4. Intracellular recording from the tactile spine neuron is possible by cutting off the top part of the spine and lowering a microelectrode down the lumen. This figure is based on a perspective view of a computer reconstruction using serial sections.

The cell body of the tactile spine sensory neuron lies in the central lumen of the spine (Fig. 4). A single sensory dendrite passes from the cell body through the wall of the spine to a mechanical attachment on the outer wall[20] and the axon passes from the lumen into the central cavity of the femur, where it joins a major nerve leading to the central nervous system. The direct electrical stimulation experiments used a preparation in which the top part of the tactile spine was amputated to make the neuron accessible to electrodes lowered down through the spine lumen. This preparation was later modified to allow microelectrodes to penetrate the neuron from above as shown in Figure 4. This figure is an accurate scale representation of the base of one tactile spine, reconstructed from serial sections of 1 μm thickness.[19]

Quantitative measurements of the rheobasic threshold current for extracellular stimulation showed that during adaptation the threshold of the neuron always increased to exceed a sustained depolarization. Therefore, adaptation can be viewed as the product of a voltage-sensitive threshold.[12] In order to test for possible mechanisms of threshold elevation and adaptation, experiments were performed with extracellular electrical stimulation of the neuron during treatment with chemical agents known to have specific effects on a variety of ionic pathways in the cell membrane.

Replacement of calcium ions in the external solution with other divalent ions that block calcium channels did not have any effects on adaptation, beyond the apparent membrane potential changes that normally accompany divalent ion concentration changes. A calcium channel ionophore was also ineffective.[11] These results make it unlikely that calcium entry, or calcium-activated potassium channels play a major role in adaptation. The agent 4-amino pyridine, which blocks A-type potassium currents in many neurons, produced significant reductions in the threshold when the neuron was initially hyperpolarized,[12] indicating that the neuron possesses an A-current.

To test the possibility of sodium channel involvement in rapid adaptation, the effects of sodium replacement and sodium channel modifiers were used. A pronounced change in both threshold behavior and rapid adaptation was produced by chloramine-T or N-chlorosuccinimide. These two chemicals are members of a group of mild oxidizing agents that have been shown to selectively modify the inactivation of voltage-activated sodium channels.[49] They are believed to act by oxidizing sulfur-containing amino acids[41] that are located in the portion of the protein responsible for inactivation.

Both of these agents strongly reduced the elevation of threshold produced by depolarization of the neuronal membrane. Neurons treated in this way no longer displayed complete adaptation, but instead continued to fire continuous trains of action potentials when depolarised.[13] This suggested that inactivation of an inward sodium current was involved in the threshold elevation and adaptation. Similar mechanisms had earlier been implicated in the adaptation of crayfish stretch receptors[35] and amphibian myelinated axons.[48]

Measurements of the dynamic behavior of the tactile spine neuron's threshold produced more evidence about the mechanisms of rapid adaptation. For any amplitude or direction of threshold change, the process was found to include two distinct components with time constants of approximately 100 ms and 1000 ms.[15] The faster process was sensitive to the mild oxidizing agents, while the slower process was sensitive to ouabain,[16] an inhibitor of the sodium-potassium pump. Based on these findings, a model of rapid adaptation was developed in which the threshold was elevated by a slow, voltage-dependent inactivation of sodium channels, combined with a voltage-activated potassium A-current and an electrogenic pump, activated by sodium influx during depolarization.

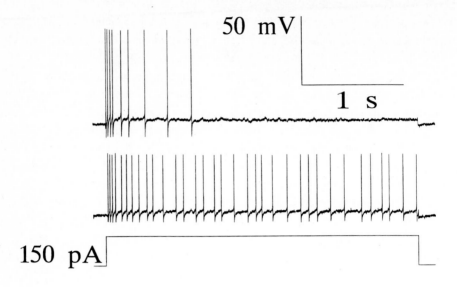

Figure 5. Step depolarizations of the tactile spine neuron produce rapidly adapting bursts of action potentials similar to those produced by mechanical stimulation (upper trace) but most of the adaptation can be removed by agents such as chloramine-T (middle trace) which are known to affect the inactivation of sodium channels.

Intracellular measurements provided a direct confirmation that the action potential encoding mechanism of the tactile spine neuron causes rapid adaptation. Figure 5 shows intracellular recordings from a tactile spine neuron during depolarization by an injected current step.[1] The adaptation seen during such step depolarizations was very similar to the results obtained from mechanical steps. This figure also shows the response in the same neuron after treatment with chloramine-T. Again, the rapid adaptation was strongly reduced, converting the neuron from completely adapting to tonically firing. The action of an electrogenic pump was indicated by a post-tetanic hyperpolarization with a time constant of several seconds. However, this effect was quite small, casting doubt on its importance in normal adaptation.

With the advent of reliable intracellular recording, attention has recently been focused on measuring the ionic currents in the tactile spine neuron under voltage clamp conditions, to produce a complete model of the ionic currents responsible for rapid sensory adaptation. As predicted by the earlier work, a slowly inactivating inward current was found. It was sensitive to sodium replacement and able to be

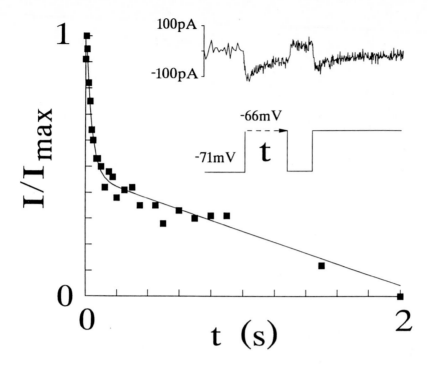

Figure 6. Two-pulse experiments under voltage clamp show that the tactile spine neuron has a slowly inactivating sodium current. The main figure shows the decrease in peak inward current after a variable length initial depolarization followed by a fixed recovery time. The inactivation curve is fitted by a double exponential function. Original inward current traces are shown inset.

blocked by tetrodotoxin.[46] Figures 6 and 7 illustrate the inactivation and recovery from inactivation of this sodium current during small depolarizations. In both cases, there are at least two time constants involved. At present, it is not known if this current is carried by the same sodium channels that cause the leading edge of the action potentials, or if it represents a separate population of channels.

Other voltage clamp work has begun to reveal the outward currents of the tactile spine neuron.[47] These include a delayed rectifier potassium current, sensitive to tetra-ethyl ammonium and activated by depolarization from rest, as well as a potassium A-current, sensitive to 4-amino pyridine, as predicted by the earlier extracellular stimulation experiments. Application of tetra-ethyl ammonium and 4-amino pyridine has recently been shown to significantly decrease the threshold for action potential production. In summary, rapid adaptation clearly involves the combined actions of several different ion channels.

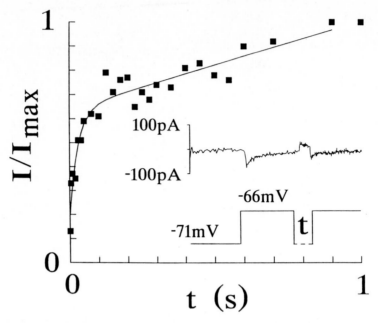

Figure 7. The recovery of peak inward current also follows a double exponential process. The main figure shows the peak current following a fixed initial depolarising pulse and a variable recovery time. Examples of original currents are shown inset.

CONCLUSIONS

Sensory transduction occurs in single cells, but there are a variety of mechanisms involved in this first level of processing sensory information. In particular, the receptor dynamics provide an initial time dependence of sensory input. None of the three stages, coupling, transduction, or encoding, are well understood in mechanoreceptors, nor in other somatic receptors such as thermoreceptors and nociceptors. Although mechanically-activated ion channels have now been widely described, it is not clear what kinds of channels are involved in the mechanical senses. Encoding of action potentials seems to play an important role in controlling the dynamic behavior of some mechanoreceptors, and probably other types of sensory receptors. Some progress has been made in identifying the ionic channels responsible for modifying the time dependence of encoding.

In the future, it will be important to identify the ion channels underlying mechanoreception. The patch clamp technique may be useful in this effort, but more biochemical approaches, such as channel protein purification, may also be helpful. Discovery of a preparation with a high density of accessible mechanoreceptors would be valuable. Relatively large and simple mechanoreceptor cells, such as the tactile spine neuron, offer one of the few ways of tackling these problems with present technology. Application of the voltage clamp technique to this or other suitable mechanoreceptors promises to yield new information about the ionic currents flowing during mechanotransduction and sensory adaptation.

ACKNOWLEDGEMENTS: Support for this work was provided by grants from the Medical Research Council of Canada and the Alberta Heritage Foundation for Medical Research. Major contributions to the work described here were made by: Trent Basarsky, Rod Gramlich, Artur Klimaszewski, Esmond Sanders, Lisa Stockbridge and Päivi Torkkeli. I am grateful to Ernst-August Seyfarth and Päivi Torkkeli for critical reading of the manuscript.

REFERENCES

1. BASARSKY, T.A. AND FRENCH, A.S. (1991) Intracellular measurements from a rapidly adapting sensory neuron. *J. Neurophysiol.* **65**, 49-56.
2. BREHM, P., KULLBERG, R. AND MOODY-CORBETT, F. (1984) Properties of non-junctional acetylcholine receptor channels on innervated muscle of *Xenopus laevis. J. Physiol.* **350**, 631-648.
3. CATTON, W.T. AND PETOE, N. (1966) A visco-elastic theory of mechanoreceptor adaptation. *J. Physiol.* **187**, 35-49.
4. CHAPMAN, K.M. AND SMITH, R.S. (1963) A linear transfer function underlying impulse frequency modulation in a cockroach mechanoreceptor. *Nature* **197**, 699-700.
5. CHAPMAN, K.M., MOSINGER, J.L. AND DUCKROW, R.B. (1979) The role of distributed viscoelastic coupling in sensory adaptation in an insect mechanoreceptor. *J. Comp. Physiol.* **A131**, 1-12.
6. ERLER, G. (1983) Reduction of mechanical sensitivity in an insect mechanoreceptor correlated with destruction of its tubular body. *Cell Tiss. Res.* **234**, 451-461.
7. ERXLEBEN, C. (1989) Stretch-activated current through single ion channels in the abdominal stretch receptor organ of the crayfish. *J. Gen. Physiol.* **94**, 1071-1083.
8. EYZAGUIRRE, C. AND KUFFLER, S.W. (1955) Processes of excitation in the dendrites and in the soma of single isolated sensory nerve cells of the lobster and crayfish. *J. Gen. Physiol.* **39,** 87-119.

9. FRENCH, A.S. (1984) Action potential adaptation in the femoral tactile spine of the cockroach, *Periplaneta americana*. *J. Comp. Physiol.* **A159**, 757-764.

10. FRENCH, A.S. (1984) The receptor potential and adaptation in the cockroach tactile spine. *J. Neurosci.* **4**, 2063-2068.

11. FRENCH, A.S. (1986) The role of calcium ions in the rapid adaptation of an insect mechanoreceptor. *J. Neurosci.* **6**, 2322-2326.

12. FRENCH, A.S. (1986) Strength-duration properties of a rapidly adapting insect sensory neuron. *J. Comp. Physiol.* **159**, 757-764.

13. FRENCH, A.S. (1987) Removal of rapid sensory adaptation from an insect mechanoreceptor neuron by oxidizing agents which affect sodium channel inactivation. *J. Comp. Physiol.* **A161**, 275-282.

14. FRENCH, A.S. (1988) Transduction mechanisms of mechanosensilla. *Annu. Rev. Entomol.* **33**, 39-58.

15. FRENCH, A.S. (1989) Two components of rapid sensory adaptation in a cockroach mechanoreceptor neuron. *J. Neurophysiol.* **62**, 768-777.

16. FRENCH, A.S. (1989) Ouabain selectively affects the slow component of sensory adaptation in an insect mechanoreceptor. *Brain Res.* **504**, 112-114.

17. FRENCH, A.S. (1992) Mechanotransduction. *Annu. Rev. Physiol.* **54**, 135-152.

18. FRENCH, A.S., HOLDEN, A.V. AND STEIN, R.B. (1972) The estimation of the frequency response function of a mechanoreceptor. *Kybernetik* **11**, 15-23.

19. FRENCH, A.S., KLIMASZEWSKI, A.R. AND STOCKBRIDGE, L.L. (1993) The morphology of the sensory neuron in the cockroach femoral tactile spine. *J. Neurophysiol.* (in press).

20. FRENCH, A.S. AND SANDERS, E.J. (1981) The mechanosensory apparatus of the femoral tactile spine of the cockroach, *Periplaneta americana*. *Cell Tiss. Res.* **219**, 53-68.

21. GRUNERT, U. AND GNATZY W. (1987) K^+ and Ca^{++} in the receptor lymph of arthropod cuticular receptors. *J. Comp. Physiol.* **A161**, 329-33.

22. GUHARAY, F. AND SACHS, F. (1984) Stretch-activated single ion channel currents in tissue-cultured embryonic chick skeletal muscle. *J. Physiol.* **352,** 685-701.

23. HAMILL, O.P. AND MCBRIDE, D.W. (1992) Rapid adaptation of single mechanosensitive channels in *Xenopus oocytes*. *Proc. Natl. Acad. Sci.* **89**, 7462-7466.

24. HILLE,, B. (1984) *Ion Channels of Excitable Membranes*. Sinauer Associates. Sunderland, Massachusetts.

25. HODGKIN, A.L. AND HUXLEY, A.F. (1952) A quantitative description of membrane current and its application to conduction and excitation in nerve. *J. Physiol.* **117**, 500-544.

26. HOLTON, T. AND HUDSPETH, A.J. (1986) The transduction channel of hair cells from the bull-frog characterized by noise analysis. *J. Physiol.* **375**, 195-227.

27. HOWARD, J., ROBERTS, W.M. AND HUDSPETH, A.J. (1988) Mechanoelectrical transduction by hair cells. *Annu. Rev. Biophys. Biophys. Chem.* **17**, 99-124.

28. HUDSPETH, A.J. (1989) How the ear's works work. *Nature* 341:397-404

29. JACK, J.J.B., NOBLE, D. AND TSIEN, R.W. (1983) *Electric Current Flow in Excitable Cells*, Oxford University Press, UK.

30. KUSTER, J.E., FRENCH, A.S. AND SANDERS, E.J. (1983) The effects of microtubule dissociating agents on the physiology and cytology of the sensory neuron in the femoral tactile spine of the cockroach, *Periplaneta americana* L. *Proc. R. Soc. Lond.* **B219**, 397-412.

31. LOEWENSTEIN, W.R. (1959) The generation of electrical activity in a nerve ending. *Ann. NY Acad. Sci.* **81**, 367-387.

32. MATTHEWS, P.B.C. (1981) Evolving views on the internal operation and functional role of the muscle spindle. *J. Physiol.* **320**, 1-30.

33. MENDELSON, M. AND LOEWENSTEIN, W.R. (1964) Mechanisms of receptor adaptation. *Science*, **144**, 544-555.

34. MORRIS, C.E. (1990) Mechanosensitive ion channels. *J. Membr. Biol.* **113**, 93-107.

35. NAKAJIMA, S. AND ONODERA, K. (1969) Membrane properties of the stretch receptor neurones of crayfish with particular reference to mechanisms of sensory adaptation. *J. Physiol.* **200**, 161-185.

36. OHMORI H (1989) Mechano-electrical transduction of the hair cell. *Jpn. J. Physiol.* **39**, 643-657.

37. PIETRAS, B. AND BOLANOWSKI, S.J. (1992) Mechanics of the Pacinian corpuscle: static and dynamic measurements. *Soc. Neurosci. Abstr.* **18**, 829.

38. PRINGL, J.W.S. AND WILSON, V.J. (1952) The response of a sense organ to a harmonic stimulus. *J. Exp. Biol.* **29**, 220-234.

39. RYDQVIS, B., SWERUP, C. AND LÄNNENGREN, J. (1990) Viscoelastic properties of the slowly adapting stretch receptor muscle of the crayfish. *Acta Physiol. Scand.* **139**, 519-527.

40. SACHS, F. (1988) Mechanical transduction in biological systems. *CRC Crit. Rev. Biomed. Eng.* **16**, 141-169.

41. SCHECHTER, Y., BURSTEIN, Y. AND PATCHORNIK, A. (1975) Selective oxidation of methionine residues in proteins. *Biochem.* **14**, 4497-4503.

42. SEYFARTH, E.-A., BOHNENBERGER, J. AND THORSON, J. (1982) Electrical and mechanical stimulation of a spider slit sensillum: outward current excites. *J. Comp. Physiol.* **A147**, 423-432.

43. STOCKBRIDGE, L.L. AND FRENCH, A.S. (1988) Stretch-activated cation channels in human fibroblasts. *Biophys. J.* **54**, 187-190.

44. STOCKBRIDGE, L.L. AND FRENCH, A.S. (1989) Ion channels in isolated mechanosensory neurons from the connective chordotonal organ in the pedicel of the american cockroach. *Soc. Neurosci. Abstr.* **15**, 1287.

45. THURM, U. AND WESSEL, G. (1979) Metabolism-dependent transepithelial potential differences at epidermal receptors of arthropods. *J. Comp. Physiol.* **134**, 119-130.

46. TORKKELI, P.H. AND FRENCH, A.S. (1992) Ionic currents underlying rapid sensory adaptation in the cockroach tactile spine. *Soc. Neurosci. Abstr.* **18**, 301.

47. TORKKEL, P.H., AND FRENCH, A.S. (1992) Ionic currents in a rapidly adapting mechanosensory neuron. *Physiol. Can.* **23**, 115.

48. VALLBO, A.B. (1964) Accommodation related to inactivation of the sodium permeability in single myelinated nerve fibres from *Xenopus laevis*. *Acta Physiol. Scand.* **61**, 429-444.

49. WANG, G.K. (1984) Irreversible modification of sodium channel inactivation in

toad myelinated nerve fibres by the oxidant chloramine-T. *J. Physiol.* **346**, 127-141.

50. WATTS, R.E. AND FRENCH, A.S. (1985) Sensory transduction in dorsal cutaneous mechanoreceptors of the frog. *J. Comp. Physiol.* **A157**, 657-665.

SIGNAL TRANSDUCTION PROCESSES IN SENSORIMOTOR NEURONS OF THE ENTERIC NERVOUS SYSTEM

Annmarie Surprenant
Vollum Institute
Oregon Health Sciences University
Portland, OR. 97201
USA

INTRODUCTION

The enteric nervous system is comprised of two distinct neural networks arranged in layers, or plexuses, along the length of the gastrointestinal (GI) tract. The largest neural network is the myenteric plexus whose major function is to control movements of the visceral smooth muscle of the GI tract; the myenteric plexus is situated within the thin longitudinal smooth muscle on the outer surface of the gut. The submucosal plexus lies within a thin connective tissue sheath between the thick circular smooth muscle of the gut and the underlying intestinal mucosa; the submucosal plexus sheath also contains the submucosal arteriolar network (Figure 1). These arterioles supply the muscle and mucosa of the GI tract. Submucosal neurons subserve two primary functions: they act to modulate water and electrolyte transport in the intestinal mucosa and they provide vasodilator innervation to the submucosal arterioles. Informative and intellectually stimulating details of the structure and function of the enteric nervous system can be found in the elegant literary style of Furness and Costa[7] with updates available in recent reviews.[12,24] This chapter will summarise evidence that suggests a population of submucosal neurons can be considered "sensorimotor" neurons in that they appear to subserve either or both an afferent as well as an efferent role. The inhibitory innervation to these sensorimotor neurons and the signal transduction processes underlying this inhibition have been studied in detail; these signal transduction mechanisms also will be reviewed. The vast majority of electrophysiological studies on submucosal

NATO ASI Series, Vol. H 79
Cellular Mechanisms of Sensory Processing
Edited by Laszlo Urban
© Springer-Verlag Berlin Heidelberg 1994

neurons have been carried out on preparations of the guinea-pig small intestine; results described in this chapter will be limited to studies of this preparation submucosal plexus.

SUBMUCOSAL "SENSORIMOTOR" VASODILATOR NEURONS

Submucosal arterioles are the final resistance vessels of the GI vasculature with outside vessel diameters ranging from 10-80 μm. Neild[16] developed an imaging analysis process that allowed on-line tracking of the outside diameter of these small arterioles; this development has allowed the functional innervation to these vessels to be determined. As is the case for all peripheral arteries and arterioles, submucosal arterioles receive vasoconstrictor innervation solely from the extrinsic sympathetic nerve supply. ATP appears to be

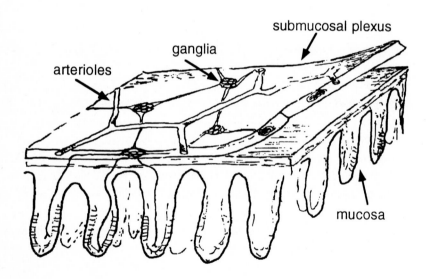

Figure 1. Diagram of isolated submucosal plexus preparation. The submucosal plexus is comprised of a thin connective tissue sheath in which lie the submucosal ganglia and the submucosal arteriolar tree. Each ganglion, or node, is composed of 4 to 15 neurons arranged in a monolayer. Fibres project to both arterioles and underlying intestinal mucosa.

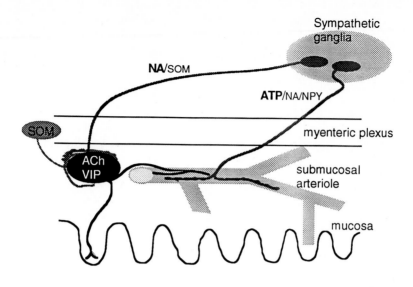

NA/SOM

ATP/NA/NPY

Sympathetic
ganglia

myenteric plexus

submucosal
arteriole

SOM

ACh
VIP

mucosa

Figure 2. Diagram of the "sensorimotor" neuron in the submucosal plexus and its inhibitory innervation by noradrenergic sympathetic neurons and somatostatin-containing myenteric neurons. The multiple excitatory synaptic input this population of neurons receives is not shown in this diagram. The sensorimotor neuron provides an efferent vasodilator innervation to submucosal arterioles and an afferent limb to intestinal mucosa. See text for details.

the only sympathetic neurotransmitter producing vasoconstriction in submucosal arterioles[6] (Figure 2). Intrinsic submucosal neurons provide a prominent vasodilator innervation to submucosal arterioles.[17] Most of the vasodilation is due to the release of acetylcholine from submucosal neurons because the neurogenic dilation is blocked by atropine and other muscarinic receptor antagonists.[2,17] The muscarinic receptor activated by neurally released acetylcholine is of the M_3 subtype.[5,17] It has been possible to directly identify individual vasodilator neurons by making intracellular microelectrode recordings from submucosal neurons while simultaneously monitoring vessel diameter.[17] In a number of submucosal neurons initiation of action potential discharge by application of intracellular depolarising pulses produces a vasodilation in the arteriole; this vasodilation produced by intracellular stimulation of a single neuron is blocked by muscarinic receptor blockers. Individual vasodilator neurons have been identified further by carrying out these types of experiments using neurobiotin-filled microelectrodes so that neurons can be located after processing for neurobiotin fluorescence and peptide immunofluorescence. Results to date have shown that such re-identified vasodilator neurons are all positive for vasoactive intestinal polypeptide (VIP) immunoreactivity. These results are quite unexpected and pose a serious interpretive dilemma because numerous immunohistochemical studies have demonstrated that submucosal neurons of the guinea-pig small intestine form two distinct, and mutually exclusive, populations: approximately 60% of all submucosal neurons are immunoreactive for VIP and the other half are immunoreactive for choline acetyltransferase (ChAT) which is a marker for cholinergic neurons (see Furness & Costa[7]). Thus, submucosal vasodilator neurons appear to be VIP-ergic based on immunohistochemical criteria but cholinergic based on physiological criteria. Currently available antibodies to ChAT stain only cell bodies in the enteric nervous system and not their processes; therefore, it has not been possible to trace cholinergic vasodilator neuronal projections using these antibodies. One explanation that might resolve these conflicting results would be if levels of ChAT in VIP-containing cells are too low (or sufficiently structurally different) to be detected by the available antibodies.

A reflex vasodilation of submucosal arterioles can be demonstrated in an isolated preparation of submucosal plexus in which the underlying mucosa is present. Mechanical or chemical stimulation of the intestinal mucosa results in arteriolar vasodilation which is neurogenic because it is blocked by tetrodotoxin or by cutting the nerve fibers running between mucosa and submucosal neurons. This reflex is also cholinergic because it is blocked by muscarinic receptor blockers[28]. Mucosal stimulation also results in increased synaptic activity in the form of nicotinic excitatory synaptic potentials (EPSPs) in a population of VIP-containing submucosal neurond for action potential discharge, vasodilation occurs. Further, the axons of many VIP-containing neurons bifurcate shortly after leaving the somata with one process passing over or around, and occasionally appearing to terminate in, an arteriole and the other process terminating in the intestinal mucosa[10]. Thus, the neuronal circuitry illustrated in Figure 2 is proposed: A population of cholinergic (VIP-containing) submucosal neurons provides dual innervation to submucosal arterioles and intestinal mucosa; this dual innervation provides an afferent limb to the mucosa and an efferent limb to the arterioles. These neurons are sensory because they can be activated by mechanical or chemical stimulation of their mucosal terminals; they are motor because action potential initiation in their cell bodies results in arteriolar vasodilation. This reflex loop is somewhat analogous to the classic axon collateral reflex in sensory dorsal horn neurons that project to both skin and skin vessels. However, these neurons also receive multiple excitatory and inhibitory input from both intrinsic enteric and extrinsic sympathetic sources (see below) and therefore cannot be considered to be solely sensory neurons possessing axon collaterals. Moreover, synaptically driven excitation of the cell body of this sensorimotor neuron will be expected to release transmitter from terminals in the intestinal mucosa as well as the vasculature. Acetylcholine released from the vascular terminals will result in vasodilation; acteylcholine and/or VIP released from the mucosal terminals will result in enhanced intestinal secretory activity (see Furness and Costa[7]). Thus, it is further proposed that the mucosal process of this sensorimotor neuron may serve both a sensory and a motor function depending on the means by which it is activated.

INNERVATION OF VASODILATOR SENSORIMOTOR NEURONS

VIP-containing submucosal neurons receive multiple excitatory and inhibitory synaptic inputs. Cholinergic innervation of these neurons provides for fast nicotinic transmission. The origin of the cholinergic innervation is two-fold, from submucosal interneurons and from cholinergic neurons located in the myenteric plexus.[4] Submucosal neurons do not receive parasympathetic vagal innervation.[11] Slow excitatory transmission is also present in these neurons; the sources of this synaptic input are most likely from sensory substance P-containing terminals and from myenteric neurons but the neurotransmitter(s) underlying this form of synaptic input have not been determined conclusively (see Mihara[12]). These neurons receive a prominent inhibitory synaptic input from extrinsic sympathetic neurons (Figure 2); the resulting inhibitory synaptic potential (IPSP) is due to the release of noradrenaline acting on postsynaptic α_2-adrenoceptors.[18,25] A less prominent inhibitory synaptic potential is due to the release of somatostatin from nerve terminals whose processes emanate from myenteric neurons (Figure 2).[3,15] However, in an impressive display of neuronal plasticity, this normally minor somatostatin input completely replaces the noradrenergic IPSP. within 3 - 5 days after removal of the sympathetic nerve supply.[20]

IONIC MECHANISM OF SYNAPTIC INHIBITION OF SENSORIMOTOR NEURONS

The somatostatin and the noradrenergic IPSP are due to identical ionic mechanisms - an increase in an inwardly rectifying potassium conductance which results in membrane hyperpolarization.[12,14,25] Opiates also mediate an identical response although there is no evidence for an opiate-mediated inhibitory synaptic potential[13]. Each of these agonists activate separate receptors to produce the same inhibition, noradrenaline acts on α_2-adrenoceptors, opiates on δ-opiate receptors and somatostatin on an as yet undetermined somatostatin receptor.

Voltage-clamp studies using both intracellular microelectrode and whole cell patch clamp methods have shown that each agonist produces an outward current at the resting potential (approximately -60 mV) with a large conductance increase; the outward current reverses at the potassium equilibrium potential (E_K) and shows a Nernstian relation for external potassium concentrations between 2.5 and 20 mM. Each agonist produces identical current-voltage responses over the potential range from -110 to -40 mV and outward currents produced by supramaximal concentrations of each agonist are not additive.[12,25,27] Moreover, each agonist can increase the activity of single potassium channels recorded from a patch of membrane.[19] These results provide very strong evidence that activation of these three distinct membrane receptors by their respective agonists results in activation of the same population of potassium channels.

The potassium conductance activated by these agonists shows strong inward rectification; that is, the inward current measured at potentials negative to E_K is greater than the outward current produced positive to E_K.[25,27] The resting membrane conductance (in the absence of inhibitory agonist) also shows similar inward rectification and both the resting and the agonist-induced inward rectification are blocked by cesium, rubidium and low micromolar concentrations of barium.[25] These results provided indirect evidence that these agonist may act by increasing the resting potassium conductance of the membrane rather than by activating a distinct set of potassium channels, as is the case for the acetylcholine-activated potassium conductance in cardiac tissue.[22] Direct evidence that this is the case comes from single channel recordings obtained from outside-out membrane patches of acutely dissociated submucosal neurons. In the absence of any inhibitory agonist, three distinct sets of unitary potassium currents are recorded from such membrane patches when the membrane is held at the normal resting potential (i.e. -60 mV), a small conductance channel (approximately 30-50 pS in equal potassium concentrations), an intermediate conductance channel (about 100 -140 pS) and a large conductance channel (215 - 260 pS). (It is unlikely that any of these "resting" unitary potassium currents were calcium-activated potassium currents because the experiments were done in the absence of calcium and in the presence of high concentrations of calcium chelators.) Activity of all three types of unitary currents was blocked by cesium, rubidium and barium. Application of somatostatin, noradrenaline and/or enkephalin to the outer surface of the membrane patch caused an increase in the activity (i.e. the open probability) of each of the unitary potassium currents that were active prior to agonist application. These agonists did not activate a potassium channel that was not already active in the absence of agonist and agonists did not cause the opening of any channels in membrane patches in which no channel activity was present prior to agonist application.[19]

SIGNAL TRANSDUCTION UNDERLYING SYNAPTIC INHIBITION TO SENSORIMOTOR NEURONS

Intracellular microelectrode and whole cell patch clamp studies have shown that a pertussis-toxin sensitive G-protein is involved in transducing inhibitory receptor activation to potassium conductance increase.[12,15,25,27] That is, intracellular injection or dialysis with the non-hydrolyzable GTP analogue, GTP-γ-S, results in an irreversible membrane hyerpolarization or outward current upon application of somatostatin, noradrenaline or enkephalin and repeated applications of these agonists produce no further response. The agonist-induced potassium conductance increase is abolished when preparations are treated with pertussis toxin or when pertussis is added directly into the cell by means of whole cell patch pipette dialysis. After pertussis toxin treatment, the agonist-induced outward current can be reconstituted by intracellular dialysis with patch pipettes containing purified G-proteins. It is not yet known which distinct G-protein subunit(s) mediate the agonist response because results obtained from reconstitution experiments in which purified G_i and G_o were added revealed that either G-protein subunit was equally effective in producing the agonist-induced response. However, these types of studies only show that exogenous application of either G-protein can be effective in signal transduction but they do not provide evidence as to which endogenous G-protein(s) are involved.

Much evidence suggests that the transduction between receptor, G-protein and potassium channel is direct and does not require a cytoplasmic second messenger system. In particular, inhibition of adenylyl cyclase does not appear to be involved in this transduction process. This is significant because biochemical studies have shown that activation of α_2-adrenoceptors, δ-opiate receptors and somatostatin receptors in every tissue in which these receptors have been demonstrated results in an inhibition of adenylyl cyclase activity providing that this enzyme has first been "turned on" by activators of this second messenger cascade (see Gilman[9]).

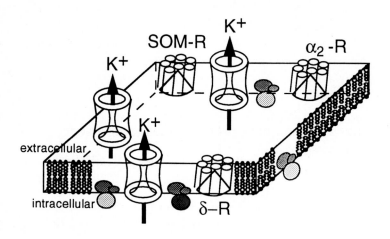

Figure 3. Diagram illustrating inhibitory receptors ($\alpha_2$adrenergic, δ-opioid and somatostatin) in submucosal neurons and their direct coupling through specific G-proteins to a family of "resting" or background potassium channels. G-proteins are depicted as trimers with the $\beta\gamma$ subunits being the same and the α subunits differing for each receptor. (Diagram is modified from Surprenant & North 1992, with permission).

Forskolin and other activators of the "cyclic AMP cascade" inhibit the prominent calcium-activated potassium conductance which is present in these submucosal neurons to produce membrane depolarization and excitation but these activators do not enhance the somatostatin, noradrenaline or opiate-induced outward current nor do they shift the dose-response curve for activation of the potassium current by these agonists[1,15,21].

Experiments in which activators or inhibitors of other second messenger transduction processes were used to examine possible involvement in the inhibitory signal transduction in submucosal neurons have all resulted in negative conclusions. That is, phorbol esters, arachidonic acid and its metabolites, or nitroprusside and inhibitors of nitric oxide synthase neither mimic, enhance nor inhibit agonist-induced outward currents in submucosal neurons (see Mihara[12]; Evans & Surprenant, unpublished observations).

Again, the most direct evidence for direct coupling between receptor, G-protein and potassium channel comes from single channel patch-clamp studies[19]. As described above, inhibitory agonists are effective in increasing single potassium channel activity when applied to the outside surface of the patch. Noradrenaline, somatostatin and enkephalin continue to increase activity of single potassium channels on repetitive applications for up to 2 hours after patch excision. However, agonist-induced increase in channel activity is only observed when GTP is included in the pipette solution bathing the inner surface of the membrane although the absence of internally applied GTP does not produce obvious changes in the appearance or activity of the potassium channels themselves. Figure 3 summarises signal transduction mechanisms mediating synaptic inhibition in sensorimotor vasodilator neurons of the submucosal plexus.

REFERENCES

1. AKASU, T. AND TOKIMASA, T. (1989). Potassium currents in submucous neurons of guinea-pig caecum and their synaptic modification. *J. Phvsiol.* **416**, 571-588.
2. ANDRIANTSITOHAINA, N. AND SURPRENANT. A. (1992) Acetylcholine released from guinea-pig submucosal neurons dilates arterioles by releasing nitric oxide from endothelium. *J. Physiol.* **453**, 493-502.
3. BORNSTEIN, J.C., COSTA, M. AND FURNESS, J.B. (1988) Extrinsic and intrinsic inhibitory synaptic inputs to submucous neurons of the guinea-pig small intestine. *J. Physiol.* **398**, 371-390.
4. BORNSTEIN, J.C., FURNESS, J.B. AND COSTA, M. (1987) Sources of excitatory synaptic input to neurochemically identified submucous neurons of guinea-pig small intestine. *J. Auton. Nerv. Syst.* **398,** 371-390
5. BUNGARDT, E., VOCKERT, E., FEIFEL, R., MOSER, U., TACKE, R., MUTSCHLER, E., LAMBRECHT, G., AND SURPRENANT, A. (1992) Characterization of muscarinic receptors mediating vasodilation in guinea-pig ileum submucosal arterioles using computer-assisted videomicroscopy. *Eur. J. Pharmacol.* **213**, 53-61.
6. EVANS, R.J. AND SURPRENANT, A. (1992) Vasoconstriction of guinea-pig submucosal arterioles following sympathetic nerve stimulation is mediated by the release of ATP. *Brit. J. Pharmacol.* **106**, 242-249.
7. FURNESS, J.B. AND COSTA, M. (1987) The Enteric Nervous System Churchill

Livingstone: New York

8. FURNESS, J.B., COSTA, M. AND KEAST, J.R. (1984) Choline acetyltransferase and peptide immunoreactivity of submucous neurons in the small intestine of the guinea pig. *Cell and Tissue Res.* **237**,328-336.

9. GILMAN, A.G. (1987) G-proteins: transducers of receptor-generated signals. *Ann. Rev. Biochemistry* **56**, 615-649.

10. JIANG, M-M., KIRCHGESSNER, A., GERSHON, M.D. AND SURPRENANT, A. (1993) Cholera toxin sensitive neurons in guinea-pig submucosal plexus. *Am. J. Physiol.* **264**, G86-G94.

11. KIRCHGESSNER, A.L. AND GERSHON, M.D. (1989) Identification of vagal efferent fibers and putative target neurons in the enteric nervous system of the rat. *J. Comp. Neurol.* **285**, 38-53.

12. MIHARA, S. (1993) Intracellular recordings from neurons of the submucous plexus. *Progress in Neurobiology* (in press)

13. MIHARA, S. AND NORTH, R.A. (1986). Opioids increase potassium conductance in submucous neurons of guinea-pig caecum by activating δ receptors. *Brit. J. Pharmacol.* **88**, 315-322 .

14. MIHARA, S., NORTH, R.A. AND SURPRENANT, A. (1987). Somatostatin increases an inwardly rectifying potassium conductance in guinea-pig submucous neurons. *J. Physiol.* **390**, 335-356.

15. MIHARA, S., NISHI, S., NORTH, R.A. AND SURPRENANT, A. (1987). A non-adrenergic, non-cholinergic slow inhibitory post-synaptic potential in neurons ofthe guinea-pig submucous plexus. *J. Physiol.* **390**, 357-366.

16. NEILD, T.O. (1989) Measurement of arteriole diameter changes by analysis of television images. *Blood Vessels* **26**, 48-52.

17. NEILD, T.O., SHEN, K-Z., AND SURPRENANT, A. (1990) Vasodilation of arterioles by acetylcholine released from single neurons in the guinea-pig submucosal plexus. *J. Physiol.* **420**, 247-265

18. NORTH, R.A. AND SURPRENANT, A. (1985) Inhibitory synaptic potentials resulting from α_2 adrenoceptor activation in guinea-pig submucous plexus neurons. *J. Physiol.* **358**, 17-32.

19. SHEN, K-Z., NORTH, R.A. AND SURPRENANT, A. (1992) Potassium channels opened by noradrenaline and other transmitters in excised membrane patches of guinea-pig submucosal neurons. *J.Physiol.* **445**, 581-699.

20. SHEN, K-Z. AND SURPRENANT, A. (1993a) Somatostatin mediates an inhibitory synaptic potential in sympathetically denervated submucosal neurons of the guinea-pig. *J. Physiol.* (in press)

21. SHEN, K-Z. AND SURPRENANT, A. (1993b) Common ionic mechanisms of excitation by substance P and other transmitters in guinea-pig submucosal neurons. *J. Physiol.* (in press)

22. SOEJIMA, M. AND NOMA, A. (1984). Mode of regulation of the ACh-sensitive K^+-channel by the muscarinic receptor in rabbit atrial cells. *Pflugers Arch.* 266, 324-334.

23. SURPRENANT, A. (1984) Slow excitatory synaptic potentials recorded from neurons of guinea-pig submucous plexus. *J. Physiol.* **351**, 343-361.

24. SURPRENANT, A. Neural control of submucosal vasculature. In: *Advances in the Innervation of the Gastrointestinal Tract.* eds. Holle, G.E. and Wood, J.D. Elsevier Sciences Publishing, Amsterdam.

25. SURPRENANT, A. AND NORTH, R.A. (1988) Mechanisms of synaptic inhibition

by noradrenaline acting at α_2 adrenoceptors. *Proc. Roy. Soc.* **234**, 85-114.

26. SURPRENANT, A. AND NORTH, R.A. (1992) Inhibitory receptors and signal transduction in submucosal neurons. In: *Advances in the Innervation of the Gastrointestinal Tract* eds., Holle, G.E. and Wood, J.D. Elsevier Sciences Publishing, Amsterdam.

27. TATSUMI, H., COSTA, M., SCHIMERLIK, M. AND NORTH, R.A. (1990) Potassium conductance increased by noradrenaline, opioids, somatostatin and G-proteins: whole cell recording from guinea-pig submucous neurons. *J. Neurosci.* **10**, 1625-1682 .

28. VANNER, S., JIANG, M-M. AND SURPRENANT, A. (1993) Mucosal stimulation evokes vasodilation in guinea-pig submucosal arterioles by neuronal and nonneuronal mechanisms. *Am. J. Physiol.* (in press)

MODULATION OF VOLTAGE DEPENDENT CALCIUM CHANNELS BY GABA$_B$ RECEPTORS AND G PROTEINS IN CULTURED RAT DORSAL ROOT GANGLION NEURONS: RELEVANCE TO TRANSMITTER RELEASE AND ITS MODULATION

Annette C. Dolphin, Anatole Menon-Johansson, Veronica Campbell, Nick Berrow and Marva I. Sweeney
Department of Pharmacology, Royal Free Hospital School of Medicine
Rowland Hill Street, London NW3 2PF
United Kingdom

INTRODUCTION

In many types of excitable cell, there are several classes of voltage-dependent calcium channel (VDCC) as determined by the characteristic properties of the single channel activity. There is a clear distinction between low conductance channels, activated by moderate depolarizations (low voltage-activated, LVA) and high conductance channels activated by large depolarizations (high voltage-activated, HVA).[2,36] In cardiac tissue these were termed T and L channels, respectively, because they were found to be pharmacologically, as well as biophysically, distinct.[2] Because of this they can also be clearly differentiated in whole-cell current recordings.[2,12] There is also evidence for a third class of single channel conductance (N type), whose biophysical properties were originally described as being intermediate between T and L, and which appears to be expressed only in cells of neuronal origin.[12,38,51] The sensitivity of N-type channels to irreversible block by ω-conotoxin GVIA (ωCgTx),[38] and the large number of ω-CgTx binding sites in neuronal tissue, indicates that they are likely to be important for neuronal function.[31] High threshold Ca^{2+} currents insensitive to both ω-CgTx and dihydropyridines have been reported,[27,38] and a selective blocker for at least part of this current is the peptide toxin from *Agelenopsis Aperta*, ω-agatoxin IVA (ω-aga IVA). The current inhibited by this toxin has been termed P current, because

NATO ASI Series, Vol. H 79
Cellular Mechanisms of Sensory Processing
Edited by Laszlo Urban
© Springer-Verlag Berlin Heidelberg 1994

Purkinje cells express calcium channel currents that are largely resistant to ω-CgTx and 1,4-dihydropyridines (DHPs),[27] and these currents are sensitive to ω-aga IVA.[35] It is difficult to distinguish these currents by biophysical means at the whole cell level,[21,35,38] and although estimates of their single channel conductances indicate differences, this is complicated by the existence of subconductance states.[53] However, the prolongation of single channel open times by DHP agonists remains diagnostic of L channels.[16]

SUBTYPES OF CALCIUM CHANNEL IN DORSAL ROOT GANGLION NEURONS

The calcium channel currents in dorsal root ganglion (DRG) neurons have been examined in a number of species, including chick and rat.[2] As well as LVA currents, DRGs express ω-CgTx sensitive, DHP sensitive and ω-aga IVA-sensitive currents.[10,35,40,47] On the basis of these pharmacological experiments, in acutely

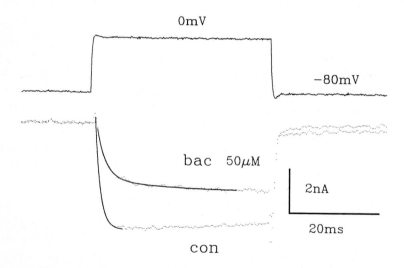

Figure 1. The effect of (-)-baclofen on I_{Ba} in cultured rat DRGs. Baclofen (50 μM) inhibits I_{Ba} within 10 s of its application. The activation of the control current can be fit by a single exponential (solid line, τ_{act}=1.4 ms), whereas the activation of the agonist-slowed I_{Ba} can be fit by a double exponential (solid line, $\tau_{f,act}$=2.3 ms; $\tau_{s,act}$=15.8 ms) (experimental details as Campbell et al, submitted). Upper trace: holding potential; lower traces: whole cell (inward) currents evoked by potential step.

dissociated DRGs, N type current represents about 50%, P type current about 25%, and L type current about 20% of the whole cell current, with a proportion of current remaining unblocked by all these antagonists. In cultured rat DRGs the proportion of L type current may be higher (about 40%)[10] but such determinations hinge on the uncertain specificity of µM concentrations of DHP antagonists for L type channels.[21,40] Interestingly, in acutely axotomised cultured DRGs, L current appears to be absent, possibly suggesting a localisation on neurites (Menon-Johannson, Berrow and Dolphin, manuscript submitted). Evidence suggests that at least for nodose sensory neurons, functional L type calcium channels appear after Na^+ and K^+ channels in development.[24]

INHIBITION OF VDCCS BY PTX SUBSTRATE G PROTEINS IN DRGS

The direct interaction of PTX substrate G proteins with ion channels is now well-established particularly for K^+ channels.[3] Initial evidence concerning VDCCs came from studies of calcium currents in DRG neurons, in which noradrenaline acting at α_2-adrenergic receptors, and GABA acting at (-)-baclofen-sensitive $GABA_B$ receptors inhibit the current (Figure 1), and this can be mimicked by GTPγS (Figure 2A) and inhibited by GDPβS and PTX.[9,19,44] It is now clear that numerous receptors on DRGs, all acting via PTX-sensitive G proteins are able to modulate VDCCs; these include adenosine A_1, µ and κ opioid, $5-HT_{1A}$ and NPY receptors.[1,7,11,30,43] Similar modulation occurs in many other neurons and neuronal cell lines, and also in neurosecretory cells, for example the pituitary cell line At-T-20, in which the calcium current is inhibited by somatostatin and by GTP analogues.[25] The most marked effect, particularly of GTP analogues, is to slow current activation[9] which has been interpreted as an inhibition of an inactivating N current (for review, see Tsien et al.[51]). However, pituitary secretory cells have not generally been shown to possess N current although a similar slowing of current activation is observed.[25,42] More recently, it has been suggested that this slowed current activation is a result of voltage-dependent interaction between the activated G protein and the calcium channel (Figure 2A and 2B).[13]

In the presence of agonist or internal GTPγS the calcium current often still has an initial rapidly activating, as well as a slowly activating component, the fast component having a similar time constant to that in control cells, and probably representing channels that are not associated with, or modified by activated G protein.[6,8,29] In support of this idea, it is found that the slowly activating component increases in proportion with time after the start of dialysis with GTPγS, at the expense of the rapidly activating component.[9,29] The slowly activating component may represent channels that are associated with activated G protein and open with a slower time course upon depolarization. In some well-perfused cells the fast component is completely lost in the presence of GTPγS,[10] indicating that all the VDCCs are potentially able to interact with activated G protein. The proportion of total current showing rapid, relative to slow, activation is not dependent on holding potential (V_H) between -30 and -90 mV.[29] In addition, Marchetti and Robello[29] have observed that the rate of activation of the slowly activating component is not

A prepulse to +40mV increases the rate
of activation of I_{Ba} in the presence of GTPγS

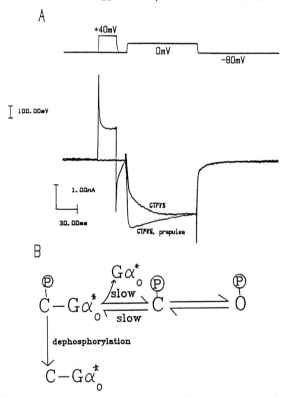

Figure 2. The effect of a 20 ms prepulse to +40 mV given 10 ms before the test pulse on the kinetics of activation of the test current. A: Recordings were performed in the presence of 200 μM GTPγS in the patch pipette. Experimental details as in Scott & Dolphin,[44]. B: Scheme of activated G protein (α•GTPγS) binding to a closed state of the channel C to form C*.

dependent on holding potential between V_H -80 and -30 mV although it is clearly dependent on test potential[9]. These results suggest that the interaction of the closed resting state of the channel (C) with activated G protein (Figure 2B) may not be voltage-dependent in this voltage range, and there is potentially a large excess of activated G protein.

We have hypothesised that activated G protein interacts with closed resting VDCCs to form a modified closed state C*, which may be unavailable to open with depolarization.[8] This complex, C*-G-GTPγS or C*-G-GTP, can dissociate with a slow rate constant, and the free closed state C is then available to open as normal (Figure 2B). Depolarization increases the rate of C→0, thus diminishing the pool of free C, and increasing the net rate of G-GTPγS-C*→C. In many cell types e.g.[13,46] a brief prepulse to a large depolarising voltage reversed the GTPγS- or agonist-induced slowing of current activation in a subsequent test pulse activated immediately afterwards (Figure 2A). During the prepulse, the equilibrium C*→C→0 is shifted towards 0. At the end of the prepulse, 0→C occurs rapidly, but the rate of C→C* is sufficiently slow that most of the channels remain as C at the time the test pulse is delivered. Subsequent current activation due to the test pulse occurs rapidly with this voltage paradigm.

It has been noted by several groups[6,13,46] that the depolarising prepulse does not restore the amplitude of the current, and it was suggested that an additional effect may be occurring.[13] We have shown that the calcium channel current in the presence of GTPγS ($I_{Ba(GTPγS)}$) is reduced in amplitude compared to the control current, and that the amplitude can be increased by agents increasing cyclic AMP such as forskolin[5] or an inhibitor of phosphatase1.[6] This finding is compatible with the hypothesis that coupling of a G protein with the Ca^{2+} channel also promotes dephosphorylation possibly of the channel itself, or of proteins associated with it.

We have also found LVA currents to be inhibited by $GABA_B$ receptor activation and by GTPγS,[23,48] although no effect was observed on the kinetics of activation of the current.

THE NATURE OF THE G PROTEIN INVOLVED IN RECEPTOR-CALCIUM CHANNEL COUPLING IN DRGs

The identification of the G protein involved in coupling receptors to Ca^{2+} current inhibition has been aided by experiments in which G proteins are included in

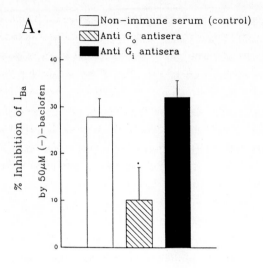

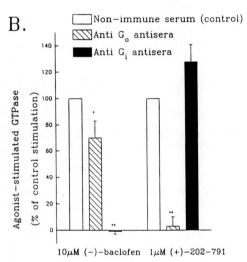

Figure 3. Effect of anti G protein antibodies on the ability of (-)-baclofen and G proteins to interact with calcium channels. A: Anti G_o antibodies but not anti G_i antibodies reduce the ability of (-)-baclofen to inhibit I_{Ba} in cultured DRGs. Experimental details as in Menon-Johansson et al (submitted). B: Anti G_i antibodies markedly inhibit $GABA_B$ activation of GTP-ase, with anti G_o antibodies having a smaller effect, whereas anti G_o antibodies completely inhibit stimulation of GTP-ase by the DHP agonist (+)-202-791. Experimental details as in Sweeney & Dolphin[50].

the patch pipette when recording Ca^{2+} currents in PTX-treated cells. Exogenously added G proteins can restore the ability of neurotransmitters to inhibit Ca^{2+} currents. These experiments have generally suggested that G_o protein mediates inhibition of neuronal calcium currents by neurotransmitters.[15,26,33] We have investigated the ability of anti-G protein antibodies to prevent the effect of the GABA$_B$ agonist (-)-baclofen and GTPγS in cultured rat DRGs. The cells were replated before use by non-enzymatic removal from the culture dish. When this was done in the presence of IgG, it resulted in the entry of antibodies into the cells by a form of scrape-loading.

This was confirmed immunocytochemically. We have shown that an anti-G_o antipeptide antibody against the C terminus of G_o (OC1, provided by G. Milligan, Glasgow), when loaded into DRGs in this way reduced the ability of (-)-baclofen to inhibit I_{Ba}. In contrast, antibodies against the N terminus of G_o or antibodies against the C terminus of G_i, recognising all G_i species, were ineffective,[34] and the anti G_o antibody OC1 was unable to prevent GTPγS from modulating the calcium channel current (Figure 3A). Additional evidence for a role of G_o was that internal application of a C terminal peptide sequence from G_o also reduced the ability of (-)-baclofen to inhibit I_{Ba}. Presumably this peptide mimics G_o and interferes with coupling between the GABA$_B$ receptor and native G_o. In these replated DRGs, in contrast to non-replated DRGs with neurites, L type Ca channels were absent and ω-CgTx inhibited approximately 30% of the current. No inhibition of the current by (-)-baclofen was observed following irreversible inhibition of the ω-CgTx-sensitive portion of the current, suggesting that only N channels are modulated by (-)-baclofen in this preparation (Menon-Johansson, Berrow and Dolphin, submitted). However, it is clear from other, secretory cell types that receptors are able to modulate L channels, again via G_o.[22] Indeed we have obtained biochemical evidence from an examination of the effects of 1,4-dihydropyridines on GTP-ase activity in cerebral cortical membranes that L type Ca channels may act as a GTP-ase activating protein or GAP for G_o since anti G_o antibodies but not anti G_i block GTP-ase activation by DHP agonists[50] (Figure 3B). Thus, G_o modulates the activity of the channel, which itself limits the temporal effectiveness of the G protein mediated signal. It is possible that other subtypes of channel may also have this effect.

Further evidence that G_o and not G_i is involved in coupling GABA$_B$ receptors to VDCCs in DRGs comes from experiments in which antisense oligonucleotides complementary to mRNA sequences for G_o and G_i were microinjected into DRGs and selectively depleted either G protein. Only depletion of G_o reduced the effectiveness of (-)-baclofen (Campbell, Berrow and Dolphin, manuscript in preparation).

WHICH TYPES OF VDCC MEDIATE TRANSMITTER RELEASE?

The release of neurotransmitters from presynaptic terminals is dependent on an influx of Ca^{2+} through VDCCs. Evidence concerning the subtype(s) of VDCC involved in transmitter release remains equivocal. It has been suggested that N channels are the most important[17,51] primarily because transmitter release is not markedly sensitive to DHP antagonists, although in some cases it is sensitive to agonists.[39] Because of the marked voltage-sensitivity of DHP antagonists,[4,16,45] they are poorly effective at hyperpolarized membrane potentials,[41] which may preclude their action on any L type channels opening briefly at the nerve terminal. However, it is likely that release of fast neurotransmitters is normally poorly sensitive to DHP antagonists because it relies on Ca^{2+} entry through channels at active zones close to synaptic vesicle docking sites, and that these channels are not L type. Nevertheless, L channels may also be involved in some systems, particularly in facilitation during trains of action potentials, and may also be involved in secretion from large-dense core vesicles which is thought to result from a less localised increase in Ca^{2+}.

The other agent that has been used extensively to dissect out the channels involved in transmitter release is ω-CgTx. This inhibits transmitter release in many, but by no means all, systems that have been investigated (for review see Tsien et al, 1988[51]). It has also been shown that ω-aga IVA inhibits the release of glutamate from rat cortical synaptosomes, whereas ω-CgTx does not.[52] In contrast the 50 mM K^+ induced release of glutamate from cerebellar granule neurones in culture is inhibited by about 20% by 1 μM ω-CgTx,[20] whereas preliminary evidence suggests that ω-aga IVA is ineffective (Cullen and Dolphin, unpublished results) and thus P channels may not be involved in release in this system.

CONTROL OF TRANSMITTER RELEASE FROM DRGs

The release of substance P from DRGs has been shown to be highly sensitive to DHP agonists and antagonists when stimulated by K^+[37,39]. In contrast, electrically stimulated substance P release was not inhibited by DHP antagonists.[39] The fast epsp recorded in cultured mouse spinal cord neurons due to stimulation of DRG neurones was enhanced by Bay K8644 in about 50% of cells[54] and was incompletely inhibited by ω-CgTx. In contrast Gruner et al.[14] showed that in a similar preparation from chick, fast DRG epsps were blocked completely by ω-CgTx. These epsps were entirely due to the release of glutamate rather than substance P, since they were blocked by the glutamate receptor antagonist CNQX. This suggests that release of fast transmitter at this synapse is N type in the avian system, but is partly non N type in mammals.

Transmitter release from DRGs, as from other neurons, is inhibited by a number of agonists that also modulate calcium currents.[14,18] Thus, it is entirely possible that modulation of transmitter release by activation of receptors such as the $GABA_B$ receptor is due to inhibition of the Ca^{2+} entry, through N and other channels required for transmitter release at the active zone, although there are other routes of modulation including K^+ channel activation, and interference with the exocytotic machinery[28] (Figure 4).

It has to be questioned whether direct modulation of the VDCCs at the active zone is likely to play any physiological role except in the cause of auto-inhibition. It is likely that adenosine would be present, close to the channels associated with release sites as it would be formed from ATP co-released with glutamate. Would the other neuromodulatory agents released in the dorsal horn of the spinal cord *in vivo* penetrate to the active zone of the primary afferent terminals to inhibit the calcium currents directly responsible for release, or are they more likely to act at more distant sites on the presynaptic terminal, for example modulating Ca^{2+} influx responsible for facilitating the movement of vesicles towards the active zone by activation of Ca^{2+}-calmodulin dependent protein kinase-II (Figure 4)? Although a number of studies have shown axo-axonic synapses onto sensory neuron terminals in the spinal cord, and these have been identified as GABA and enkephalin-containing among others,[32] nevertheless the transmitter released by these axo-axonic terminals would have to diffuse some distance to reach the active zones of the primary afferent terminals (Figure 4).

There are clearly $GABA_B$ as well as $GABA_A$ receptors on sensory neuron terminals, because (-)-baclofen produces a substantial inhibition of synaptic transmission. However, synaptically released GABA is thought to mediate presynaptic inhibition of primary afferents to the spinal cord largely by $GABA_A$ receptor activation. Evidence for a substantial physiological inhibitory effect of GABA via $GABA_B$ receptors remains elusive in the absence of any studies with potent $GABA_B$ antagonists.[49] It is possible that $GABA_B$ receptor activation only comes into play in presynaptic inhibition over a period of prolonged activation when $GABA_A$ receptors have desensitised, and sufficient GABA has been released to activate $GABA_B$ receptors.

Possible Routes of Presynaptic Modulation
by GABA

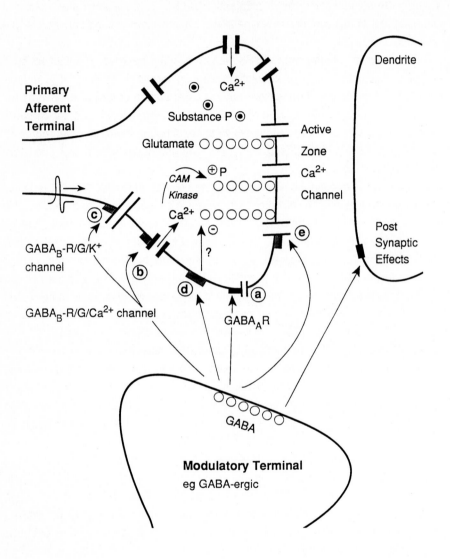

Figure 4. Scheme of presynaptic inhibition by GABA, showing a sensory terminal in the spinal cord, with an associated GABA-ergic axo-axonic synapse, illustrating the possible means by which GABA inhibits transmission at the primary afferent-spinal cord synapse.

Possible GABA effects on sensory terminal

a) $GABA_A$ activation of Cl^- channel, shunting the invasion of an action potential into the terminal.

b) $GABA_B$ inhibition of Ca^{2+} channels distant from primary afferent active zone, reducing Ca^{2+} influx into the terminal. These Ca^{2+} channels may (i) mediate substance P release, (ii) activate CAM kinase II or C kinase, increasing the availability of small synaptic vesicles for release, but will not directly affect release of small synaptic vesicles at the active zone induced by single action potentials.

c) $GABA_B$ activation of K^+ channels, hyperpolarising terminal.

d) $GABA_B$ activation of a second messenger system, reducing vesicle availability for release.

e) Diffusion of GABA to subsynaptic region to directly inhibit VDCCs at the active zone by activation of $GABA_B$ receptors.

Key

1. Ca^{2+} channels at active zone (largely non L type).
2. Ca^{2+} channels distant from active zone (may be L type).

• Small synaptic vesicles releasing fast transmitter for which glutamate is the major contender.

o Large vesicles releasing peptides including substance P.

CONCLUSION

The modulation of calcium channel current in cultured rat DRGs by $GABA_B$ receptors involves the GTP binding G_o and may, if it occurs at presynaptic terminals *in vivo* due to synaptically released GABA, provide a mechanism of primary afferent inhibition.

ACKNOWLEDGEMENTS: The work in this laboratory was supported by the Wellcome Trust and MRC. M.I. Sweeney was a Canadian MRC Fellow.

REFERENCES

1. AOSAKI, T. AND KASAI, H. (1989) Characterization of two kinds of high-voltage-activated Ca-channel currents in chick sensory neurons. *Pflugers Arch.* **414**, 150-156.
2. BEAN, B.P. (1985) Two kinds of calcium channels in canine atrial cells. *J. Gen. Physiol.* **86**, 1-30.

3. BREITWIESER, G.E. AND SZABO, G. (1985) Uncoupling of cardiac muscarinic and ß-adrenergic receptors from ion channels by a guanine nucleotide analogue. *Nature* **317**, 538-540.

4. BROWN, A.M., KUNZE, D.L. AND YATANI, A. (1986) Dual effects of dihydropyridines on whole cell and unitary calcium currents in single ventricular cells of guinea-pig. *J. Physiol.* **379**, 495-514.

5. DOLPHIN, A.C. (1991) Ca^{2+} channel currents in rat sensory neurones: Interaction between guanine nucleotides, cyclic AMP and Ca^{2+} channel ligands. *J. Physiol.* **432**, 23-43.

6. DOLPHIN, A.C. (1992) The effect of phosphatase inhibitors and agents increasing cyclic-AMP-dependent phosphorylation on calcium channel currents in cultured rat dorsal root ganglion neurones: Interaction with the effect of G protein activation. *Pflügers Arch.* **421**, 138-145.

7. DOLPHIN, A.C., FORDA, S.R. AND SCOTT, R.H. (1986) Calcium-dependent currents in cultured rat dorsal root ganglion neurones are inhibited by an adenosine analogue. *J. Physiol.* **373**, 47-61.

8. DOLPHIN, A.C., HUSTON, E. AND SCOTT, R.H. (1990) Direct and indirect modulation of neuronal calcium currents by G-protein activation. *Biochem. Soc. Symp.* **56**, 45-60.

9. DOLPHIN, A.C. AND SCOTT, R.H. (1987) Calcium channel currents and their inhibition by (-)-baclofen in rat sensory neurones: modulation by guanine nucleotides. *J. Physiol.* **386**, 1-17.

10. DOLPHIN, A.C. AND SCOTT, R.H. (1989) Interaction between calcium channel ligands and guanine nucleotides in cultured rat sensory and sympathetic neurones. *J. Physiol.* **413**, 271-288.

11. EWALD, D.A., PANG, I.-H., STENWEIS, P.C. AND MILLER, R.J. (1989) Differential G protein-mediated coupling of neurotransmitter receptors to Ca^{2+} channels in rat dorsal root ganglion neurons *in vitro*. *Neuron* **2**, 1185-1193.

12. FOX, A.P., NOWYCKY, M.C. AND TSIEN, R.W. (1987) Kinetic and pharmacological properties distinguishing three types of calcium currents in chick sensory neurones. *J. Physiol.* **394**, 149-172.

13. GRASSI, F. AND LUX, H.D. (1989) Voltage-dependent GABA-induced modulation of calcium currents in chick sensory neurons. *Neurosci. Lett.* **105**, 113-119.

14. GRUNER, W., SILVA, L.R. AND DUNLAP, K. (1992) ω-Conotoxin-sensitive calcium current mediates presynaptic inhibition at the sensory neuron-spinal cord synapse. *Soc. Neurosci.* **18**, 247P.

15. HARRIS-WARWICK, R.M., HAMMOND, C., PAUPARDIN-TRITSCH, D., HOMBURGER, V., ROUOT, B., BOCKAERT, J. AND GERSCHENFELD, H.M. (1988) An $\alpha 40$ subunit of a GTP binding protein immunologically related to G_o mediates a dopamine-induced decrease of a Ca^{2+} current in snail neurones. *Neuron* **1**, 17-32.

16. HESS, P., LANSMAN, J.B. AND TSIEN, R.W. (1984) Different modes of Ca channel gating behaviour favoured by dihydropyridine Ca agonists and antagonists. *Nature* **311**, 538-544.

17. HIRNING, L.D., FOX, A.P., MCCLESKEY, E.W., OLIVERA, B.M., THAYER, S.A., MILLER, R.J. AND TSIEN, R.W. (1988) Dominant role of N-type Ca^{2+}

channels in evoked release of norepinephrine from sympathetic neurons. *Science* **239**, 57-60.

18. HOLZ, G.G., KREAM, R.M., SPIEGEL, A. AND DUNLAP, K. (1989) G proteins couple α-adrenergic and GABAb receptors to inhibition of peptide secretion from peripheral sensory neurons. *Neuroscience* **9**, 657-666.

19. HOLZ, G.G., RANE, S.G. AND DUNLAP, K. (1986) GTP binding proteins mediate transmitter inhibition of voltage-dependent calcium channels. *Nature* **319**, 670-672.

20. HUSTON, E., CULLEN, G., SWEENEY, M.I., PEARSON, H.A., FAZELI, M.S. AND DOLPHIN, A.C. (1993) Pertussis toxin treatment increases glutamate release and dihydropyridine binding sites in cultured rat cerebellar granule neurones. *Neuroscience* **52**, 787-798.

21. JONES, S.W. AND JACOBS, L.S. (1990) Dihydropyridine actions on calcium currents of frog sympathetic neurons. *J. Neurosci.* **10**, 2261-2267.

22. KLEUSS, C., HESCHELER, J., EWEL, C., ROSENTHAL, W., SCHULTZ, G. AND WITTIG, B. (1991) Assignment of G-protein subtypes to specific receptors inducing inhibition of calcium currents. *Nature* **353**, 43-48.

23. KOBRINSKY, E.M., PEARSON, H.A. AND DOLPHIN, A.C. (1993) Pharmacological properties of low-voltage activated calcium channel currents in the dorsal root ganglion cell x neuroblastoma hybrid cell line, ND7-23. *J. Physiol.* **459**, 403P.

24. LARMET, Y., DOLPHIN, A.C. AND DAVIES, A.M. (1992) Intracellular calcium regulates the survival of early sensory neurons before they become dependent on neurotrophic factors. *Neuron* **9**, 563-574.

25. LEWIS, D.L., WEIGHT, F.F. AND LUINI, A. (1986) A guanine nucleotide binding protein mediates the inhibition of voltage-dependent calcium current by somatostatin in a pituitary cell line. *Proc. Natl. Acad. Sci. USA* **83**, 9035-9039.

26. LLEDO, P.M., HOMBURGER, V., BOCKAERT, J. AND VINCENT, J.-D. (1992) Differential G protein-mediated coupling of D_2 dopamine receptors to $K+$ and Ca^{2+} currents in rat anterior pituitary cells. *Neuron* **8**, 455-463.

27. LLINÁS, R., SUGIMORI, M., LIN, J.-W. AND CHERKSEY, B. (1989) Blocking and isolation of a calcium channel from neurons in mammals and cephalopods utilizing a toxin fraction (FTX) from funnel-web spider poison. *Proc. Natl. Acad. Sci. USA* **86**, 1689-1693.

28. MAN-SON-HING, H., ZORAN., M.J., LUKOWIAK, K. AND HAYDON, P.G. (1989) A neuromodulator of synaptic transmission acts on the secretory apparatus as well as on ion channels. *Nature* **341**, 237-239.

29. MARCHETTI, C. AND ROBELLO, M. (1989) Guanosine-5'-0-(3-thiotriphosphate) modifies kinetics of voltage-dependent calcium current in chick sensory neurons. *Biophys. J.* **56**, 1267-1272.

30. MARSZALEC, W., SCROGGS, R.S. AND ANDERSON, E.G. (1988) Serotonin-induced reduction of the calcium-dependent plateau in frog dorsal root ganglion cells is blocked by serotonergic agents acting at 5-hydroxytryptamine1A sites. *J. Pharm. &. Exp. Therap.* **247, No.2**, 399.

31. MARTIN-MOUTOT N., SEAGAR M. AND COURAUD F. (1990) Subtypes of voltage-sensitive calcium channels in cultured rat neurons. *Neuroscience Lett.* **115**, 300-306.

32. MAXWELL, D.J., CHRISTIE, W.M., SHORT, A.D. AND BROWN, A.G. (1990) Direct observation of synapses between GABA-immunoreactive boutons and muscle afferent terminals in lamina VI of the cat's spinal cord. *Brain Res.* **530**, 215-222.

33. MCFADZEAN, I., MULLANEY, I. AND BROWN, D.A. (1989) Antibodies to the GTP binding protein, G_0, antagonize noradrenaline-induced calcium current inhibition in NG108-15 hybrid cells. *Neuron* **3**, 177-182.

34. MENON-JOHANSSON, A. AND DOLPHIN, A.C. (1992) Inhibition of GABA$_B$ modulation of cultured rat dorsal root ganglion neurones by loading replated cells with anti G protein antibodies. *J.Physiol.* **452**, 117P(Abstract).

35. MINTZ, I.M., ADAMS, M.E. AND BEAN, B.P. (1992) P-type calcium channels in rat central and peripheral neurons. *Neuron* **9**, 85-95.

36. NILIUS, B., HESS, P., LANSMAN, J.B. AND TSIEN, R.W. (1985) A novel type of cardiac calcium channel in ventricular cells. *Nature* **316**, 443-446.

37. PERNEY, T.M., HIRNING, L.D., LEEMAN, S.E. AND MILLER, R.J. (1986) Multiple calcium channels mediate neurotransmitter release from peripheral neurons. *Proc.Natl.Acad.Sci.USA* **83**, 6656-6659.

38. PLUMMER, M.R., LOGOTHETIS, D.E. AND HESS, P. (1989) Elementary properties and pharmacological sensitivities of calcium channels in mammalian peripheral neurons. *Neuron* **2**, 1453-1463.

39. RANE, S.G., HOL, G.G. AND DUNLAP, K. (1987) Dihydropyridine inhibition of neuronal calcium current and substance P release. *Pflugers Arch.* **409**, 361-366.

40. REGAN, L.J., SAH, D.W.Y. AND BEAN, B.P. (1991) Ca2+ channels in rat central and peripheral neurons: High-threshold current resistant to dihydro-pyridine blockers and ω-conotoxin. *Neuron* **6**, 269-280.

41. SANGUINETTI, M.C. AND KASS, R.S. (1984) Voltage-dependent modulation of Ca channel current in the calf cardiac purkinje fiber by dihydropyridine calcium channel antagonists. *Circ.Res.* **55**, 336-348.

42. SCHMIDT, A., HESCHELER, J., OFFERMANNS, S., SPICHER, K., HINSCH, K.-D., KLINZ, F.-J., CODINA, J., BIRNBAUMER, L., GAUSEPOHL, H., FRANK, R., SCHULTZ, G. AND ROSENTHAL, W. (1991) Involvement of pertussis toxin-sensitive G-proteins in the hormonal inhibition of dihydropyridine-sensitive Ca2+ currents in an insulin-secreting cell line (RINm5F). *J.Biol.Chem.* **266**, 18025-18033.

43. SCHROEDER, J.E., FISCHBACH, P.S., ZHENG, D. AND MCCLESKEY, E.W. (1991) Activation of μ opioid receptors inhibits transient high- and low-threshold Ca2+ currents, but spares a sustained current. *Neuron* **6**, 13-20.

44. SCOTT, R.H. AND DOLPHIN, A.C. (1986) Regulation of calcium currents by GTP analogue: potentiation of (-)-baclofen-mediated inhibition. *Neuroscience Lett.* **69**, 59-64.

45. SCOTT, R.H. AND DOLPHIN, A.C. (1987) Activation of a G protein promotes agonist responses to calcium channel ligands. *Nature* **330**, 760-762.

46. SCOTT, R.H. AND DOLPHIN, A.C. (1990) Voltage-dependent modulation of rat sensory neurone calcium channel currents by G Protein activation: effect of a dihydropyridine antagonist. *Br. J. Pharmacol.* **99**, 629-630.

47. SCOTT, R.H., DOLPHIN, A.C., BINDOKAS, V.P. AND ADAMS, M.E. (1990) Inhibition of neuronal Ca2+ channel currents by the Funnel Web spider toxin x-Aga-1A. *Mol. Pharmacol.* **38**, 711-718.

48. SCOTT, R.H., WOOTTON, J.F. AND DOLPHIN, A.C. (1990) Modulation of neuronal T-type calcium channel currents by photoactivation of intracellular guanosine 5'-0(3-THIO) triphosphate. *Neuroscience* **38**, 285-294.

49. STUART, G.J. AND REDMAN, S.J. (1992) The role of GABA$_A$ and GABA$_B$ receptors in presynaptic inhibition of Ia EPSPs in cat spinal motoneurones. *J.Physiol.* **447**, 675-692.

50. SWEENEY, M.I. AND DOLPHIN, A.C. (1992) 1,4-Dihydropyridines modulate GTP hydrolysis by G$_0$ in neuronal membranes. *FEBS Lett.* **310**, 66-70.

51. TSIEN, R.W., LIPSCOMBE, D., MADISON, D.V., BLEY, K.R. AND FOX, A.P. (1988) Multiple types of neuronal calcium channels and their selective modulation. *Trends Neurosci.* **11, No.10**, 431-438.

52. TURNER, T.J., ADAMS, M.E. AND DUNLAP, K. (1992) Calcium channels coupled to glutamate release identified by omega-Aga-IVA. *Science* **258**, 310-313.

53. USOWICZ, M.M., SUGIMORI, M., CHERKSEY, B. AND LLINÁS, R. (1992) P-type calcium channels in the somata and dendrites of adult cerebellar Purkinje cells. *Neuron* **9**, 1185-1199.

54. YU, C., LIN, P.-X., FITZGERALD, S. AND NELSON, P. (1992) Heterogeneous calcium currents and transmitter release in cultured mouse spinal cord and dorsal root ganglion neurons. *J.Neurophysiol.* **67**, 561-575.

SIGNAL INTEGRATION IN THE AXON TREE DUE TO BRANCH POINT FILTERING ACTION

S. David Stoney, Jr.
Department of Physiology and Endocrinology
Medical College of Georgia
Augusta, Georgia 30912-3000
USA

INTRODUCTION

The often extravagant branching of axons into numerous collateral and even more numerous terminal branches is one of the most distinctive morphological features of neurons. It is not surprising then, that the possibility of signal integration in the axon tree, i.e., one or another form of filtering action, which may degrade, enrich or focus the neural signal as it propagates through the axon tree, has been suggested since the early days of analytical neurophysiological research.[1] In fact, evidence for filtering action at branch points of dorsal column fibers and at intramuscular branch points of phrenic motor neuron axons was soon forthcoming.[14,15,41] Subsequently however, very little addition information on the nature and frequency of occurrence of branch point filtering action in *vertebrate* neurons has been obtained, due no doubt in large part to the practical difficulties of monitoring activity in the parent and daughter branches of their small diameter, relatively inaccessible axons. On the other hand, convincing evidence for such action at axon branch points of *invertebrate* neurons, as well as the development of a thorough mathematical understanding of some of the basic mechanisms accounting for this phenomenon, became available for invertebrate nerve cells.[7,8,26,27,45]

This paper considers the question of what types of branch point filtering action are likely to occur in the axon tree of vertebrate neurons and whether or not they are likely to be a common phenomenon in the vertebrate nervous system. A number of excellent reviews[18,40,42] have dealt with the question of branch point filtering action

NATO ASI Series, Vol. H 79
Cellular Mechanisms of Sensory Processing
Edited by Laszlo Urban
© Springer-Verlag Berlin Heidelberg 1994

in invertebrate neurons and considered the early results on vertebrate neurons, so no attempt will be made for inclusiveness, especially with respect to the older material. Instead, the coverage will first focus on the occurrence of branch point filtering action in the dorsal root ganglion, one of the few sites in the vertebrate nervous system where conduction from a single parent axon into each of its daughter branches can be unequivocally measured. The results of experiments carried out there will be compared to results of computer simulations of action potential conduction at regions of axonal inhomogeneity, especially branch points.

VARIETIES OF BRANCH POINT FILTERING ACTION

It appears useful to distinguish between several types of branch point filtering action. Evidence suggestive of one or another type of branch point filtering action in the axonal tree of vertebrate neurons has been reported for dorsal column fibers conveying somatic sensory information,[1,41] for motor neuron axon terminal branches,[14,15] for dorsal root ganglia (DRG) neurons,[6] for thalamocortical fiber terminals[5] and for Group Ia afferent fiber terminals in the spinal cord.[21,22] Barron and Matthews[1] described an intermittent *blocking* of discharges in dorsal column fibers which they ascribed to excitation in the central grey which, via collateral branches, produced an "electrotonic block" of activity at the bifurcation points of the entering afferent fibers. This form of filtering action is, in fact, a form of *inhibition* due to conduction blockade where the entering afferent activity is temporarily prevented from accessing higher levels of the neuraxis. Subsequently, Wall and his colleagues[41] observed that a conditioning volley in the same or neighboring peripherally activated dorsal column fibers caused a reduction in the area of a test response over at least a 25 msec CT interval. They suggested that the branch point of each primary afferent might act like a "valve," limiting the maximum frequency of centrally conducting impulses to values well below what could be sustained in unbranched portions of the same axons. This *bandpass limiting* form of branch point filtering action was also observed by Dun[6] for pairs of compound action potentials conducting across the frog DRG.

Both of these types of branch point filtering action are simple, providing that the conduction block or bandpass limiting effect applies to both daughter branches. However, perhaps they could operate together or separately for individual branches to produce a *differential* effect, where activity is confined to one or another subset of daughter branches in the axonal tree. Such a possibility would provide for much more flexible influences on signal processing in the axon tree, especially if the filtering action arises as a consequence of excitability changes associated with activity,[8,26] i.e. after a period of stimulation or only at certain frequencies of stimulation. For vertebrate neurons, the best example of this type of filtering action appears to be the asynchronous failure of endplate potentials recorded simultaneously from two endplates of the same motor unit during 64 Hz stimulation.[14,15] The suggestion by Luscher and his colleagues,[21,22] that differences in the extent of post-tetanic potentiation of Group Ia EPSPs in large compared to small motor neurons is due to more extensive relief of branch point conduction block in the GIa terminal arbors supplying larger cells, is a more contemporary example of a hypothesised role for spatio-temporal filtering action. The possibility that such *spatio-temporal* filtering action plays a major role in signal processing has been championed by Lettvin and his colleagues[4]. Indeed, a general "rule" has been proposed[30] that "the connectivity between an axon and its post-synaptic elements is a dynamic property that depends on the temporal pattern of impulses it carries."

FILTERING ACTION IN FROG DRG

The dorsal root ganglion (DRG) is a propitious place to test for the occurrence of branch point filtering action in the vertebrate nervous system. Each DRG neuron connects, via its stem process, to an intraganglionic branch point from which arises the dorsal root process and the peripheral nerve process.[20] While it is impracticable to record from the branch point itself, recordings can be made from the DRG neuron cell body, which allows for monitoring of conduction into the stem process and cell body. Whether or not conduction occurs for the dorsal root portion of the fiber every time there is invasion of the stem process which can be assessed by applying an appropriately timed stimulus to the dorsal root. If the propagating action potential also invaded the dorsal root process then it will collide with the impulse evoked by dorsal root stimulation and no antidromic response will be recorded from the cell body. In this manner the success or failure and the pattern of conduction through the branch point can be measured.

Stoney[37,39] took advantage of this preparation and measured conduction at the branch point of frog DRG neurons for pairs of impulses at short intervals and for short trains of impulses at various frequencies. The frog was chosen for study because it provides such a robust *in vitro* preparation and because invasion of the stem process is often reliably signalled by small electrotonic potentials (NM and M spikes) that can be recorded from the cell body even when the cell body itself is not invaded by the conducting action potential.[11,12] Figure 1 illustrates the experimental setup and shows the intracellularly recorded responses of three different neurons to pairs of suprathreshold stimulating pulses at decreasing intervals applied to the

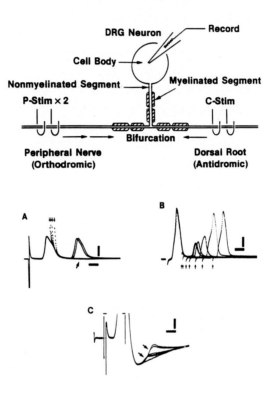

Figure 1. Setup for recording from frog DRG neurons and results of double pulse stimulation of peripheral nerve. **Top** schematic diagram of a DRG neuron (not to scale). Certain features of neuron structure, location of electrodes and direction of impulse travel are shown. Myelinated internodes near the branch point are stippled; others are not shown. **A-C** responses of different neurons to suprathreshold double pulse stimulation of the peripheral nerve; each trace is 4-7 superimposed oscilloscope sweeps with the interval approaching (**A, B**) or at (**C**) the ARP. When the response to the 2nd stimulus failed, a baseline trace appeared (bottom arrow in **A**). Often, due to conduction failure prior to reaching the soma, the 2nd response decomposed into a smaller component before failing. **B** shows an NM spike produced by spike failure in the nonmyelinated portion of the stem process. **C** shows a small multicomponent M spike produced by spike failure in the myelinated segment; spike potential is truncated. Time = 1 msec (**B,C**), 2 msec (**A**). Voltage = 50, 20, 5 mV for **A, B, C**. T = 22 °C. (Adapted from Stoney[39], with permission)

peripheral nerve. Two measurements were made from such records. First, the absolute refractory period (ARP), the minimal *interpulse* interval at which two orthodromic responses would successfully invade the stem process, was measured. The occurrence of a full-blown or of a partial spike (NM or M spike) was taken as "successful" invasion. Second, the least conduction interval (LCI), the interval between responses recorded at the ARP was measured. This inter-response interval is close to the minimum interval at which conducted responses can occur and was always measured between the foot of the first spike and the foot of the second response. These values, which averaged ARP = 1.7±.04 msec and LCI = 2.4±.04 msec for DRG *neurons* with fast somatic action potentials and rapidly conducting axons, were significantly longer than values for ARP (1.1±.03 msec) and LCI (1.6± .07 msec) for a sample of afferent *fibers* recorded from just distal to the ganglion (Figure 2). This result shows that the second response was not failing in the peripheral nerve itself (or at the stimulating electrodes) and indicates that there are limitations on the minimum interval between impulses that can conduct into the stem process.

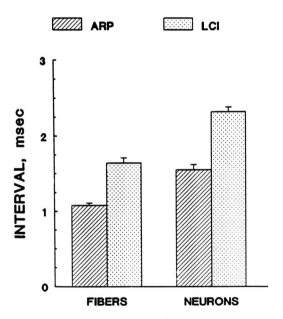

Figure 2. Histograms showing ARP and LCI (mean ± SEM) for DRG neurons and for afferent fibers in the peripheral nerve just distal to the ganglion. Responses of afferent fibers were recorded with glass microelectrodes. Fiber ARP and LCI were significantly longer than ARP and LCI measured for DRG neurons. (Adapted from Stoney[39])

The question remained as to whether or not the limitation on conduction into the stem process also applied for impulses conducting into the dorsal root. This question was answered unequivocally using the collision method. In only 2 instances in 71 cases tested was there evidence that the second response successfully conducted into the dorsal root at the same or shorter interval at which it failed to invade the stem process. In these cases the stem process response to the second stimulus disappeared without the expected appearance of the antidromic response from dorsal root stimulation (Figure 3C). In fact, only two other instances of differential conduction by the second impulse were found, where conduction into the dorsal root process failed at a longer interval than conduction into the stem process. It is clear, at least for pairs of impulses at the LCI, that differential conduction is rare at the intraganglionic axon branch point of frog afferent nerve fibers. In the great majority of cases (almost 95%) they act as a two position switch, either conducting the impulse into each of the branches or into neither of them.

The ARP has traditionally been taken as the interval corresponding to the maximum frequency of firing (ARP^{-1} x 1000) that a fiber will support. A number of workers, perhaps most notably Paintal[25], have pointed out that the actual interval between conducting impulses, i.e., the LCI, is a more accurate measure of a fiber's maximum frequency of firing. This certainly appears to also be the case, in exaggerated form, for conduction at intraganglionic axon branch points. The long LCIs for conduction through the branch point indicate a low safety factor for conduction and a significant degree of bandpass filtering action, i.e. a reduction in the maximum frequency of action potentials that can propagate through the ganglion and access the CNS. What was not clear is how the frequency following capability based on ARP and LCI measurements compared with actual measurements of the branch point's maximum frequency of firing for repetitive trains of impulses. In order to determine this, the actual frequency at which all-or-none response failure in the stem process first occurred during trains of impulses was measured for a sample of neurons for which ARP and LCI were also measured. The results are clear: comparison of maximum branch point firing frequency based on ARP and LCI with actually measured values (Figure 4) shows that the actual maximum firing frequency was always very much lower than predicted by *fiber* ARP or LCI and substantially lower than the predicted on the basis of *branch point* ARP. On the contrary, the branch point LCI is by far and away the best predictor of the actual maximum branch point firing frequency. What was still uncertain, however, was whether the both-or-neither pattern of impulse conduction failure observed for pairs of impulses would hold during a high frequency train of impulses. This was tested for in 18 instances using the collision method during short (11-41 msec) trains at frequencies ranging from 130-909 Hz. Not a single instance of differential conduction was found, so it is clear that the LCI for two impulses is a valid and reliable measure of phasic maximum firing frequencies.

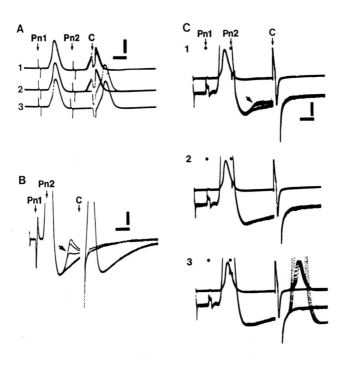

Figure 3. Responses recorded during collision testing. **A.** Three sets of responses recorded at progressively shorter peripheral nerve stimulation (Pn1, Pn2) intervals with dorsal root stimulation at C. Each trace is 5 superimposed sweeps. When the 2nd response failed (traces **A2, 3**) the antidromic response always appeared. Therefore, the 2nd impulse was not failing to invade the stem process while continuing to invade the dorsal root process. **B.** Collision between the antidromic response and the 2nd response occurred even when all that remained of the 2nd response in the stem process was a small M spike. **C.** A rare (2/71) instance of differential conduction. Each trace is 8 superimposed sweeps the top at low the bottom at high gain. The antidromic response due to dorsal root stimulation failed to appear (trace **C2**) when the 2nd response dropped out. At a shorter interval (**C3**), the antidromic response appeared. (Adapted from Stoney[39], with permission)

MAXIMUM FREQUENCY OF FIRING

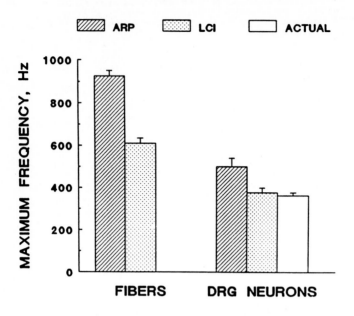

Figure 4. Maximum firing frequencies for fibers and for axon branch points in the DRG. Maximum firing frequencies based on average (± SEM) ARP and LCI for 47 afferent fibers and for 6 DRG neurons for which ARP, LCI and the actual maximum firing frequency for peripheral nerve stimulation were also measured. (Adapted from Stoney[39])

The degree of branch point bandpass filtering action was different for different types of DRG neurons and the shape of the somatic action potential was its most reliable predictor. Neurons with slowly rising and falling action potentials with a shoulder on their falling phase (C neurons and H neurons) had branch points with the lowest maximal rates of firing. For example, based on average LCI values, C neurons could reliably transmit action potential trains to the CNS only at frequencies up to about 90 Hz, H neurons only up to 270 Hz. F neurons, which had brief, smooth action potentials, could reliably conduct action potential trains up to almost 420 Hz. These neurons tended to have fast peripheral axonal conduction velocity (CV), but had low LCI (i.e., relatively high maximum firing frequency) regardless of CV. In fact,

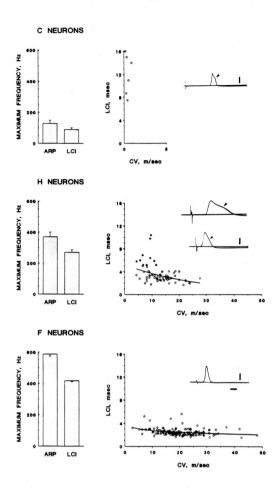

Figure 5. Distribution of branch point LCI and axonal CV along with maximum firing frequency for the three different types of neurons encountered in frog DRG. Cells were classified as C, H or F neurons on the basis of somatic spike shape. Examples of spikes are shown in the insets along right margin. Voltage =50 mV; Time =1 msec, except for C neurons =10 msec. Maximum firing frequencies were based on average (± SEM) ARP and LCI values. C neurons (n = 6) had CV < 1 m/sec. Some H neurons (filled circles) had very long duration spikes and long LCI values. All C and H neurons had a discernible shoulder on the falling phase of their action potentials. F neurons had fast, smooth spikes although an inflection was visible on the dv/dt record of the falling phase for about half of them. LCI was weakly correlated with peripheral axonal CV for H (r = -0.43) and for F (r = -0.30), both with exponential curve fits. (Adapted from Stoney[39])

MAXIMUM FREQUENCY OF FIRING

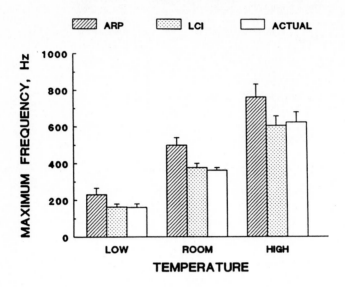

Figure 6. Maximum branch point firing frequency at different temperatures based on ARP and LCI and actual measurements. ARP, LCI and actual maximum firing frequency was measured for 6-7 F neurons at low (average 12.6 °C), room (average 22.1 °C) and high (average 31.1 °C) temperature. (Adapted from Stoney[39])

there was a modest correlation between axonal CV and LCI for the whole sample (r = -0.78), but it arose mainly because of the high LCI and low conduction velocity of the C and H neurons. F neurons seemed to have found a way to minimise branch point filtering action that was practically independent of CV (r = -0.30).

The last question addressed by Stoney[37,39] was the effect of changes in temperature on branch point filtering action in frog DRG. For these experiments, F neurons with relatively rapidly conducting axons were used and the temperature of the perfusion solution changed in 5-8°C steps over a range of 12-35°C. The results were quite similar to the effects temperature changes on impulse conduction in ordinary myelinated nerve fibers[25], i.e., the ARP and LCI were indirectly proportional and the maximum firing frequency directly proportional to the temperature, at least within the limits of 12-35°C (Figure 6). ARP and LCI value converged as the temperature approached 36 °C. It is very clear, therefore, that, over a fairly wide range of temperatures warming *decreases* bandpass filtering action at the DRG branch point of frog afferent axons. The kind of filtering action which entails conduction block of a single impulse and whose likelihood is *increased* by warming[29,43] was observed in 4/17 neurons studied at temperatures up to 37-41°C. For these neurons, which had an average LCI of 4.3 msec at room temperature, the M spike due to a single orthodromic action potential was reversibly lost at an average temperature of 38°C. Ten of these 17 neurons reversibly lost the somatic component of their action potentials at an average temperature of about 36°C. As is well known,[23,29,43] temperature sensitive conduction failure of this type arises only at sites which had a very high Geometrical Ratio[39] or a very low safety factor for conduction to begin with.

These results show that branch points of afferent axons in frog DRG act as 2 position switches with low-pass filtering action. Orthodromic impulses approaching the branch point either invade the branch point and both daughter branches or they fail to invade the branch point at all and thus invade neither branch. By reducing the maximum frequency of firing, they reduce the bandwidth and maximum information content of the neural signals that can access the CNS. DRG neurons with slowly conducting axons *and* a broad somatic spike with a shoulder on the falling phase appear to be poor neural signalers (average high frequency cut-off at 90-270Hz) relative to neurons with brief, smooth action potentials (high frequency cut-off at 417 Hz). Within limits, warming decreases this bandpass limiting form of branch point filtering action. This suggests that the evolution of homeothermy has conferred a previously unsuspected advantage, namely an increase the bandwidth and information content of neural signals that can access and be processed in the warmer brains of the homeotherms.

TYPES OF DRG NEURONS

In many respects, the shape of the somatic action potentials of different types of frog DRG neurons[39] is remarkably similar to the shape of somatic action potentials of cat[2,13,17,31] and rat[9,10,16] and mouse[46] DRG neurons. Examples of action potentials of cat DRG neurons and the relationship between duration and axon CV for neurons subserving different modalities is illustrated in Figure 7. Because LCI is well correlated with spike duration in frog DRG neurons, Figure 7 may be usefully compared to Figure 5. The qualitative similarities in somatic spike shape across different animals stands in considerable contrast to very diverse neurochemical properties of DRG neurons even in one animal[44]. In frogs, cats and rats, cells giving rise to unmyelinated axons have very broad somatic spikes with a distinct shoulder on the falling phase. Furthermore, all three animals have a class of cell with a brief, smooth spike that had axonal CVs spanning the Aδ-Aα range. Finally, all three animals had cells with broad spikes with an inflection on the falling phase that had axonal CVs in the Aβ range. In the case of cat,[13,31] the cells with broad spikes and axonal CV in the Aδ-Aβ range were identified as high threshold mechanoreceptors, i.e. nociceptors. In the case of the rat[9,10] all the cells with axonal CV in the Aδ range had brief, smooth spikes and were shown in a separate study[16] to be a subset of the "large light" type of DRG neuron that reacts well to the monoclonal antibody (RT97) to the high molecular weight subunits of neurofilaments. It will be interesting to find out for the rat whether, like the cat, mechanical nociceptive afferents span the Aδ-Aβ range and whether, like the snake,[19] some of those nociceptive neurons exhibit brief, smooth and others shouldered spikes. For the cat, it will be interesting to see if, as is the case for rats,[16] the Aδ-Aβ nociceptive afferents are RT97 positive. Regardless, however, of how action potential shape ends up correlating with different functional groups of DRG neurons in different animals, two facts relating to the size of DRG neurons are now very clear. The first is that DRG neurons with small somata cannot be assumed to represent a homogeneous population. The second is that, except at the highest (Aα fiber) range, the conduction velocity of primary afferent fibers, cannot safely be used to infer functional grouping.

What ions determine spike shape in DRG neurons? This question can only be partially answered. Stoney[38] showed that tetraethylammonium (TEA) prolonged the falling phase of frog DRG neuron spikes. For F and rapidly conducting H neurons which already had an inflection on the falling phase of their spikes, TEA caused the appearance of or accentuated a shoulder on the falling phase of the spikes. The fast, smooth spikes of F neurons only exhibited a modest spike broadening in TEA and did not develop a shoulder on their falling phase. The shoulder on rapidly conducting H type neurons was accentuated in TEA with high calcium (Ca) and eliminated in TEA with low Ca or with manganese (Mn). Mn alone also eliminated the inflection on the falling phase of rapidly conducting H neurons. This data is entirely compatible with the finding by Scroggs and Fox[32] of a 1:1 mix of L-type (nimodopine sensitive) and N-type (ω-conotoxin sensitive) calcium channel currents activated from holding potentials of -60 mV in *small* DRG neurons acutely isolated from frogs. N-type calcium channels carried 96% of the Ca current in large neurons isolated in the same fashion[32]. The variability in the shoulder on the spike falling phase that was apparent across the F and rapidly conducting H neuron population probably reflects the ratio of L-type to N-type calcium channels in the soma membrane in these neurons. The F neurons with brief, smooth spikes may have more N-type channels which are not strongly activated by the brief action potential at the resting potential. Other factors, such as TTX-resistant Na channels and K channels with slow kinetics, which have been reported by Campbell[3] for about 75% of small DRG neurons of frogs, will certainly contribute to the spike broadening and will allow for greater activation of calcium channels in those neurons. A differential distribution of L-, N- and T-type calcium channels has been reported[33] for rat DRG neurons of different sizes, so it is likely that a Ca influx also contributes to spike shape in some of those neurons.

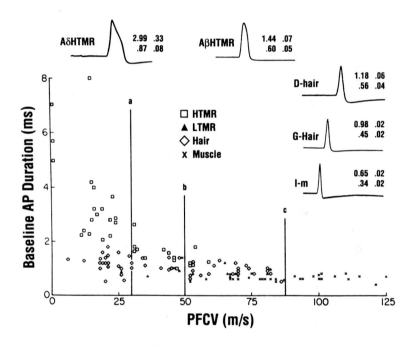

Figure 7. Relationship between spike duration and peripheral axon CV for cat DRG neurons sensitive to different submodalities of somatosensory input. Examples of the shape of the somatic action potentials from different neurons are shown at the top and to the right. Numbers to the right of each spike give the duration at baseline (above) and the duration of the rising phase (below) ± SEM. Very slowly conducting neurons had slow spikes with a shoulder on the falling phase. HTMRs had long duration spikes and axon CV in the Aδ and Aβ range. Some low threshold mechanoreceptors, especially those responsive to down-hair (D-hair) stimulation, had brief smooth spikes even though their CV was in the Aδ range. (Adapted with permission from Rose et al[31])

COMPUTER SIMULATIONS OF IMPULSE CONDUCTION AT POINTS OF LOW SAFETY FACTOR

Early results of mathematical modelling and computer simulations of action potential conduction in bifurcating axons[7,27] indicated that there was no geometrical arrangement of parent and daughter branch axon diameter that would produce differential conduction of impulses. That is, the branch point behaved as a two position switch, either on or off for both branches, just like the branch points in frog dorsal root ganglion studied by Stoney,[39] *provided the length of the daughter branches was relatively long*. Under these circumstances, the behavior of the action potential at such branch points was shown to depend on ratio of the diameters of the parent and daughter branches, the Geometrical Ratio:

$$GR = (d_1{}^{3/2} + d_2{}^{3/2})/ d_p{}^{3/2}$$

where, d_1 and d_2 are the diameters of the two daughter branches being invaded and d_p is the electrophysiological parent branch along which the propagating impulse is approaching. The GR is directly proportional to the electrical load that the approaching impulse encounters at the branch point. For GR < 1, which occurs when the daughter branches are relatively small compared to the parent branch, the electrical load is less than that of the parent fiber in which the impulse is conducting; the situation is analogous to conduction through a step *decrease* in diameter. Action potential amplitude and conduction velocity increase at and immediately before (within ~ 0.5 λ) the branch point. For GR = 1, the input impedance of the parent and daughter branches are equal and the branch point has no influence on the success of conduction. For GR > 1, the daughter branches are relatively large and the electrical load seen by the approaching impulse is large. In this situation, which for an unmyelinated fiber is analogous to conduction through a step increase in diameter, action potential amplitude and velocity decrease at and immediately before the branch point. The safety factor for conduction at the branch point is reduced and the ARP is increased[28]. When excitation of the branch point is sufficiently delayed due to high GR, an antidromically conducting ("reflected") action potential can be produced in the parent axon as it recovers its excitability before the orthodromic impulse exits the branch point. With a higher GR, conduction failure occurs as the impulse fails to invade the branch point and either of the daughter branches. It should be noted that changes seen in spike amplitude and CV during conduction failure at a demyelinated internode are identical to those shown when an impulse propagates through a region of low safety factor due to high branch point GR for unmyelinated fibers. Figure 8 illustrates such changes for conduction failure in a myelinated fiber. The similarity of the results on limitations on impulse conduction at frog DRG neuron axon branch points[39] and computer simulations dealing with conduction through regions with high GR[7,27,28] strongly suggests that *geometrical properties alone are likely to produce a bandpass limiting type of filtering action at branch points with long daughter branches.*

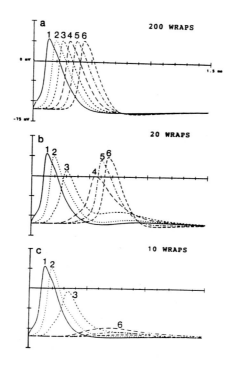

Figure 8. Computer simulation of conduction block in demyelination. **a** normal myelination. The membrane potential across six successive nodes of Ranvier are plotted. An action potential was initiated at node 1 and propagated toward the right with a constant velocity. **b** when the number of myelin wraps was reduced to 20 in the internode between nodes 3 and 4, conduction between these nodes was delayed. **c** demyelination of the internode between nodes 3 and 4 to 10 wraps caused conduction to be blocked. (From Quandt and Davis[28], with permission)

The above conclusion, which applies for branch points with long daughters, may not be true for branch points in the terminal arborizations of axons where one or both of the daughter branches is electrotonically short. Experiments[36] and computer simulations[34,35] of conduction at squid axon branch points where the daughter branches were of different electrotonic length revealed that differential conduction could occur for pairs of impulses at short intervals and for trains of impulses at different frequencies. In computer simulations,[34,35] the necessary conditions for observing differential conduction were that one branch was short (< ~ 0.6 λ), the temperature was relatively high (32 °C in order to decrease the safety factor for conduction) and the Geometrical Ratio was neither too low (> ~ 1.5) or too high (< ~ 3.0). As illustrated in Figure 9, the pattern of successful conduction into the daughter branches under these conditions was quite variable depending on action potential frequency and the GR.

Subsequent simulations[23,24] added realism by including large (4 μm diameter, 5-6 μm length) cylindrical terminal enlargements ("boutons") as well as varicosities, "synapses en passant," at or close to the branch points of small (0.1 μm diameter) unmyelinated axons. Antidromic (reflected) spikes were found to play an important role in the simulations, probably due to the high GR of the large boutons and the increase in spike amplitude near the sealed end of the boutons[7]. Figure 10 illustrates how varying the length of one of the daughter branches causes marked changes in the probability of the action potential successfully invading both branches. In Figure 10A, with the A branch at 6.5 μm and the B branch at 19 μm, the conducting action potential failed to invade the branch point but its electrotonic spread was sufficient to excite the bouton of branch A which generated a antidromic spike that also failed to invade the branch point. The electrotonic spread from the A branch antidromic spike activated the bouton in branch B. This second antidromic spike also failed to invade the branch point. Interestingly, bouton activation may occur even without branch point invasion if both branches are short. Different patterns of activation could occur when the length of the A branch was varied relative to the B branch which remained at 19 μm. There was differential conduction over a narrow range of A branch lengths (6.5-12 μm, Figure 10B); simultaneous failure over a short range (12-26 μm, Figure 10C) and success for both branches over all longer lengths (27-100 μm, Figure 10D). Conduction failure that occurred for both branches at certain critical branch length ratios (Figure 10C) could be changed to successful invasion by placing the branch point at a varicosity[23].

Simulations were also carried out using different patterns of terminal arborization[24]. In complex arborizations, many boutons were uninvaded and the number of

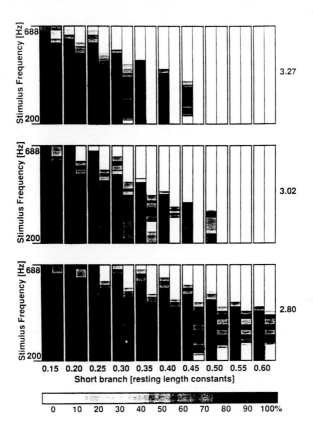

Figure 9. A series of simulations were run with branched cables in which the length of the short branch was varied from 0.15 to 0.6 λ. Each simulation run was a 1-s train of regularly spaced suprathreshold stimuli applied to the sealed end of the parent branch. The number of action potentials was counted ~0.5 λ from the bifurcation. Action potentials in the two daughter branches were counted at their distal ends. Bar on the left corresponds to the activity in the short daughter branch, and the bar on the right to that of the long daughter branch. The number of action potentials in the daughter branch as a percentage of the activity shown was used to compute a grey scale value. As showing the scale at the bottom, white areas correspond to complete conduction block and black areas to 100% propagation success. Values to the right of the figure give the geometric ratio at the branch. (From Stockbridge[35], with permission)

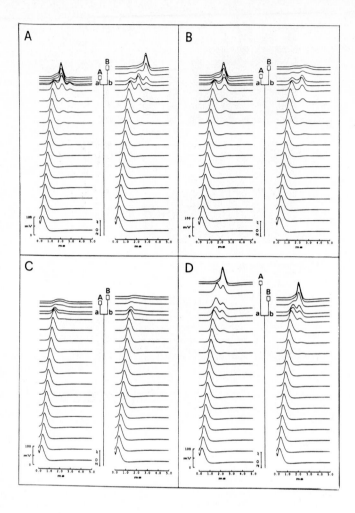

Figure 10. Action potential propagation along a bifurcating axon with short collaterals carrying synaptic boutons. A drawing of the axon structure is given in the middle of each panel. On the left side in each panel, the action potentials are illustrated for each compartment of the structure as it propagates along the main axon and into collateral *a*; on the right, as it propagates into collateral *b*. The action potential is always initiated at the first compartment of the main axon. The length of collateral *b* is constant (19 μm). The length of collateral *a* is 6.5 μm in **A**, 9.5 μm in **B**, 12 μm in **C**, and 40 μm in **D**. The activation pattern of synapse *A* and *B* is different for different lengths of collateral *a*. (From Luscher and Shiner[23], with permission)

successfully invaded boutons could be increased by increasing the safety factor for conduction (by lowering the temperature). A kind of frequency dependence, with one or another branch dropping out earliest as the frequency was raised, was also shown. Luscher and Shiner[24] concluded that "Whereas the simulation study...clearly indicates that the presynaptic arborization may offer a broad range of possibilities for information processing...the available experimental evidence information on these questions is not sufficient to decide whether the structure of the terminal arborizations are designed for optimal and safe impulse conduction, or whether the central nervous system takes advantage of the possibilities offered by the structural complexity for presynaptic information processing."

CONCLUSIONS

Results from contemporary experiments and computer simulations of impulse conduction at axon branch points support new conclusions about the possibility of integration due to branch point filtering action in the axonal arborizations of vertebrate neurons. One of the conclusions is that complex forms of *spatio-temporal* filtering action at main or collateral branch points, typically points of branching where both daughter branches are relatively long (> 0.5-1.0 λ), is an unlikely possibility on the basis of geometrical factors alone. This conclusion, which is supported by direct experimental evidence[39] and computer simulation studies,[7,23,24,27,34] follows directly from fact that impulse conduction failure at this type of branch point is *all-or-none for both branches* because the propagating action potential either invades or fails to invade the branch point itself. Thus, any influence onto one of the branches which lowers the safety factor of the branch point sufficiently to prevent its activation by an approaching impulse will, in fact, prevent invasion of both daughter branches.

A second conclusion is that the possibility of spatio-temporal filtering action at axon branch points where at least one daughter branch is short ($< \sim 0.5$ λ), a variety which is especially numerous in the terminal arborizations of axons, appears to be more likely. Experimental[36] and computer simulation[23,24,34,35] results are concordant. Frequency dependent invasion of the two branches can be achieved over a physiologically relevant range of frequencies and terminal branch lengths. The possibility that such filtering action occurs, while intriguing, is by no means established. The fact that the experiments and simulations which so far have demonstrated this type of filtering action have made use of branch points with relatively high GRs (> ~ 2 - 3, perhaps considerably larger) and low safety factors raises some question about how much predictive power the results should be given. Furthermore, the sheer number of terminal boutons, numbering in the hundreds or thousands for individual neurons, makes the idea of individual control almost unimaginable. For example, there are about 10^{30} ways of controlling the activity of 100 boutons by regulating conduction at branch points in a symmetrical 2 x 2 axonal arborization[40]. It is clearly desirable to obtain direct evidence for impulse conduction failure at these sites in the terminal arborization. Until such evidence is available it seems best to regard the possibility of such filtering action as speculative.

The third and final conclusion that can be drawn is that the *bandpass limiting* form of branch point filtering action is likely to be a common occurrence in the axonal arborization. In homeotherms, warmer brain temperature will ameliorate this form of filtering action. Nevertheless, it will almost certainly occur to some degree at any branch point where GR > 1 and may be especially significant for branch points of certain types of neurons. For primary afferent neurons, cells with slowly conducting axons *and* a high concentration of L-type calcium channels in the somatic membrane are likely to exhibit the greatest amount of lowpass filtering action at their axon branch points.

REFERENCES

1. BARRON, D. H. AND MATTHEWS, B. H. C. (1935) Intermittent conduction in the spinal cord. *J. Physiol.* **85**, 73-103.
2. CAMERON, A. A., LEAH, J. D. AND SNOW, P. J. (1986) The electrophysiological and morphological characteristics of feline dorsal root ganglion cells. *Brain Res.* **362**, 1-6.
3. CAMPBELL, D. T. (1992) Large and small vertebrate neurons express different Na and K channel subtypes. *Proc. Natl. Acad. Sci. U.S.A.* **89**, 9569-9573.
4. CHUNG, S. H., RAYMOND, S. A. AND LETTVIN, J. Y. (1970) Multiple meaning in single visual units. *Brain Behav. Evol.* **3**, 72-101.
5. DESCHENES, M. AND LANDRY, P. (1980) Axonal branch diameter and spacing of nodes in the terminal arborization of identified thalamic and cortical neurons. *Brain Res.* **191**, 538-544.
6. DUN, F. T. (1955) The delay and blockage of sensory impulses in the dorsal root ganglion. *J. Physiol.* **127**, 252-264.
7. GOLDSTEIN, S. S. AND RALL, W. (1974) Changes in action potential shape and velocity for changing core conductor geometry. *Biophy. J.* **14**, 731-757.
8. GROSSMAN, Y., SPIRA, M. E. AND PARNAS, I. (1973) Differential flow of information into branches of a single axon. *Brain Res.* **64**, 379-386.

9. HARPER, A. A. AND LAWSON, S. N. (1985) Conduction velocity related to morphological cell type in rat dorsal root ganglion neurones. *J. Physiol.* **359**, 31-46.

10. HARPER, A. A. AND LAWSON, S. N. (1985) Electrical properties of rat dorsal root ganglion neurones with different peripheral nerve conduction velocities. *J. Physiol.* **359**, 47-63.

11. ITO, M. AND SAIGA, M. (1959) The mode of impulse conduction through the spinal ganglion. *Jpn. J. Physiol.* **9**, 33-42.

12. ITO, M. AND TAKAHASHI, I. (1960) Impulse conduction through spinal ganglion. In: *Electrical Activity of Single Cells*, ed. Y. Katsuki. Tokyo: Ikagu Shoin.

13. KOERBER, H. R., DRUZINSKY, R. E. AND MENDELL, L. M. (1988) Properties of somata of spinal dorsal root ganglion cells differ according to peripheral receptor innervated. *J. Neurophysiol.* **60**, 1584-1596.

14. KRNJEVIC, K. AND MILEDI, R. (1958) Motor units in the rat diaphragm. *J. Physiol.* **140**, 427-439.

15. KRNJEVIC, K. AND MILEDI, R. (1958) Failure of neuromuscular propagation in rats. *J. Physiol.* **140**, 440-461.

16. LAWSON, S. N. AND WADDELL, P. J. (1991) Soma neurofilament immunoreactivity is related to cell size and fibre conduction velocity in rat primary sensory neurons. *J. Physiol.* **435**, 41-63.

17. LEE, K. H., CHUNG, K., CHUNG, J. M. AND COGGESHALL, R. E. (1986) Correlation of cell body size, axon size and signal conduction velocity for individually labeled dorsal root ganglion cells in the cat. *J. Comp. Neurol.* **243**, 335-346.

18. LEVY, R. A. (1980) Presynaptic control of input to the central nervous system. *Can. J. Physiol. Pharmcol.* **58**,751-766.

19. LIANG, Y.-F. AND TERASHIMA, S.-I. (1993) Physiological properties and morphological characteristics of cutaneous and mucosal mechanical nociceptive neurons with A-δ peripheral axons in the trigeminal ganglia of crotaline snakes. *J. Comp. Neurol.* **328**, 88-102.

20. LIEBERMAN, A. R. (1976) Sensory ganglia. In: *The Peripheral Nerve,* ed. D.N. Landon. New York: Halstead.

21. LUSCHER, H. R. (1990) Transmission failure and its relief in the spinal monosynaptic reflex arc. In: *The Segmental Motor System,* ed. M. D. Binder, and L.M. Mendell. New York: Oxford.

22. LUSCHER, H. R., RUENZEL, P. W. AND HENNEMAN, E. (1983) Effects of impulse frequency, PTP, and temperature on responses elicited in large populations of motoneruons by impulses in single Ia fibers. *J. Neurophysiol.* **50**, 1045-1058.

23. LUSCHER, H. R. AND SHINER, J. S. (1990) Computation of action potential propagation and presynaptic bouton activation in terminal arborizations of different geometries. *Biophys. J.* **58**, 1377-1388.

24. LUSCHER, H. R. AND SHINER, J. S. (1990) Simulation of action potential propagation in complex terminal arborizations. *Biophys. J.* **58**, 1389-1399.

25. PAINTAL, A. S. (1973) Conduction in mammalian nerve fibres. In: *New Developments in Electromyography and Clinical Neuophysiology,* Vol. 2, ed. J.E. Desmedt. Basel: Karger.

26. PARNAS, I. (1972) Differential block at high frequency of branches of a single axon innervating two muscles. *J. Neurophysiol.* **35**, 903-914.

27. PARNAS, I. AND SEGEV, I. (1979) A mathematical model for conduction of action potentials along bifurcating axons. *J. Physiol.* **295**, 323-343.

28. QUANDT, F. N. AND DAVIS, F. A. (1992) Action potential refractory period in axonal demyelination: a computer simulation. *Biol. Cybern.* **67**, 545-552.

29. RASMINSKY, M. (1973) The effects of temperature on conduction in demyelinated single nerve fibers. *Arch. Neurol.* **28**, 29-47.

30. RAYMOND, S. A (1979) Effects of nerve impulses on threshold of frog sciatic nerve fibres. *J. Physiol.* **290**, 273-303.

31. ROSE, R. D., KOERBER, H. R., SEDIVEC, M. J. AND MENDELL, L. M. (1986) Somal action potential duration differs in identified primary afferents. *Neurosci. Lett.* **63**, 259-264.

32. SCROGGS, R. S. AND FOX, A. P. (1991) Distribution of dihydropyridine and ω-conotoxin-sensitive calcium currrents in acutely isolated rat and frog sensory neuron somata: Diameter-dependent L channel expression in frog. *J. Neurosci.* **11**: 1334-1346.

33. SCROGGS, R. S. AND FOX, A. P. (1992) Calcium current variation between acutely isolated adult dorsal root ganglion neurons of different size. *J. Physiol.* **445**, 639-658.

34. STOCKBRIDGE, N. (1988) Differential conduction at axonal bifurcations. II. Theoretical basis. *J. Neurophysiol.* **59**, 1286-1294.

35. STOCKBRIDGE, N. (1988) Theoretical response to trains of action potentials of a bifurcating axon with one short daughter branch. *Biophys. J.* **54**, 637-641.

36. STOCKBRIDGE, N. AND STOCKBRIDGE, L. L. (1988) Differential conduction at axonal bifurcations. I. Effect of electrotonic length. *J. Neurophysiol.* **59**, 1277-1285.

37. STONEY, S. D. Jr. (1985) Unequal branch point filtering action in different types of dorsal root ganglion neurons of frogs. *Neurosci. Lett.* **59**, 15-20.

38. STONEY, S. D. Jr. (1987) Differential effects of potassium and calcium channel blockers on action potentials of frog dorsal root ganglion neurons. *Soc. Neurosci. Abstr.* **13**, 780.

39. STONEY, S. D. Jr. (1990) Limitations on impulse conduction at the branch point of afferent axons in frog dorsal root ganglion. *Exp. Brain Res.* **80**, 512-524.

40. SWADLOW, H. A., KOCSIS, J. D. AND WAXMAN, S. G. (1980) Modulation of impulse conduction along the axonal tree. *Ann. Rev. Biophys. Bioeng.* **9**, 143-179.

41. WALL, P. D., LETTVIN, J. Y., MCCULLOCH, W. S. AND PITTS, W. H. (1956) Factors limiting the maximum impulse transmitting ability of an afferent system of nerve fibers. In: *Information Theory. Third London Symposium,* ed. C. Cherry. London: Butterworths.

42. WAXMAN, S. G. (1975) Integrative properties and design principles of axons. *Int. Rev. Neurobiol.* **18**, 1-40.

43. WESTERFIELD, M., JOYNER, R. W. AND MOORE, J.W. (1977) Temperature-sensitive conduction failure at axon branch points. *J. Neurophysiol.* **41**, 1-8.

44. WILLIS, W. D., JR. AND COGGESHALL, R. E. (1991) *Sensory Mechanisms of the Spinal Cord,* New York: Plenum.
45. YAU, K.-W. (1976) Receptive fields, geometry and conduction block of sensory neurones in the central nervous system of the leech. *J. Physiol.* **263**, 513-538.
46. YOSHIDA, S., MATSUDA, Y. AND SAMEJIMA, A. (1978) Tetrodotoxin-resistant sodium and calcium components of action potentials in dorsal root ganglion cells of the adult mouse. *J. Neurophysiol.* **41**, 1096-1106.

POLYMODALITY IN NOCICEPTIVE NEURONS: EXPERIMENTAL MODELS OF CHEMOTRANSDUCTION

Carlos Belmonte, Juana Gallar, Laura G. Lopez-Briones and Miguel A. Pozo
Departamento de Fisiologia and Instituto de Neurociencias
Universidad de Alicante, 03080 Alicante
Spain

INTRODUCTION

Transduction of chemical changes in the environment is present in all levels of living organisms, from protozoa to man. In bacteria, chemotransduction mediates a modification of flagellar motion that biases the individual cell's random displacement, leading to an accumulation if the chemical cue is an attractant or to a dispersion in the case of a repellent. Likewise, in metazoans chemotransduction is involved in chemical detection of nutrients and mates, and triggers also behavioral mechanisms to approach or escape the stimulus[72].

Sensory transduction of chemical stimuli in vertebrates involves taste, smell, detection of blood pO_2 and pCO_2 changes and also the "common chemical sense," originally defined as the sense mediating irritation aroused by the action of noxious chemicals on exposed and semiexposed mucosal membranes[37]. This chemosensitivity allows aquatic vertebrates to detect contact with noxious chemicals and is mediated through solitary chemoreceptive cells in the epidermis. In terrestrial vertebrates, such specialisation does not seem to occur and chemotransduction of irritant stimuli takes place in free nerve terminals of primary sensory neurons that distribute widely in the organism and may also transduce other forms of energy, thus being polymodal. Silver and Finger[66], proposed the term "chemesthesis" to distinguish chemical sensitivity mediated by free nerve endings in humans and other terrestrial vertebrates, from other forms of chemotransduction.

In mammals, free terminals of sensory neurons detecting irritant stimuli are called polymodal nociceptors. They belong to the group of unmyelinated (C) or thin

NATO ASI Series, Vol. H 79
Cellular Mechanisms of Sensory Processing
Edited by Laszlo Urban
© Springer-Verlag Berlin Heidelberg 1994

myelinated (A-delta) nerve fibers and were named for the fact that they respond to chemical irritants, but also to mechanical and thermal noxious stimuli[6]. The proportion of polymodal nociceptors varies among tissues, but are the most abundant subpopulation of nociceptive afferents. For example, they comprise 52%-79% of all C fibers with cutaneous fields in the saphenous nerve of the rat[50] and reach an 80% of skin nociceptors in monkey[46]. Recently, a population of 'silent nociceptors', with a prominent chemical sensitivity has also been described[64].

A characteristic feature of polymodal nociceptors is sensitisation. After a heat trauma, nociceptors respond to repetitively applied suprathreshold heating stimulus with an enhancement of the firing rate and a lower threshold; furthermore, they usually develop a spontaneous, on-going activity at rest. Sensitisation has been observed in nociceptors innervating the skin, joints, muscle, cornea, and various viscerae[5,11,27,46,53,63] and extends often to the firing responses to other stimulus modalities[67].

Under normal conditions, sensitisation of nociceptors occurs during tissue inflammation, through the release by injured tissues of chemical agents. Therefore, polymodal nociceptors not only respond to exogenous chemical agents but also to endogenous mediators produced by inflammatory processes. Endogenous chemicals include substances that directly activate nociceptive nerve terminals (ATP, protons, bradykinin, 5-HT, acetylcholine, histamine) as well as others that modify membrane excitability and sensitise nociceptive endings (prostaglandins, leukotrienes and hydroxy-acids, cytokines)[18].

The response pattern of nociceptors to mechanical and thermal stimulation is fairly well known. Several studies have also determined the characteristics and time course of nociceptor's discharge during inflammation of somatic and visceral tissues, and have attempted to identify the various chemical agents contributing to excitation and/or sensitisation of nociceptors[28,29]. However, information on the cellular mechanisms involved in chemosensitivity of nociceptive terminals is scarce. This is due mainly to the small size of nerve endings, that precludes the use of conventional biophysical and biochemical methods to explore this property. Another contributing factor is the complexity of the tissues where nociceptive endings locate, that in most cases include autonomic nerves, blood vessels, several subpopulations of sensory fibers and many different types of cells. The use of 'in vitro' preparations has reduced but not eliminated some of these problems[28,60]. An alternative is to employ tissues with a minimal structural heterogeneity. The cornea of the eye is an avascular organ of relatively simple structure, chiefly innervated by sensory fibers. Only sensations of irritation and pain have been evoked by suprathreshold mechanical, thermal or chemical stimulation of the corneal surface[7,14,39]. Thus, the cornea appears to be an advantageous model to explore the response of nociceptors to various forms of stimulating energies.

A different approach to study mechanisms of nociceptive transduction, is based upon the assumption that the membrane of the soma of nociceptive primary sensory neurons possess some of the transducing properties of peripheral terminals[3]. This strategy has been employed to study membrane currents and ionic fluxes in a subpopulation of cultured dorsal root ganglion cells, that were classified as nociceptive, based upon their sensitivity to capsaicin[8,75]. Another option to explore membrane mechanisms of nociceptive neurons is the use of lower animal species, where neurons can more easily be identified and recorded.

Finally, peripheral neural signals evoking pain are also elicited from neuromas of severed sensory nerves[9]. Nerve sprouts of neuromas possess chemosensitivity to some of the algogenic substances[77] and may thus be used to explore the membrane mechanisms underlying chemosensitivity of nociceptive neurons.

POLYMODALITY IN CORNEAL NOCICEPTORS

The cornea is composed by 5-6 layers of epithelium cells, a stroma formed by parallel sheets of collagenous material and an internal, single layered endothelium, facing the aqueous humor. It is sensorily innervated by neurons located in the trigeminal ganglion. The peripheral axons of corneal ganglion cells enter the eye with the ciliary nerves; they reach the cornea as about 30 radial trunks, that penetrate the stroma and branch continually to form just beneath or within the basal cell layer of the epithelium, a subepithelial plexus. Fine branches of this plexus ramify and ascend perpendicularly, ending as unspecialized nerve terminals in the superficial layers of the epithelium[13].

Types of corneal nociceptors

Functional properties of sensory units innervating the cornea have been studied chiefly in the cat[4,5,22]. They are either thin myelinated (A-delta, conduction velocity: 5-10 m/s) or unmyelinated (C, conduction velocity: <2m/s). Within the cornea, all axons loose their myelin sheath and become unmyelinated. Depending on their responses to mechanical probes, thermal stimulation with a contact

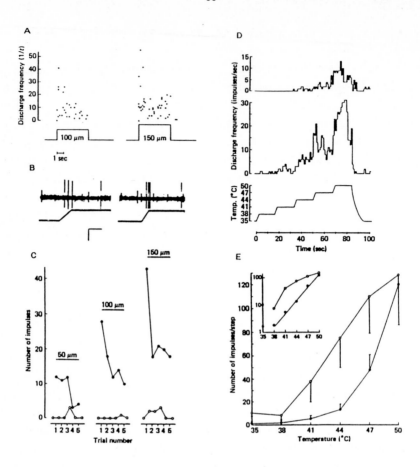

Figure 1. Response of corneal polymodal nociceptors to mechanical and thermal stimulation. A. Instantaneous frequency changes in a single unit, evoked by two mechanical indentations of the cornea (lower traces). B. Response of a polymodal unit to stimulation with two different indentation rates, represented in the lower trace (vertical calibration: 200µm; horizontal calibration: 20 msec). C. Fatigue of the mechanical response to three different series of square-wave indentations. The number of impulses evoked per stimulus (5 sec duration, black circles) is plotted versus the stimulus order. The number of impulses evoked during the 5 sec interestimulus period (open circles) is also plotted in a similar way. D. Peristimulus time histograms showing the first (upper) and the second (lower) response to two identical stepwise heatings separated by 3 min. The lower trace shows the stimulus waveform. E. Mean stimulus-response relation of eight corneal units in response to the first (black circles) and the second (open circles) stepwise heatings. Bars are S.E.M. Inset: the same data plotted in log-linear coordinates. (Modified, from Belmonte and Giraldez[5])

thermode (5-50°C) and application of acid solutions (pH 3.0 to 7.0), corneal nociceptors have been classified as high threshold mechano-receptors, corresponding to thin myelinated fibers that are excited exclusively by mechanical indentation of the epithelium; A-delta and C polymodal nociceptors that are sensitive to mechanical stimuli, but also to noxious heat (over 41.5 °C), and to application of acid and hypertonic saline; and mechano-heat nociceptors, similar to polymodals but not responding initially to chemicals, although chemosensitivity develops after sensitisation. Also, a population of C-'cold' nociceptors has been identified, that respond to low temperatures and to irritant chemicals but are insensitive to mechanical stimuli.

Functional properties

Functional characteristics of corneal polymodal nociceptors are essentially similar to those of cutaneous polymodal afferents[5]. Thin myelinated and unmyelinated polymodal fibers of the cornea respond to mechanical stimulation with a threshold of about 0.6 mN. Receptive fields are large and continuous, particularly those of A-delta fibers, which often cover a quadrant of the cornea and a fringe of neighboring sclera. The same units also respond to heating of the corneal surface over 41-43°C, with a discharge that increases in a regular manner with increasing temperatures. In most fibers, repeated heating sensitises the unit, as evidenced by a decreased thermal threshold, an enhanced response to temperature increments and the appearance of ongoing background activity[4,5,22] (Figure 1).

Responses to chemical stimulation

Corneal polymodal nociceptors are excited by various exogenous and endogenous chemical agents.

Protons: Decrease of tissue pH to values down to 4.7has been repeatedly proposed as a mechanism of activation of nociceptors during inflammation or ischemia[48,67]. The accessibility of corneal nociceptive terminals to exogenously applied acidic solutions make them particularly suitable to study in detail[4] the stimulatory effects of pH changes on polymodal nociceptors.

Topical application of acidic solutions containing protons at different concentration (pH 4.5-7.0) elicits a firing response in corneal polymodal fibers that is roughly proportional to pH values. This effect of H+ appears to be extracellular, since the magnitude of the response is similar when stimulation is carried out with permeable and non-permeable buffers[4] (Figure 2).

The stimulatory action of acid on corneal nociceptors can also be evidenced by application on the cornea of a gas stream containing CO_2 at different concentrations. Pain has been elicited by application of brief CO_2 pulses to the nasal mucosa of volunteer subjects[1]. Furthermore, cutaneous nociceptors 'in vitro' respond in a dose-response manner to superfusion with CO_2 saturated solutions[67]. Likewise, application of CO_2 pulses to the cornea of humans elicits pain sensations when a threshold concentration of about 40% CO_2 is reached. A correlation exists between CO_2 concentration and corneal sensations of pain. This relationship closely reflects activation of polymodal nociceptors by CO_2[14], as evidenced by the correspondence between curves of firing frequency and intensity of sensation shown in Figure 3.

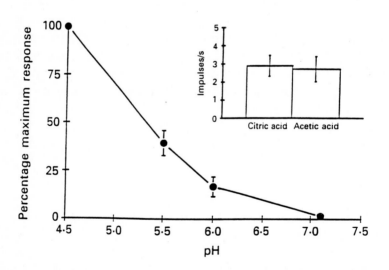

Figure 2. Influence of pH changes on the discharge rate of corneal polymodal fibers. Acetic acid solutions, buffered to pH values of 4.5, 5.5, 6.0 and 7.3 were applied to the receptive field of 12 corneal units. The variation in firing frequency has been expressed as percentage of the discharge rate elicited by a pH 4.5 solution. Inset: mean discharge rates elicited in eight polymodal fibers by application of pH solutions made with citric acid and with acetic acid. Data are means ± S.E.M. (From Belmonte et al.,[4])

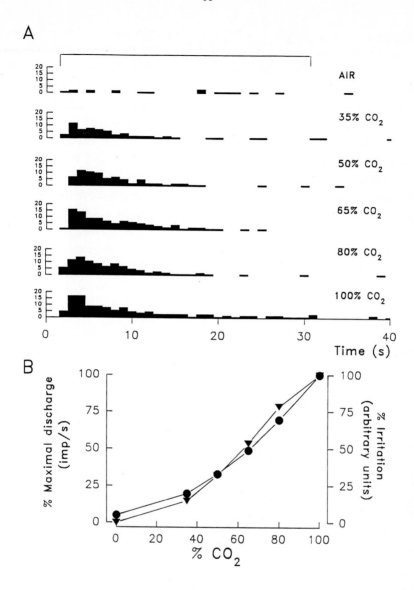

Figure 3. Effects of CO_2 administration to the cornea. A. Peristimulus histograms of a corneal polymodal unit in response to pulses of CO_2 of increasing concentration, applied to the corneal surface during the time indicated by the upper bar. Interval between CO_2 pulses was 5 min. B. Stimulus-response relation obtained by CO_2 pulses of increasing concentration. Circles, mean firing response of 13 corneal polymodal units. Triangles, mean sensation of irritation measured with a visual analog scale in 7 human volunteers. In both cases, data are represented as percent of maximal response. (Unpublished data from Chen, Pozo, Baeza, Gallar & Belmonte).

Inflammatory substances: Direct effects of inflammatory mediators on nociceptors are usually masked by their simultaneous action on vascular smooth muscle and capillary permeability[19,69]. In the cornea, the absence of blood vessels permits the testing of the actions of inflammatory mediators on nociceptive endings, without the interference of tissue pressure changes or extravasation of blood-borne substances.

Bradykinin (BK), is an inflammatory mediator with well known effects on membrane currents of primary sensory neurons[10,16]. It excites consistently polymodal nociceptive endings in the skin, muscle, joints and testis[34,41,45,47]. In agreement with this observation, 10^{-5}M BK applied to the cornea elicits a discharge of impulses in about 80% of A-delta and C-polymodal fibers; the response of corneal nociceptors to BK outlasts the stimulation period and has a long latency and slow onset compared with other chemical stimuli (acetic acid, for instance). Although a certain degree of tachyphylaxis is present, it does not seem to be as prominent in corneal nociceptors as in nociceptors of other tissues[45] (Figure 4).

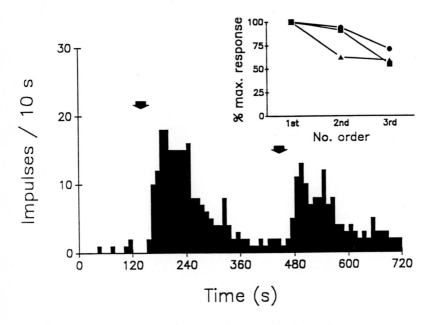

Figure 4. Response of corneal polymodal units to bradykinin. Spike density histogram of a polymodal nociceptive unit stimulated with two consecutive applications to the corneal receptive field (arrows) of 10^{-5} M bradykinin (60 µl). Inset: Response (represented as percentage of maximal discharge rate of each unit) of three corneal polymodal fibers to consecutive instillations of 10^{-5} M bradykinin, applied with a 5 min interval. (Unpublished data from Gallar & Belmonte).

Prostaglandins (notably PGE_2) are substances that do not activate directly nociceptors but contribute to sensitisation to other mediators of inflammation[26,54,65]. In the cornea, PGE_2 or its analogue 19(R) OH-PGE_2, applied at 10^{-7} to 10^{-4}M, increases in most cases spontaneous activity of A-delta and C-polymodal nociceptors in a dose-dependent manner. Furthermore, responses to topical application of 10 mM acetic acid are significantly enhanced after PGE_2 administration (Figure 5)[20].

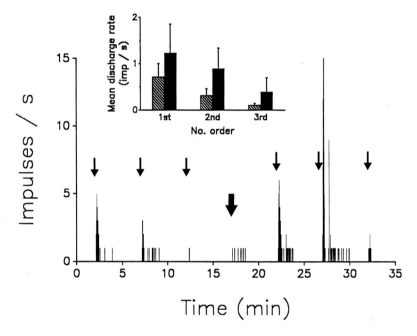

Figure 5. Enhancement by PGE_2 of the responses to chemical irritants in corneal polymodal nociceptors. Spike density histograms of an A-delta polymodal unit have been represented for three consecutive applications to the cornea of 10 mM acetic acid (60 µl, thin arrows), before and after instillation of 60 µl of 10^{-5} M PGE_2 (large arrow). Inset: Mean discharge values of the response to 10 mM acetic acid of six corneal polymodal fibers, before (hatched bars) and after (filled bars) application of 10^{-5} M PGE_2. Data are means ± S.D. (Unpublished data from Gallar & Belmonte).

It has been hypothesised that neuropeptides may contribute to sensitisation of peripheral nociceptors[12]. Corneal nerves contain Substance P (SP) and calcitonin-gene-related peptide (CGRP)[68]. When tested in A-delta and C polymodal nociceptive fibers of the cornea, topical substance P (10^{-3} to 10^{-5} M) does not evoke any impulse activity. Responses to mechanical and chemical stimuli or sensitisation to heat are not changed by pretreatment with SP. Moreover, SP-antagonists spantide and SP-150 do not alter neural activity or responsiveness of corneal nociceptors to acidic stimulation. CGRP is equally ineffective in modifying spontaneous or evoked discharges of corneal polymodal units[59].

Inflammatory soup: Inflammatory exudates contain a mixture of various endogenous mediators, as well as an elevated concentration of K+ ions and low pH. The excitatory effects of acute inflammatory exudates on nociceptors have been reproduced in a nerve-skin preparation 'in vitro'[40] with a mixture of BK, 5-HT, histamine, PGE_2 and SP (all at 10^{-5}M)and K+ (7×10^{-3}M), at a pH of 7.0, called "inflammatory soup" (IS). Application of IS to the cornea also excites polymodal nociceptors (Figure 6), in a more consistent and vigorous manner than when BK alone is applied[24].

Hypertonic saline: Hypertonic saline has been used to test polymodal nociceptors in muscle and scrotum[44,45]. In the cornea, 660 mM NaCl elicits a sustained excitation of polymodal nociceptors[4,22]. The mechanism of this activation is obscure, because solutions of equivalent osmolarity made with sucrose do not evoke a similar firing response[21]. Excitation of nociceptors by hypertonic NaCl may be associated to direct membrane potential changes that are more prominent in nociceptive terminals due to their very small size.

Capsaicin: Capsaicin (8-methyl N-vanillyl-6-nonenamide) is an irritant substance with selective excitatory effects on polymodal nociceptors. Pioneering experiments by Jancsó et al.[33] showed that capsaicin, applied topically to the rat's cornea evokes eye scratching movements suggestive of pain. This was followed by insensitivity to ocular application of other irritant chemicals, although mechanical sensitivity remained unaltered. Selective stimulating effects of capsaicin have been demonstrated electrophysiologically in cutaneous C-polymodal nociceptors[38,69,70]. This excitatory effect has been confirmed in the cornea, where application of 0.33 mM capsaicin excites thin myelinated and unmyelinated-polymodal units. This is followed by a complete inactivation of C fibers to all stimulus modalities, while A-delta units lose their responsiveness to thermal and chemical stimuli but maintain mechanical sensitivity[4,22].

It can be concluded that, because its structural simplicity, the cornea of the eye may serve as an adequate model to study some of the mechanisms involved in the excitation of nociceptive terminals. A-delta and C, corneal polymodal nociceptors respond to mechanical, thermal and chemical stimuli as do polymodal nociceptive fibers of other somatic territories (skin, joint, muscle). Likewise they become sensitized after repeated heating and following topical application of prostaglandins or of a mixture of inflammatory mediators (inflammatory soup). The absence of blood vessels in the cornea and the accessibility of its nerve terminals to exogenous substances, has made this tissue particularly suitable to study chemosensitivity of nociceptive endings.

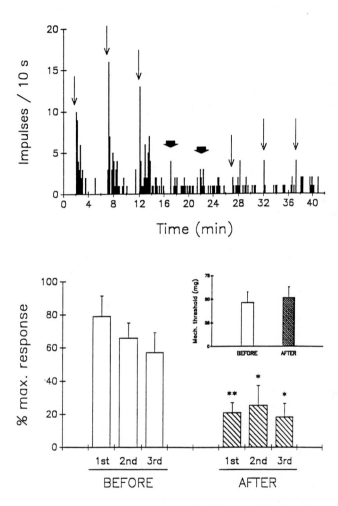

Figure 6. Response of corneal nociceptors to 'inflammatory soup' (IS, see text). A. Spike density histogram of a corneal polymodal unit stimulated with three consecutive applications of IS, (60 µl, thin arrows), before and after corneal instillation of 1 mM diltiazem (20 µl, thick arrows). B. Average response of nine polymodal nociceptive fibers (represented as percentage of maximal frequency of each unit) to three consecutive applications of IS with a 5 min interval, before (empty bars) and 10 min. after (hatched bars) topical application of 1 mM diltiazem. Inset: Mean mechanical threshold of units, before (empty bar) and after (hatched bar) diltiazem treatment. Data are means ± S.E.M. (Unpublished data from Gallar & Belmonte).

Ionic basis for transduction of chemical stimuli

The existence in nociceptive terminals of separate mechanisms for transduction of mechanical, thermal and chemical stimuli was suggested by behavioral data showing the selective effects of capsaicin on noxious sensibility to chemical irritants[33]. As noted above, this possibility has been confirmed in the cornea, where topical capsaicin blocks impulse responses of corneal polymodal nociceptors to acid and to heat, without affecting mechanosensitivity of the same nerve fiber (Figure 7). The reduced dimensions of nociceptive terminals precludes a direct biophysical characterization of ion channels. Therefore, information on membrane mechanisms associated with polymodality and sensitisation of nociceptive nerve endings has been obtained with ion substitution experiments and with drugs that interfere with ionic conductances. The problem has also been addressed using the soma of nociceptive neurons as a model for peripheral transduction, in spite of the fact that it is not established whether the cell body of sensory neurons possess the same ion channels as the peripheral terminals[42].

The effects of chemical agents on the membrane of nociceptive terminals are finally mediated through ionic channels. These can be gated directly, by coupling of the stimulating substance to the channel protein or be activated indirectly, through a second-messenger system.

Voltage- and calcium-activated K^+ channels present in cutaneous sensory nerve terminals may play a role in controlling nerve excitability of nociceptive endings and presumably contribute also to the sensitizing effects of opioid and of some inflammatory mediators like PG's[42,58], but do not seem to be essential for chemosensory transduction.

Another family of membrane channels, the voltage-sensitive Ca^{2+} channels, participate in some ligand-gated responses and in the release of neuropeptides by nociceptive nerve terminals[51,58], but they apparently do not mediate direct chemical excitation of nociceptors by protons or capsaicin (see below). Nevertheless, Ca^{2+} ions, through their ubiquitous effects, play a critical role in some components of the response of nociceptive terminals to noxious chemical stimuli, such as sensitisation and efferent secretion of neuropeptides. In general terms, effects of Ca^{2+} are exerted through membrane depolarization, either by Ca^{2+} entrance or by surface potential changes, and also through the activation of second messenger systems. In testicular nociceptive endings, suppression of extracellular Ca^{2+} does not eliminate responses to direct depolarising stimuli (high external K^+ or hypertonic NaCl) but inhibits the stimulating effects of BK[62]; moreover, the absence of $[Ca^{2+}]_o$ does not prevent nociceptor excitation by capsaicin in this tissue. Ruthenium red, an inorganic dye with Ca^{2+} entry blocking properties, inhibits capsaicin-induced nociceptor stimulation as well as the concomitant neuropeptide release in the skin. However, ruthenium red suppresses excitatory effects of capsaicin presumably by a direct blocking action on either the cationic channel or the capsaicin receptor itself, while its elimination of neuropeptide secretion is the consequence of the reduced Ca^{2+} entrance[51].

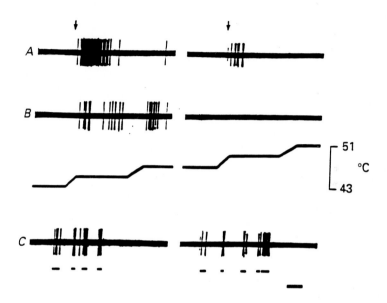

Figure 7. Effects of capsaicin on the responsiveness of corneal polymodal nociceptors. Impulse discharges evoked by 10 mM acetic acid (arrow, A), stepwise heating (recorded in the lower trace, B), and mechanical indentation (indicated by the horizontal bars, C) before (left) and after a 5 min pretreatment with 0.33 mM capsaicin (right) (From Belmonte et al.,[4]).

In the cornea, it is feasible to perfuse the anterior chamber with a Ca^{2+} free, 1mM EGTA solution while the external surface is bathed continuously with the same solution. In this way, Ca^{2+} can be effectively removed from the extracellular fluid in the intact cornea 'in situ'. Under these circumstances, acidic stimulation with CO_2 pulses or with topical 10 mM acetic acid still produces a normal or an even slightly enhanced response, as can be expected from the increased excitability of nervous membranes in absence of $[Ca^{2+}]_o$. When a heating pulse is applied, a distinct firing response is also obtained; however, repetition of this thermal stimulus evokes only a few spikes or no response at all; this situation is reversed in most cases when returning to normal $[Ca^{2+}]_o$ (Figure 8). These data indicate that Ca^{2+} ions are not necessary for nociceptive responses to protons but they are required for thermal responsiveness and sensitisation of nociceptors. The site (epithelium cells, nerve terminals) at which Ca^{2+} ions are needed was not established in these experiments.

Transduction by nociceptive neurons of at least some exogenous and endogenous chemical noxious stimuli, seems to depend on non-selective cation channels, whose gating allows movement of Na^+, K^+ and Ca^{2+} ions along their concentration gradients[2]. This is the type of cation channel that responds to protons and may be also coupled to the receptor of capsaicin and perhaps of other algogenic substances.

The characteristics of these non-selective cation channels in polymodal nociceptive neurons are still poorly defined. It has been suggested[43] that the cation channel activated by protons in the soma of sensory neurons is a 'transformed' Ca^{2+} channel, whose permeability is transiently modified by hydrogen ions, so that the channel becomes briefly, permeable to Na^+. In sensory ganglion cells, Bevan & Yeats[8] described another specific, sustained inward current elicited by protons that, according to these authors, flows through a different cation channel, the same that is activated by capsaicin. In single polymodal nociceptors of the cornea[57], experimental manoeuvres that in sensory neurons altered the gating of the 'transformed' Ca^{2+} channel also modify the firing response of nerve fibers to protons. For instance, Ca^{2+} channel blockers Cd^{2+} and diltiazem, as well as elevated $[Ca^{2+}]_o$, attenuate nociceptive discharges to acid without affecting mechanosensitivity of the fibers (Figure 9). Moreover, excitatory effects of protons are partly inactivated by high $[Ca^{2+}]_o$ or by hydrogen ion concentrations that by themselves fail to excite nociceptive endings. These data indicate that in nociceptive terminals, ion channels opened by protons exhibit some of the properties attributed to the 'transformed' Ca^{2+} channels of the cell soma; however, information is still insufficient to define the type of cation channel(s) involved in nociceptive transduction to algogenic chemicals. It is interesting to note that in photoreceptors and olfactory receptors, cyclic nucleotide-activated ionic channels (gated by cGMP and cAMP, respectively) mediate sensory transduction[36]. Cyclic nucleotide channels are cation selective channels that do not discriminate well between monovalent alkali cations. They are also permeable for divalent cations but differ from voltage-gated Ca^{2+} channels in the fact that Ca^{2+} channels allow permeation of monovalent cations only in the complete absence of Ca^{2+} ions, and they discriminate better by several orders of magnitude between Ca^{2+} and monovalent ions. Cyclic nucleotide channels are selectively blocked by l-cis-diltiazem, that binds and alters the gating of the channel[31]. It has been proposed[36] that cyclic nucleotide-gated channels are primordial channel chimeras which might combine features of voltage-gated channels with those of ligand-gated channels. Although available evidence is scarce, the possibility that a type of ion channel similar to cyclic nucleotide-gated channels is involved in transduction of noxious chemical stimuli deserves experimental attention.

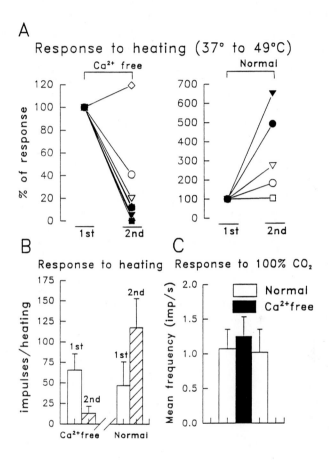

Figure 8. Effects of removal of extracellular Ca^{2+} on impulse discharges of corneal polymodal units to thermal and chemical stimuli. A. Response of 8 polymodal units to heating pulses from 35°C to 49°C in two different conditions: a Ca^{2+} free medium with 1 mM EGTA (left) and a 2.2 mM Ca^{2+} solution (right). Data are expressed as percentage of the total number of impulses evoked by the first heating cycle. B. Average number of impulses per heating cycle of the units represented in A. C. Average response to CO_2 pulses in normal and Ca^{2+} free media of the units depicted in A and B. (Unpublished data from Chen, Pozo, Gallar & Belmonte)

Diltiazem as a blocker of chemosensitivity in polymodal nociceptors

The selective blocking effects of diltiazem on chemosensory responses are particularly interesting, because diltiazem, a benzothiazepine described as a voltage-sensitive Ca^{2+} channel antagonist, also blocks at higher doses non-selective cation channels[35]. Thus, the possibility exists that diltiazem acts as a specific channel blocker for non-selective cation channels mediating the action of protons and perhaps of other chemical agents on nociceptors. This interpretation is supported by the observation that diltiazem greatly reduces sensitisation of corneal polymodal nociceptors to repeated heating (Figure 10); responses to inflammatory substances are also attenuated by pretreatment with diltiazem (Figure 6). In both cases mechanically-evoked discharges are not altered by the drug.

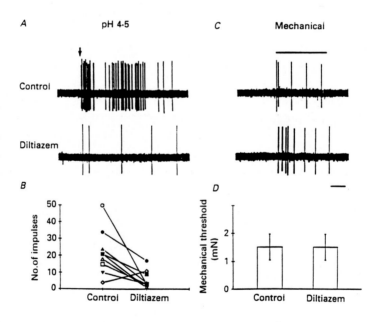

Figure 9. Reduction by diltiazem of the response of corneal polymodal nociceptors to chemical but not to mechanical stimulation. A and C, sample records of the impulse discharge evoked by a pH 4.5 solution and by mechanical stimulation with a brush, before and 10 min after bathing the cornea with a solution containing 1 mM diltiazem. B. Change in total number of impulses elicited by acid during a 30 sec period, before and after 1 mM diltiazem, in 9 separate units. D. Average mechanical threshold of the units depicted in B, before and after diltiazem. Bars are S.E.M. Time scale in A and C, 5 sec. (From Pozo et al.,[57]).

The reduction by diltiazem of chemosensory responses to exogenous and endogenous inflammatory agents makes this drug a potential tool as analgesic and anti-inflammatory agent. There is indirect evidence suggesting that this is the case. Expression of the proto-oncogene *c-fos* protein, that has been associated with neuronal activation by natural stimuli[32] can be detected in corneal trigeminal nucleus neurons a few hours after noxious stimulation of the cornea by acids. Pretreatment with diltiazem, significantly reduced the number of neurons expressing the proto-oncogene protein product after acidic stimulation[52]. Furthermore, diltiazem decreases the signs of ocular irritation and neurogenic inflammation evoked by topical instillation in the eye of irritant agents (capsaicin, nitrogen mustard) or exposure of the anterior segment to ultraviolet radiation[23,25]. These effects may be due to a diminished release of neuropeptides, consecutive to the reduction by diltiazem of nociceptor's excitation.

In summary, stimuli acting on nociceptive terminals are ultimately transduced into membrane currents, which are mediated by changes in the properties of ion channels. Chemical substances may act directly on ion channel proteins or bind to a receptor molecule that in turn will modulate ion channel gating, either directly or through a second messenger system. There is still a very incomplete knowledge of the role played by the various receptor/ion channel systems found in other excitable cells on the activation and sensitization of nociceptive terminals. Indirect evidence obtained in the cornea suggests that chemical stimuli use a transduction mechanism different from that of chemical and thermal stimuli. Furthermore, excitation by protons and other chemical substances appears to be mediated by a non-selective cation channel that can be blocked by capsaicin and diltiazem. Calcium ions may play an important role in the sensitization process of nociceptors.

THE SOMA OF PRIMARY SENSORY NEURONS AS A MODEL OF POLYMODALITY

Cultured trigeminal neurons

Cultured primary sensory neurons, or hybrid cell lines derived from neonatal dorsal root ganglion (DRG) neurons fused with neuroblastoma cells, have been used to analyse molecular and cellular mechanisms of nociceptor's activation[8,17,74,75].

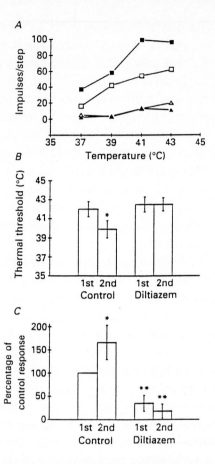

Figure 10. The effects of diltiazem on the response of corneal nociceptors to noxious heating. A. Stimulus response relation of corneal polymodal units in response to a first (open symbols) and a second (filled symbols) stepwise heating, before (squares) and after (triangles) application of 1 mM diltiazem. B. Average thermal thresholds of 6 corneal polymodal units at successive stepwise heatings, before and after diltiazem. C. Change in total number of impulses per heating cycle, expressed as percentage of the first cycle, in the same fibers as in B, before and after administration of diltiazem. Bars are S.E.M. (* P <0.05; ** p <0.01). (From Pozo et al.,[57])

Capsaicin (0.5 µM), applied to the soma of DRG neurons increases membrane permeability to Na+, Ca2+ and K+, leading to cell depolarization in about 50% of the cells. Protons are also excitatory when applied to the soma of nociceptive neurons.

As commented above[8], two distinct inward currents evoked by protons have been distinguished in cultured DRG cells: a rapidly inactivating inward sodium current and a sustained, slowly inactivating inward current, that is present only in capsaicin-sensitive neurons and appears to be due to an increase in non-selective cation conductance. These data have been interpreted as suggestive that in nociceptive neurons, capsaicin and protons activate the same non-selective cation channel.

Another approach to explore membrane mechanisms activated by protons and capsaicin is to measure changes in cytoplasmic free calcium concentration ($[Ca^{2+}]_i$) with Indo-1 fluorescence, in cultured trigeminal ganglion neurons of new-born rabbits[49]. Resting values of $[Ca^{2+}]_i$ (about 100 nM) increased rapidly with depolarization induced by exposure to 30-60 mM K^+. Eighty-three percent of these cells also respond to protons, showing a transient increase in $[Ca^{2+}]_i$ with sudden changes in extracellular pH values from 7.0 to 5.0; maximal responses appear at pH's of 5.5 to 6.5. As shown in figure 11, repeated exposure to low pH reduces the amplitude of the response. Moreover, the magnitude of $[Ca^{2+}]_i$ increase was related to the size of the pH step.

In 72% of neurons that are sensitive to protons, capsaicin also evokes a sustained elevation of $[Ca^{2+}]_i$, to values up to 4 times the control. The response to capsaicin is more sustained than to acid (figure 12). Furthermore, repeated acidic stimulation reduces the magnitude of the response to protons but not to capsaicin, thus suggesting that different mechanisms are used for the $[Ca^{2+}]_i$ increases induced by each stimulus. This possibility is further supported by experiments where extracellular Ca^{2+} concentration is changed or Ca^{2+} channel antagonists are employed; proton-induced Ca^{2+} transients are reduced or abolished both by zero or by 20 mM$[Ca^{2+}]_o$ (Figure 13); 5 mM Ni^{2+} and the organic Ca^{2+} channel blockers diltiazem (0.5-1mM) and nitrendipine (10 µM) also decrease or eliminate $[Ca^{2+}]_i$ elevations induced by acid (Figure 14). In contrast, only zero $[Ca^{2+}]_o$ abolishes responses to capsaicin, while nifedipine attenuates the response of only some of the cells and high $[Ca^{2+}]_o$ and diltiazem are ineffective (Figure 14). Thus, these observations speak against a common mechanism for the increase in $[Ca^{2+}]_i$ induced by H^+ and capsaicin in primary sensory neurons.

The N neuron of the leech

One of the main limitations in studying cellular mechanisms for nociceptive transduction in primary neurons of sensory ganglia is the difficulty in identifying those neurons that specifically detect noxious stimuli among the heterogeneous population of ganglion cells.

Simple organisms have been often used as a model of behavioral responses more easily accessible to electrophysiological techniques. For instance, neural mechanisms of behavioral sensitisation to noxious stimuli have been studied in Aplysia as a simple form of learning[76]. Detection of noxious stimuli is the first step of

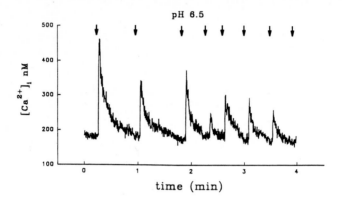

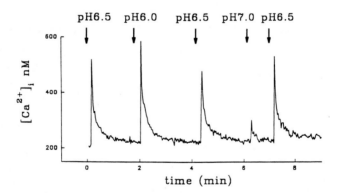

Figure 11. A. Changes in intracellular free Ca^{2+} induced by application of acid to cultured new-born rabbit trigeminal neurons, measured with indo-1 fluorescence. Desensitization develops after repeated applications of a pH 6.5 solution. B. $[Ca^{2+}]_i$ increases, evoked by solutions at different pH values (6.0, 6.5, 7.0), applied for 3 seconds (arrows). (Unpublished data from Lopez-Briones, Garcia-Hirschfeld, Valdeolmillos & Belmonte).

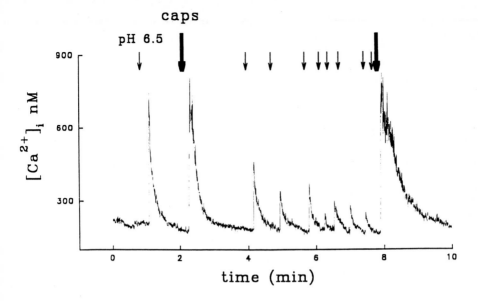

Figure 12. Changes in intracellular free Ca^{2+} induced by application of acid and capsaicin to cultured new-born rabbit trigeminal neurons. Repeated pH 6.5 stimulation reduced the magnitude of the response to protons but not to 1 μM capsaicin. (Unpublished data from Lopez-Briones, Garcia-Hirshfeld, Valdeolmillos & Belmonte).

a very primitive biological response directed to the defence of physical integrity. Thus, the possibility exist that some of the transducing membrane mechanisms present in lower species are preserved in mammals.

The leech has a nervous system that possess several advantages for studying nociception. The skin of each segment of the animal is innervated by a number of mechanosensitive neurons, including the N neurons, whose cell bodies are located in the segmental ganglion in a stereotyped position. Each N cell can be recognised individually and impaled with microelectrodes; they can be activated by controlled stimuli to the skin or by electrical stimuli to the cell body. N neurons have been considered "nociceptive" because of their high mechanical threshold compared to other mechanosensitive ganglion cells[55]. Recently, it has been explored whether N neurons of the leech exhibit functional properties similar to polymodal nociceptive neurons of mammals, i.e. responsiveness to different stimulus modalities and

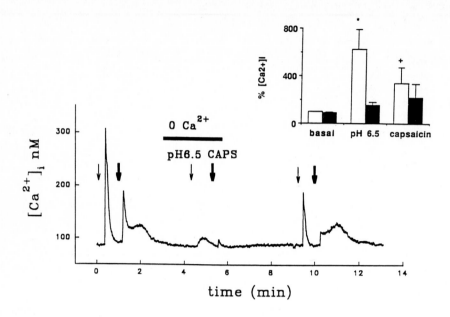

Figure 13. Influence of extracellular Ca^{2+} on intracellular free Ca^{2+} changes induced by application of acid and capsaicin to new born rabbit cultured trigeminal neurons. During the period indicated by the horizontal bar, cells were superfused with a zero Ca^{2+} medium containing EDTA, instead of 2.2 mM Ca^{2+}. Applications of 1 µM capsaicin and pH 6.5 solutions are indicated by thick and thin arrows, respectively. Inset, the effects of zero $[Ca^{2+}]_o$ on the pH 6.5 and capsaicin-induced $[Ca^{2+}]_i$ rises (filled bars), expressed as percentage of basal $[Ca^{2+}]_i$ (empty bars: 2.2 mM Ca^{2+}). Data are means ± S.E.M. Number of neurons: Basal $[Ca^{2+}]_i$, n = 17; pH 6.5, n = 17; 1 µM capsaicin, n = 10 (+ $p < 0.02$; * $p < 0.01$). (Unpublished data from Lopez-Briones, Garcia-Hirschfeld, Valdeolmillos & Belmonte).

sensitisation to repeated noxious stimuli[56]. In an 'in vitro' preparation of the segmental ganglion
 attached to the skin, it is possible to record intracellularly in the soma of the lateral and medial N neurons while the skin is stimulated. A train of nerve impulses is evoked in N-neurons by application to the cutaneous surface of high threshold mechanical indentation but also of acetic acid solutions, capsaicin or NaCl crystals. Impulse discharges are also elicited by heat, with a mean thermal threshold of about 38°C. Repeated heating pulses sensitise the firing response, as evidenced by a significant reduction of thermal threshold and enhanced responses to each heating pulse (Figure 15). Discharges evoked by chemicals are also augmented after exposure to noxious heat. Furthermore, sensitivity to acid and to capsaicin is present

also in the soma of N neurons. Therefore, N neurons of the leech may be an alternative model for biophysical studies of membrane mechanisms involved in chemotransduction by nociceptors.

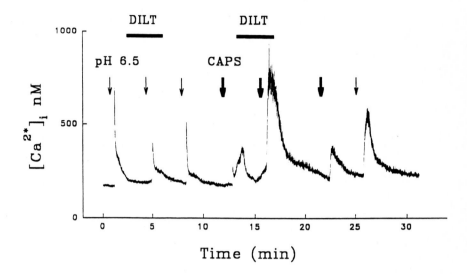

Figure 14. Influence of Ca^{2+} antagonist diltiazem on intracellular free Ca^{2+} responses to acid and capsaicin in cultured new-born rabbit trigeminal neurons. $[Ca^{2+}]_i$ rises induced by pH 6.5 but not by 1 µM capsaicin were inhibited by 0.5 mM diltiazem (Unpublished data from Lopez-Briones, Garcia-Hirschfeld, Valdeolmillos & Belmonte)

CHEMICAL SENSITIVITY OF NEUROMAS

Severed sensory axons form swelled end bulbs shortly after injury. Channel and receptor proteins synthesised in the cell soma are transported anterogradely down the nerve and presumably accumulate in axonal swellings[15]. Injured axons exhibit sensitivity to stimuli that normally excite nociceptive terminals, including protons, BK, histamine, adrenaline and capsaicin[30,73]. The rat saphenous nerve neuroma 'in vitro'[77], is a promising preparation to analyse under controlled conditions the response characteristics of single fibers to chemical agents that excite intact nociceptors[61]. As shown in Figure 16, regenerating nerve terminals are excited by many of the chemical mediators of peripheral nociception. Dissociated regenerating nerve terminals may become accessible to patch clamp and isolation techniques, thus offering another alternative model to study in greater detail membrane properties of nociceptive terminals.

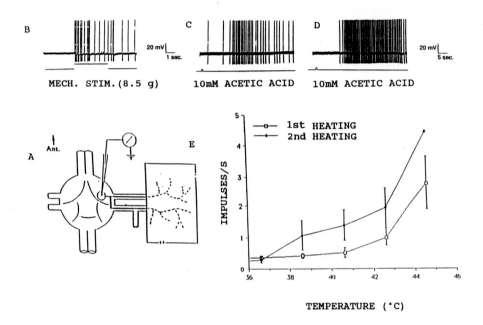

Figure 15. Polymodal responses of the N neuron of the leech segmental ganglion. A. Schematic diagram of the ganglion-body wall preparation, showing the location of the N neuron and the innervation of the skin by branches of its peripheral axon (modified from 71). Impulse response recorded intracellularly in the soma of a N medial cell during mechanical indentation (C) and after application of a drop of 10 mM acetic acid before (C) and after (D) three stepwise heating cycles up to 46°C. E. Mean stimulus-response relation of 5 N neurons in response to a first (open symbols) and a second (filled symbols) stepwise heating cycles (from 36°C to 45°C), separated by a 10 min. interval (Unpublished data from Pastor, Soria and Belmonte).

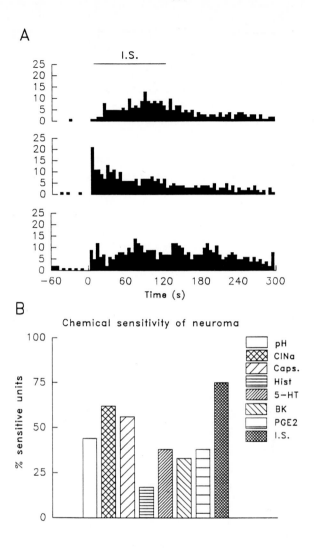

Figure 16. The effects of chemical stimulation on regenerating nerve fibers of a neuroma. A.. Peristimulus histogram of the impulse response of a mechanosensitive unit of a saphenous nerve neuroma to three successive superfusions with inflammatory soup (I.S., see text) for 2 min, separated by a 15 min interval. B. Percentage of response of mechano- and/or chemosensitive units of saphenous and sciatic nerve neuromas, to each of the chemical stimuli indicated on the right side of the figure. NaCl: hypertonic NaCl; Caps: capsaicin; Hist: Histamine; 5-HT: Serotonin; BK: Bradykinin; PGE_2: Prostaglandin E_2; I.S.: Inflammatory soup. (Unpublished data from Rivera, Gallar, Pozo & Belmonte).

In summary, the soma of mammalian sensory neurons presumed as nociceptive, can be employed to study cellular mechanisms associated with nociceptor activation and sensitization. These cellualar mechanisms appear to be already present in invertebrates, where nociceptive neurons can be identified by their position in the ganglia and therefore they are more accessible to biophysical manipulations.

Finally, the enlarged nerve endings of the neuroma constitute a potential source of putative nociceptive terminals to study transduction mechanisms in nociceptors.

CONCLUDING REMARKS

Mechanisms for transduction of exogenous and endogenous chemical stimuli by peripheral nociceptors have resisted experimental analysis at cellular and molecular level, in part due to the reduced accessibility of nerve terminals. In spite of these limitations, several models are available to advance in the knowledge of membrane processes associated to excitation of nociceptive terminals by chemical stimuli. These include sensory terminals in simple tissues, cultured primary sensory cells, invertebrate nociceptive neurons or regenerating nociceptive endings. Each of these experimental preparations can be useful to extend our knowledge about membrane processes triggered off by lesive stimuli in peripheral terminals of nociceptive neurons. It is attractive to speculate that membrane mechanisms developed to respond to irritant chemicals in the environment, the most primitive form of protective behavior, have been preserved for other forms of chemical transduction in sensory cells, as olfaction or photoreception. If the same type of ion channels were employed for the different types of peripheral chemosensitivity, it would be possible to extend the more advanced understanding of mechanisms of transduction and sensitivity adjustment in these sensory cells to the field of nociception. Here, a better knowledge of the excitatory mechanisms present in peripheral nociceptive terminals will have the additional interest of being important for pain therapy.

REFERENCES

1. ANTON, F., EUCHNER, I. AND HANDWERKER, H.O. (1992) Psychophysical examination of pain induced by defined CO_2 pulses applied to the nasal mucosa. *Pain* **49**, 53-60.

2. AKAIKE, N., KRISHTAL, OA. AND MARUYAMA, T. (1990) Proton-induced current in frog isolated dorsal root ganglion cells. *J. Neurophysiol.* 805-813.

3. BACCAGLINI, P.I. AND HOGAN, P.G.(1983) Some rat sensory neurons in culture express characteristics of differentiated pain sensory cells. *Proc. Natl. Acad. Sci. USA.* **80**, 594-598.

4. BELMONTE, C., GALLAR, J., POZO, M.A. AND REBOLLO, I. (1991) Excitation by irritant chemical substances of sensory afferent units in the cat's cornea. *J. Physiol.* **437**, 709-725.

5. BELMONTE, C. AND GIRALDEZ, F. (1981) Responses of cat corneal sensory receptors to mechanical and thermal stimulation. *J. Physiol.* **321**, 355-368.

6. BESSOU, P. AND PERL, E.R. (1969) Response of cutaneous sensory units with unmyelinated fibers to noxious stimuli. *J. Neurophysiol.* **32**,1025-1043.

7. BEUERMAN, R.W. AND TANELIAN, D.L. Corneal pain evoked by thermal stimulation. *Pain* 1979; 7:1-14.

8. BEVAN, S. AND YEATS, J. (1991) Protons activate a cation conductance in a sub-population of rat dorsal root ganglion neurones. *J. Physiol.* **433**, 145-161.

9. BLUMBERG, H. AND JÄNIG, W. (1984) Discharge pattern of afferent fibers from a neuroma. *Pain* **20**, 335-353.

10. BURGESS, G.M., MULLANEY, I., MCNEILL, M., DUNN, P. AND RANG, H.P. (1989) Second messengers involved in the action on bradykinin on cultured sensory neurons. *J. Neurosci.* **9**, 3314-3325.

11. CERVERO, F. (1982) Afferent activity evoked by natural stimulation of the biliary system in the ferret. *Pain* **13**, 137-151.

12. CHAHL, L.A. (1991) Antidromic vasodilatation and neurogenic inflammation. In: *Novel Peripheral Neurotransmitters.* ed. C. Bell. Pergamon Press.

13. CHANG-LING, T. (1989) Sensitivity and neural organization of the cat cornea. *Invest. Ophthalmol. Vis. Sci.* **30**, 1075-1082.

14. CHEN, X., POZO, M.A., BAEZA, M., GALLAR, J. AND BELMONTE, C. (1993) Stimulation of corneal nerve fibers by CO_2: a method to measure corneal sensitivity. *Invest. Ophthalmol. Vis. Sci. (suppl. ARVO Meeting).*

15. DEVOR, M. (1991) Neuropathic pain and injured nerve: peripheral mechanisms. *Br. Med. Bull.* **47**, 619-630.

16. DRAY, A., BETTANEY, J., FOSTER, P. AND PERKINS, M.N. (1988) Bradykinin-induced stimulation of afferent fibres is mediated through protein kinase C. *Neurosci. Lett.* **91**, 301-307.

17. DRAY, A., FORBES, C.A. AND BURGESS, G.M. (1990) Ruthenium red blocks the capsaicin-induced increase of intracellular calcium and activation of membrane currents in sensory neurons as well as the activation of peripheral nociceptors in vitro. *Neurosci. Lett.* **110**, 52-59.

18. DRAY, A. AND WOOD, J.N. (1991) Nonopioid molecular signaling mechanisms involved in nociception and antinociception. In: *Towards a New Pharmacotherapy of Pain*. eds. A.I. Basbaum, J.M. Besso. John Wiley & Sons Ltd.

19. FJÄLLBRANT, N. AND IGGO, A. (1961) The effect of histamine, 5-hydroxytryptamine and acetylcholine on cutaneous afferent fibres. *J. Physiol.* **156**, 5788-590.

20. GALLAR, J. AND BELMONTE, C.(1990) Modulation by prostaglandins of nervous activity in corneal nociceptors. *Invest. Ophthalmol. Vis. Sci.* **31**, (suppl):514.

21. GALLAR, J., POZO, M.A. AND BELMONTE, C. Unpublished results.

22. GALLAR, J., POZO, M.A., TUCKETT R.P. AND BELMONTE, C. (1993) Response of unmyelinated fibres to mechanical, thermal and chemical stimulation of the cat's cornea. *J. Physiol.* **468**, 609-622.

23. GARCIA DE LA RUBIA, P., GONZÁLEZ, G.G., GALLAR, J. AND BELMONTE, C. (1993) Attenuation of anterior segment inflammation by blockade of sensory nerves with calcium antagonist diltiazem. *Invest. Ophthalmol. Vis. Sci* (in press).

24. GONZALEZ, G.G., GALLAR, J. AND BELMONTE, C. (1992) Polymodal nociceptors and neurogenic inflammation in the cornea. *Exp Eye Res.* **55** (suppl. 1), S53.

25. GONZÁLEZ, G.G., GARCIA, DE LA RUBIA, P., GALLAR, J. AND BELMONTE, C. Reduction of capsaicin-induced ocular pain and neurogenic inflammation. Invest. *Ophthalmol. Vis. Sci.* (submitted).

26. GRUBB, B.D., BIRRELL, G.J., McQUENN, D.S. AND IGGO, A. (1991) The role of PGE_2 in the sensitization of mechanoreceptors in normal and inflamed ankle joints of the rat. *Exp. Brain Res.* **84**, 383-392.

27. HÄBLER, H.J., JÄNIG, W. AND KOLTZENBURG, M. (1990) Activation of unmyelinated afferent fibres by mechanical stimuli and inflammation of the urinary bladder in the cat. *J. Physiol.* **425**, 545-562.

28. HANDWERKER, H.O. (1991) What peripheral mechanisms contribute to nociceptive transmission and hyperalgesia?. In: *Towards a New Pharmacology of Pain*. eds. A.I. Basbaum, J.-M. Besson. John Wiley & Sons.

29. HANDWERKER, H.O. AND REEH, P.W. (1991) Pain and inflammation. Proc. VIth World Congress on Pain. 59-70.

30. HARTUNG, M., LEAH, J. AND ZIMMERMANN, M. (1989) The excitation of cutaneous nerve endings in a neuroma by capsaicin. *Brain Res.* **499**, 363-366.

31. HAYNES, L.W. (1992) Block of the cyclic GMP-gated channel of vertebrate rod and cone photoreceptors by l-cis-diltiazem. *J. Gen. Physiol.* **100**, 783-801.

32. HUNT, S.P., PINI, A. AND EVAN, G. (1987) Induction of *c-fos*-like protein in spinal cord neurons following sensory stimulation. *Nature* **328**, 632-634.

33. JANCSÓ, N., JANCSÓ-GABOR, A., SZOLCSÁNYI, J. (1968) The role of sensory nerve endings in neurogenic inflammation induced by human skin and in the eye and paw of the rat. *Br. J. Pharmacol. Chemother.* **33**, 32-41.

34. KANAKA, R., SCHAIBLE, H.G. AND SCHMIDT, R.F. (1985) Activation of fine articular afferent units by bradykinin. *Brain Res.* **327**, 81-90.

35. KAUPP, U.B. (1991) The cyclic nucleotide-gated channels of vertebrate photoreceptors and olfactory epithelium. *Trends Neurosci.* **14**, 150-157.
36. KAUPP, U.B. AND KOCK, K.W. (1992) Role of cGMP and Ca^{2+} in vertebrate photoreceptor excitation and adaptation. *Ann. rev. Physiol.* **54**, 153-175.
37. KEELE, C.A. (1962) The common chemical sense and its receptors. *Arch. Int. Pharmacodyn.* **139**, 547-57.
38. KENINS, P. (1982) Response of single nerve fibers to capsaicin applied to the skin. *Neurosci Lett.* 29, 83-88.
39. KENSHALO, D.R. (1960) Comparison of thermal sensitivity of the forehead, lip, conjunctiva and cornea. *J. Appl. Physiol.* **15**, 987-991.
40. KESSLER, W., KIRCHHOFF, C., REEH, P.W. AND HANDWERKER, H.O. (1992) Excitation of cutaneous afferent nerve endings in vitro by a combination of inflammatory mediators and conditioning effect of substance P. *Exp. Brain Res.* **91**, 467-476.
41. KIRCHHOFF, C., JUNG, S., REEH, P.W. AND HANDWERKER, HO. (1990) Carragenaan inflammation increases bradykinin sensitivity of rat cutaneous nociceptors. *Neurosci. Lett.* **111**, 206-210.
42. KIRCHHOFF, C., LEAH, J.D., JUNG, S. AND REEH, P.W. (1992) Excitation of cutaneous sensory nerve endings in the rat by 4-aminopyridine and tetraethylammonium. *J. Neurophysiol.* **67**, 125-131.
43. KONNERTH, A., LUX, H.D. AND MORAD, M. (1987) Proton-induced transformation of calcium channel in chick dorsal root ganglion cells. *J. Physiol.* **386**, 603-633.
44. KUMAZAWA, T. AND MIZUMURA, K. (1977) Thin-fibre receptors responding to mechanical, chemical and thermal stimulation in the skeletal muscle of the dog. *J. Physiol.* **273**, 179-194.
45. KUMAZAWA, T. AND MIZUMURA, K. (1980) Chemical responses of polymodal receptors of the scrotal contents in dogs. *J. Physiol.* **299**, 219-232.
46. KUMAZAWA, T, AND PERL, E.R. (1977) Primate cutaneous sensory units with unmyelinated (C) afferent fibers. *J. Neurophysiol.* **40**, 1325-1338.
47. LANG, E., NOVAK, A., REEH, P. AND HANDWERKER, H.O. (1990) Chemosensitivity of fine afferents from rat skin in vitro. J. *Neurophysiol.* **63**, 887-901.
48. LINDAHL O. (1961) Experimental skin pain induced by injection of water-soluble substances in humans. *Acta Physiol. Scand.* **179,** (suppl.), 1-89.
49. LÓPEZ-BRIONES, L.G., GARCÍA-HIRSCHFELD, J., VALDEOLMILLOS, M. AND BELMONTE, C. (1993) Calcium transients produced by pH changes and capsaicin in cultured trigeminal neurons. (in preparation).
50. LYNN, B. AND BARANOWSKI, R.A. (1987) Comparison of the relative numbers and properties of cutaneous nociceptive afferents in different mammalian species. In: Fine afferent nerve fibers and pain. eds. R.F. Schmidt et al. VCH Publishers.
51. MAGGI, C.A. (1991) Capsaicin and primary afferent neurons: from basic science to human therapy?. *J. Auton Nerv. Sys.* **33**, 1-14.
52. MARTINEZ, S. AND BELMONTE, C. C-fos expression in trigeminal nucleus neurones after chemical irritation of the cornea: reduction by selective blockade of nociceptor's chemosensitivity. *Eur. J. Neurosci.* (submitted).
53. MENSE, S. (1977) Nervous outflow from skeletal muscle following chemical noxious stimulation. *J Physiol.* **267**, 75-88.

54. MIZUMURA, K., SATO, J. AND KUMAZAWA, T. (1987) Effects of prostaglandins and other putative chemical intermediaries on the activity of canine testicular polymodal receptors studied in vitro. *Pflügers Arch.* **408**, 565-572.

55. NICHOLLS, J.G. AND BAYLOR, DA. (1968) Specific modalities and receptive fields of sensory neurons in CNS of the leech. *J. Neurophysiol.* **31**, 740-756.

56. PASTOR, J.E., SORIA, B. AND BELMONTE, C. (1993) Nociceptive responses in the N neuron of the leech. Proc. 16th Meeting of the European Neuroscience Association, Madrid.

57. POZO, M.A., GALLEGO, R., GALLAR, J. AND BELMONTE, C. (1992) Blockade by calcium antagonists of chemical excitation and sensitization of polymodal nociceptors in the cat's cornea. *J. Physiol.* **450**, 179-189.

58. RANG, H.P., BEVAN, S. AND DRAY, A. (1991) Chemical activation of nociceptive peripheral neurones. *Br. Med. Bull.* **47**(3), 534-548.

59. REBOLLO, I. AND BELMONTE, C. (1988) Effects of substance P and SP-antagonists on the neural activity of corneal sensory fibers.Proc. 8th International Congress of Eye Research. 110.

60. REEH, P.W. (1986) Sensory receptors in mammalian skin in an in vitro preparation. *Neurosci. Lett.* **66**, 141-146.

61. RIVERA, L., GALLAR, J., POZO, M.A. AND BELMONTE, C. (1993) Chemical responses of sensory neuromas: an 'in vitro' study. Proc. 16th Meeting of the European Neuroscience Association.

62. SATO, J., MIZUMURA, K. AND KUMAZAWA, T. (1989) Effects of ionic calcium on the response of canine testicular polymodal receptors to algesic substances. *J. Neurophysiol.* **62**, 119-125.

63. SCHAIBLE, H.G. AND SCHMIDT, RF. (1985) Effects of an experimental arthritis on the sensory properties of fine articular nerves. *J. Neurophysiol.* **54**, 1109-1122.

64. SCHAIBLE, H.G. AND SCHMIDT, R.F. (1988) Direct observation of the sensitization of articular afferents during an experimental arthritis. In: *Pain Research and Clinical Management,* vol 3, Proc. VIth World Congress on Pain. eds. R. Dubner et al. Elsevier.

65. SCHAIBLE, H.G. AND SCHMIDT, R.F. (1988) Excitation and sensitization of fine articular afferents from cat's knee joint by prostaglandin E_2. *J. Physiol.* **403**, 91-104.

66. SILVER, W.L. AND FINGER, T.E. (1991) The trigeminal system. In: *Smell and Taste in Health and Disease.* eds. T.V. Getchell et al. Raven Press.

67. STEEN, K.H., REEH, P.W., ANTON, F. AND HANDWERKER, H.O. (1992) Protons selectively induce lasting excitation and sensitization to mechanical stimulation of nociceptors in rat skin, in vitro. *J. Neurosci.* **12**, 86-95.

68. STONE, R.A., KUWAYAMA, Y. AND LATIES, A.M. (1987) Regulatory peptides in the eye. *Experientia* **43**, 791-800.

69. SZOLCSÁNYI, J. (1987) Selective responsiveness of polymodal nociceptors of the rabbit ear to capsaicin, bradykinin and ultra-violet irradiation. *J. Physiol.* **388**, 9-23.

70. SZOLCSÁNYI, J., ANTON, F., REEH, P. AND HANDWERKER, H.O. (1988) Selective excitation by capsaicin of mechano-heat sensitive nociceptors in rat skin. *Brain Res.* **446**, 262-268.

71. VAN ESSEN, D.C. (1973) The contribution of membrane hyperpolarization to adaptation and conduction block in sensory neurones of the leech. *J. Physiol.* **230**, 509-534.

72. VAN HOUTEN, J. (1991) Chemosensory transduction in Paramecium. In: Biology of chemotactic response. eds. J. Armitage and J. Lackie. Cambridge University Press.

73. WEELK, E., LEAH, J.D. AND ZIMMERMANN, M. (1990) Characteristics of A- and C-fibers ending in a sensory nerve neuroma in the rat. *J. Neurophysiol.* **63**, 759-766.

74. WOOD, J.N., BEVAN, S.J., COOTE, P.R., DUNN, P.M., HARMAR, A., HOGAN, P., LARCHMAN, D.S., MORRISON, C., ROUGON, G., THEVENIAU, M. AND WHEATLEY, S. (1990) Novel cell lines display properties of nociceptive sensory neurons. *Proc. R. Soc. Lond.* B. **241**, 187-194.

75. WOOD, J.N., WINTER, J., JAMES, I.F., RANG, H.P., YEATS, J. AND BEVAN, S. (1988) Capsaicin-induced ion fluxes in dorsal root ganglion cells in culture. *J. Neurosci.* **8**, 3208-3220.

76. WOOLF, C.J. AND WALTERS, E.T. (1991) Common patterns of plasticity contributing to nociceptive sensitization in mammals and Aplysia. *Trends Neurosci.* **14**(2), 74-78.

77. ZIMMERMANN, M. AND KORSCHORKE, G.M. (1987) Chemosensitivity of nerve sprouts in experimental neuroma of cutaneous nerves of the cat. In: Fine afferent nerve fibers and pain. EDS. r.f. Schmidt RF et al. VCH Publishers.

CHEMICAL EXCITATION AND SENSITIZATION OF NOCICEPTORS

Peter W. Reeh
Institute of Physiology and Biocybernetics
University of Erlangen-Nürnberg
8520 Erlangen
F.R.G.

INTRODUCTION

Sensory capacities of nociceptors have been extensively characterised using noxious mechanical and thermal stimuli. Apart from interesting exceptions, nociceptor responsiveness correlated reasonably well with human sensation or animal behavior.[1] These sensory capacities, however, fail to explain pain that outlasts the acute injury, e.g. post traumatic and inflammatory pain, or pain that results from harmless physical actions as in the case of hyperalgesia. To understand the ongoing discharge and sensitization of nociceptors in these conditions, it is necessary to know about chemical influences on the peripheral nerve endings. This knowledge has been considerably advanced by the introduction of *in vitro* techniques in primary afferent physiology.[2,4,11,18] In our hands, it is a superfused rat skin-nerve preparation that provides differentiated and well categorised populations of cutaneous nociceptors and allows treatment of their receptive fields directly with chemicals in controlled concentrations. The following data in this brief review result from a number of studies on this preparation using the single fiber recording method.

CONSTITUENTS OF THE INFLAMMATORY MILIEU

We have tested a number of endogenous chemicals involved in inflammations or in other painful diseases and investigated their interactions in exciting and

NATO ASI Series, Vol. H 79
Cellular Mechanisms of Sensory Processing
Edited by Laszlo Urban
© Springer-Verlag Berlin Heidelberg 1994

sensitising nociceptors. Herein, we have focused on the most numerous sub population of the "polymodal", i.e. mechano-heat sensitive nociceptor that proved to provide the widest spectrum of chemosensitivity (Figure 1). In terms of prevalence, i.e. number of units excited, bradykinin (10^{-5}M) and low pH (6.1) are the most effective agents each driving about 60% of the polymodals.[12,23] At equal and pathophysiologically relevant concentration (10^{-6}M), however, the hydrogen ions were more potent than bradykinin and even than an ample combination of inflammatory mediators.[7,17] In addition, pH 6.1 elicits significantly higher discharge rates and produces long-lasting non-adapting activities while the inflammatory mediators lose their excitatory action due to tachyphylaxis within minutes. However, combining low pH with bradykinin, histamine, serotonin and prostaglandin E_2 in one "inflammatory soup" (10^{-6}M) prevents the tachyphylaxis and further increases the algogenic potency (Figure 1). This combination has also been used to recruit part of the "sleeping" nociceptor/s that were found in a recent study using electrical search techniques in sympathectomised skin (Kress et al. 1992). The chemicals combined in "inflammatory soup" have all been shown to be present in inflammatory exudates or in pathological tissues (for review see Handwerker and Reeh[5]) and to act on nociceptors in one way or the other.

Serotonin (5-HT) alone excites only a small proportion of the polymodals (Figure 1), but reliably increases their responsiveness to bradykinin[12] (Lang et al. 1990). It can emerge in inflamed or injured tissue through degranulation of mast cells (rat and human respiratory tract) and of **blood platelets**, the latter being activated either by collagen, by catecholamines or by prostaglandin E_2. Platelets as a whole, however, are more potent than 5-HT alone in exciting nociceptors. This turned out from recent experiments when cutaneous receptive fields were first incubated with human "platelet rich plasma", ineffective by itself, that was then activated with 10^{-5}M ADP, again ineffective by itself (Figure 2). Within 2-4 min, about 70% of the nerve terminals developed sustained activity which, in first trials, could not be prevented by various antagonists nor by treatment of the blood donor with acetylsalicylic acid (unpublished).

A potentiation of the bradykinin effect was also to be expected from the ubiquitous **prostaglandin E_2**, as reported from joint and from visceral nociceptors[14,20]. In the cat knee joint, even an excitatory and mechanically sensitizing effect of prostaglandins in high dosage was accomplished[15]. In the skin, *in vitro*, prostaglandin E_2 fails completely to excite or sensitise nociceptors to physical stimulation, and its amplification of the bradykinin responsiveness is

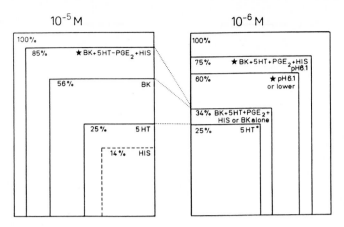

Effective: carbachol (ACh analog) 10^{-6} M ⟶ 32%

Relatively
ineffective: noradrenaline, prostaglandin E$_2$*, leukotrien D$_4$, ATP, CGRP, NKA,
                substance P*, oxygen radicals (O$_2^-$, H$_2$O$_2$).

*can increase nociceptor sensitivity to inflammatory mediators
★can induce sustained activity

Figure 1. Prevalence of chemosensitivity among polymodal nociceptors in rat skin, *in vitro.* Receptive fields were superfused at the corium side with defined aqueous solutions of bradykinin (BK), serotonin (5HT), prostaglandin E$_2$ (PGE$_2$), histamine (HIS), and other substances named in the figure. The size of each rectangle displays the relative proportion of saphenous C-fiber endings that were significantly activated by a given substance or a combination of substances applied at high concentration (10^{-5} M) and at a more patho-physiological concentration (10^{-6} M), respectively. The areas are containing each other as to illustrate that, indeed, histamine- and 5-HT-sensitive neurons are a subpopulation of the BK-responsive nerve endings. The intensities of discharge evoked by chemicals in 10^{-6}M concentration follow a similar rank order as displayed in the present graph; the only difference is that BK alone produces weaker responses than the combination of inflammatory mediators, while both chemical stimuli recruit about the same proportion of C-fibers. Histamine is ineffective at 10^{-6}M concentration and evokes only a minute amount of discharge at 10^{-5}M. In combination with BK and 5HT; histamine and PGE$_2$ do not significantly contribute to the combined excitatory effect on average (see text below).
Acetylcholine (Ach) and carbachol are quite effective in selecting exciting nociceptors but not included in the graphs since a role in inflammation can not yet be evaluated (see text below).
Chemicals rubrified "relatively ineffective" have been tested up to at least 10^{-5} M concentration; details on PGE$_2$, substance P (SP) and the oxygen radicals are communicated in the text below. The footnotes on nociceptor sensitization (by 5HT, PGE$_2$ and SP) and on sustained activation are detailed in the text. The latter refers to constant superfusions of receptive fields for at least 30 min.
Data are compiled from unpublished work and from different publications[7,12,17,21,23].

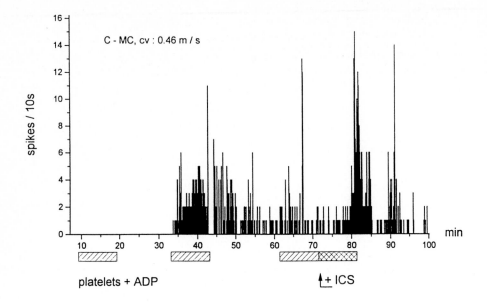

Figure 2. Human platelets excite nociceptors when activated *in vitro* by ADP. Spike density histogram from a mechano-cold sensitive C-fiber that was typically excited by a second application to its receptive field of freshly activated human platelets in "platelet rich plasma" (PRP). A $5HT_3$-antagonist (ICS 205930, 10^{-6}M) was unable to block the sustained discharge and to prevent a newly provoked response, as were methiotepin, ketanserin and a combination of all three 5HT-antagonists in other cases.

Mechano-heat sensitive ("polymodal") nerve endings, in contrast to the above C-MC-fiber, show their response to activated platelets regularly during first application; no tachyphylaxis occurs upon repeated applications. ADP alone are ineffective in exciting nociceptors (during 20min of incubation of their receptive fields).

inconsistent: "Responders" seem to be balanced by "non-responders" among the nociceptive units[12]. Accordingly, inhibition of prostaglandin synthesis has a very limited effect on cutaneous nociceptor sensitization[4]. Recent experiments took into account that e.g. bradykinin can stimulate endogenous prostaglandin release (Figure 3). Even so, during cyclooxygenase block with flurbiprofen, nociceptor responses to combined inflammatory mediators (10^{-6}M) did not measurably depend on the presence or absence of PGE_2 in the "inflammatory soup" (Brehm and Reeh: ongoing work).

Histamine, the substance released from mast cells and from basophilic leukocytes, plays an enigmatic role in cutaneous sensation, in that it produces marked itching in smallest doses but hardly excites any primary afferent in human microneurography studies[6]. In rat skin *in vitro*, only a minute proportion of the polymodals is weakly driven by histamine in high concentration[12]. The picture changes, however, when the units are pretreated (and stimulated) with bradykinin. Then, 75% of the nociceptors respond to histamine[12], and the amount of discharge is no longer significantly different from the bradykinin response (Figure 4). Accordingly, in human skin pretreated with a bradykinin injection (10^{-7}M), histamine iontophoresis no longer produces itch but a sensation of burning pain[9]. A recent hypothesis on the mechanisms of itch is based on these observations[6]. In respect to pain, however, histamine cannot be counted as an algogenic constituent of the "inflammatory soup", since its excitatory effect is not additive to the combined action of the other mediators.

Another enigmatic substance is **acetylcholine** that specifically activates a considerable number of nociceptors but leaves them with a marked desensitization to mechanical stimulation[21,22]. Thus, acetylcholine could either be interpreted as an algogenic agent or as an anti-nociceptive. In any case, to our knowledge no evidence is available on the appearance of acetylcholine in inflammation or in other painful diseases.

In view of the multiplicity of agents affecting nociceptors it might be interesting to recognise a number of substances that are ineffective, at least in exciting nociceptors (Figure 1). Among them, **substance P**, the neuropeptide tachykinin, plays a special role. It is released, together with CGRP and NKA, from the nociceptive nerve endings themselves whenever they are excited, and is assumed to cause "neurogenic inflammation", i.e. vasodilatation and plasma extravasation[13].
Substance P does not excite nociceptors nor sensitise them to physical stimulation but it has a conditioning, sensitising effect on their responsiveness to inflammatory mediators[7]. This effect disappears when the "inflammatory soup" has built up an ongoing nociceptor discharge, but it is present in the very beginning of the response. This agrees well with the assumption that neuropeptides are the first mediators to be released after cutaneous injury.
In contrast, late agents to appear, e.g. in inflammation, are the oxygen radicals that are secreted by invading macrophages and neutrophilic leukocytes and that are assumed to contribute to tissue destruction. The latter holds true even for the nociceptors which are only weakly activated by highest concentrations (>1mM) of hydrogen peroxide but afterwards left with complete desensitization to natural stimuli

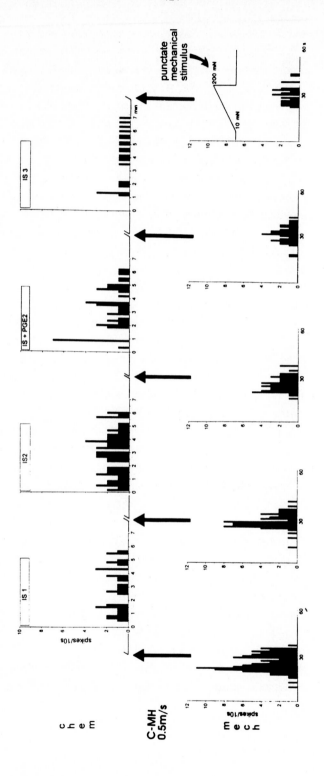

Figure 3. BK+5HT+HIS+/-PGE$_2$ stimulate nociceptors in spite of cyclooxygenase block.
Spike density histograms from a polymodal C-fiber responding repeatedly (10 min interval) to a combination of bradykinin, serotonin and histamine (10^{-6}M: IS 1, IS 2, IS 3). Addition of prostaglandin E$_2$ (10^{-6}M) appears ineffective although cyclooxygenase is blocked by flurbiprofen given systematically and contained in the superfusate over the skin preparation.
The lower row of inserts shows responses to standardised electromechanical stimulation (see last insert for stimulus shape). No sensitization is revealed.

(unpublished). A smaller but still high concentration of hydrogen peroxide sometimes shows a facilitatory effect on the nociceptor discharge induced and sustained by inflammatory mediators, and this is not followed by desensitization (Figure 5). These results may explain the widespread disappointment about the use of superoxide

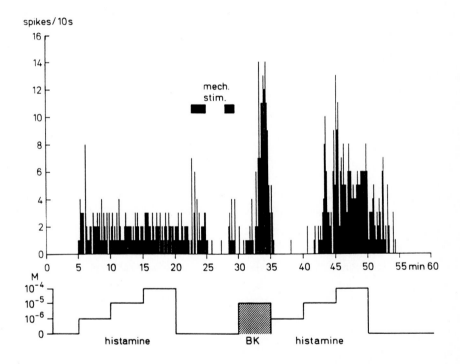

Figure 4. Bradykinin can enhance histamine responsiveness. Spike density histogram from a polymodal C-fiber that is weakly activated by histamine in a dose-independent manner. After treatment and response with bradykinin, the fiber shows an increased and dose-dependent response to histamine superfusion.

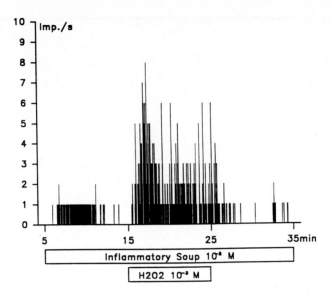

Figure 5. Hydrogen peroxide can enhance nociceptor response to inflammatory mediators. Spike density histogram of a polymodal C-fiber responding to a combination of bradykinin, histamine, prostaglandin E2, serotonin (10-5M) at pH7.0. Addition of hydrogen peroxide (1 mM) interrupts the adaptation in this case and enhances the response. H_2O_2 alone has weak excitatory effects only at even higher concentration (10 mM) which leaves the nerve endings with total desensitization.

dismutase in the therapy of painful arthritis. Another chemical radical, **nitric oxide** (NO), has recently gained major scientific interest as a short distance messenger released e.g. from macrophages in inflamed tissue. In first experiments, gaseous NO (0.126% in N_2) dissolved in the superfusate over receptive fields caused a mild but significant activation and sensitization of nociceptors (Kress, Riedl and Reeh: ongoing work). Further work using controlled NO solutions and related agonists and antagonists is in progress.

A relatively high osmotic pressure is a frequent constituent of inflammatory exudates,[19] and hyperosmolar solutions are clinically known to be painful when injected into human tissue. However, pure osmotic stimuli (sucrose, distilled water) are relatively weak excitants to a small proportion of nociceptors only and produce a marked desensitization to mechanical stimulation (Wedekind and Reeh, in preparation). Yet, if the hyperosmolarity is created by dissolved salts, predominantly by sodium chloride, a strong and dose-dependent excitation of 82% of all nociceptors results, but this is again followed by marked transient desensitization

(Figure 6). Osmotic effects from either source are non-specified in that they affect not only nociceptive but also different types of mechanoreceptive primary afferents with rapidly conducting fibers.

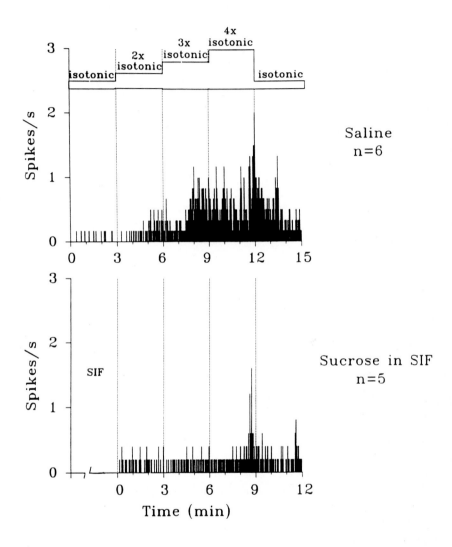

Figure 6. Nociceptors show poor sensitivity to osmotic stimuli. Averaged spike density histograms recorded from C-fiber nociceptors during superfusion of their receptive fields with different anisotonic solutions. Note that only the hyperionic solutions produce graded responses. Hypertonic sucrose, however, was dissolved in a physiological salt solution ("SIF").

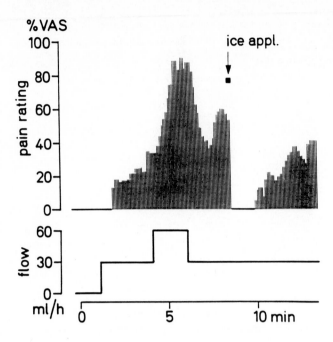

Figure 7. Low pH infusion causes sustained graded pain in human skin. Continuous subepidermal infiltration of isotonic phosphate buffer (pH 5.2) using a syringe pump leads to localised burning pain as rated by the subject every 10s on a visual analogue scale (VAS). Cooling the very surrounding of the intracutaneous cannula with a piece of ice causes abrupt pain relief.

SENSITIZATION AND HYPERALGESIA

Chemical sensitivity of nociceptors can explain ongoing, though low-frequent discharge that may contribute to pain under resting conditions. To most patients in pain, however, the hyperalgesia to daily life stimuli seems to be more of a problem. The neuro-biological mechanisms of this hypersensitivity are complex, and the relative weights of its constituents cannot yet be evaluated. Certainly, part of the phenomenon is located in peripheral nociceptors that are able to increase their sensitivity to physical stimulation markedly. So, bradykinin produces a strong nociceptor **sensitization to heat** by which the intracutaneous threshold temperature can drop sufficiently so as to be in the range of body temperature[8]. Thus, theoretically pain could result from thermal stimuli at temperatures reached directly by the inflamed tissue or via inflammatory hyperaemia. This speculation gains some support from the analgesic effect of cooling regions of inflammation (Figure 7).

Hyperalgesia to mechanical stimulation is somewhat puzzling from the viewpoint of peripheral nociception. Only a small, specialised sub population of high-threshold mechanoreceptive nociceptors has yet been shown to become **sensitised to mechanical stimuli** after injury to the skin[16]. The polymodals, the majority of nociceptors, however, remain unsensitised in a variety of inflammatory models which readily produce behavioral signs of mechanical hyperalgesia (see Steen et al.[23] for discussion). This apparent contradiction cannot yet be resolved but, at least, a chemical condition can be reported that enhances the mechanical sensitivity of nociceptors in the skin: Prolonged or repeated treatment of their receptive fields with pH 6.1 effectively lowers their thresholds to mechanical stimulation[23]. This is supported by a work on human subjects (Figure 7) who show a prominent cutaneous hyperalgesia to mechanical stimulation when low pH buffer is slowly but continuously infused into their skin[21,22]. However, those subjects also present with the phenomenon of allodynia, aversive unpleasant sensations evoked by light stroking of the acidotic skin with a soft brush. Such stimuli cannot excite most nociceptors, even when sensitised. This points higher up to the central nervous system that integrates somatosensory input and finally decides whether nociceptor discharge is perceived as painful or not.

AKNOWLEDGEMENT: This work is supported by the DFG (SFB 353).

REFERENCES

1. CAMPBELL, J.N., RAJA, S.N., COHEN, R.H., MANNING, A.A.K. AND MEYER, R.A. (1989) Peripheral Neural Mechanisms of Nociception. In: *Textbook of Pain,* eds. P.D. Wall and R. Melzack. Churchill Livingston, Edinburgh.

2. CERVERO, F. AND SANN, H. (1989) Mechanically Evoked Responses of Afferent Fibres Innervating the Guinea-Pigs Ureter - An In vitro Study. *J. Physiol.* **412**, 245-266.

3. COHEN, R.H. AND PERL, E.R. (1988) Chemical factors in the sensitization of cutaneous nociceptors. *Prog. Brain Res.* **74**, 201-206.

4. COHEN, R.H. AND PERL, E.R. (1990) Contributions of arachidonic acid derivatives and substance P to the sensitization of cutaneous nociceptors. *J. Neurophysiol.* **64**, 457-464.

5. HANDWERKER, H.O. AND REEH, P.W. (1991) Pain and Inflammation. In: *Proceedings of the VIth World Congress on Pain*, eds. M.R. Bond, J.E. Charlton and C.J. Woolf. Elsevier, Amsterdam.

6. HANDWERKER, H.O., FORSTER, C. AND KIRCHHOFF, Ch. 1991) Discharge patterns of human C-fibers induced by itching and burning stimuli. *J. Neurophysiol.* **66**, 307-315.

7. KESSLER, W., KIRCHOFF, Ch., REEH, P.W. AND HANDWERKER, H.O. (1992) Excitation of cutaneous afferent nerve endings in vitro by a combination of inflammatory mediators and conditionsing effect of substance P. *Exp. Brain Res.* **91**, 467-476.

8. KOLTZENBURG, M., KRESS, M. AND REEH, P.W. (1992) The nociceptor sensitization by bradykinin does not depend on sympathetic neurones. *Neuroscience* **46**, 465-473.

9. KOPPERT, W., REEH, P.W., HANDWERKER, H.O. (1993) Conditioning of histamine by bradykinin alters responses of rat nociceptors and human itch sensation.*Neurosci. Lett.* **152**, 117-120.

10. KRESS, M., KOLTZENBURG, M., REEH, P.W., HANDWERKER, H.O. (1992) Responsiveness and functional attributes of electrically localized terminals of cutaneous C fibers, in vivo and in vitro. *J. Neurophysiol.* **68**, 581-595.

11. KUMAZAWA, T. AND MIZUMURA, K. (1983) Temperature dependency of the chemical responses of the polymodal receptor units in vitro. *Brain Res.* **278**, 305-307.

12. LANG, E., NOVAK, A., REEH, P.W. AND HANDWERKER, H.O. (1990) Chemosensitivity of fine afferents from rat skin in vitro. *J. Neurophysiol.* **63**, 887-901.

13. LEMBECK, F. (1983) Sir Thomas Lewis nocifensor system, histamine and substance-P-containing primary afferent nerves. *Trends Neursoci.* **6**, 106-108.

14. MIZUMURA, K., SATO, J., AND KUMAZAWA, T. (1987) Effects of prostaglandins and other putative chemical intermediaries on the activity of canine testicular polymodal receptors studied in vitro. *Pflugers Arch.* **408**, 565-572.

15. NEUGEBAUER, V., SCHAIBLE, H.-G., AND SCHMIDT, R.F. (1989) Sensitization of articular afferents to mechanical stimuli by bradykinin. *Pflugers Arch.* **415**, 330-335.

16. REEH, P.W., BAYER, J., KOCHER, L., AND HANDWERKER, H.O. (1987) Sensitization of nociceptive cutaneous nerve fibers from the rat's tail by noxious mechanical stimulation. *Exp. Brain Res.* **65**, 505-512.

17. REEH, P.W., STEEN, K.H., HANISCH A. (1991) A dominant role of acid pH in inflammatory excitation of nociceptors in rat skin. *Soc. Neurosci. Abstr.* **17**, 537.

18. REEH, P.W. (1986) Sensory receptros in mammalian skin in an in vitro preparation. *Neurosci. Lett.* **66**, 141-146.
19. SCHADE, H. (1923) Die physikalische Chemie in der Inneren Medizin. Th. Steinkopff, Dresden und Leipzig.
20. SCHAIBLE, H.-G. AND SCHMIDT, R.F. (1988) Excitation and sensitization of fine articular afferents from cat's knee joint by prostaglandin E2. *J. Physiol.* **403**, 91-104.
21. STEEN, K.H. AND REEH, P.W. (1993) Actions of cholinergic agonists and antagonists on sensory nerve endings in rat skin, in vitro. *J. Neurophysiol.* **70**, 397-405.
22. STEEN, K.H. AND REEH, P.W. (1993)Sustained graded pain and hyperalgesia from harmless experimental tissue acidosis in human skin. *Neurosci. Lett.***154**, 113-116.
23. STEEN, K.H., REEH, P.W., ANTON, F. AND HANDWERKER, H.O. (1992) Protons selectively induce lasting excitation and sensitization to mechanical stimulation of nociceptors in rat skin, in vitro. *J. Neurosci.* **12**, 86-95.

LOCAL EFFECTOR FUNCTIONS OF PRIMARY AFFERENT NERVE FIBRES

Peter Holzer
Department of Experimental and Clinical Pharmacology
University of Graz
Universitätsplatz 4, A-8010 Graz
Austria

INTRODUCTION

More than a century ago it was discovered that under certain experimental conditions primary afferent nerve fibers can behave as if they were axons of autonomic neurons. Stricker[54] was the first to observe that stimulation of the peripheral ends of cut dorsal roots induced hyperaemia in the corresponding skin area. This increase in blood flow results from antidromic conduction of nerve impulses in afferent nerve fibers[1] and, in the rat, is associated with an increase in vascular permeability.[24] These reactions are embodied in the term "neurogenic inflammation" which denotes inflammatory responses that depend on the afferent innervation of the tissue.[5,24] We now know that neurogenic inflammation is due to the release of vasoactive peptide transmitters from the peripheral endings of fine, mostly unmyelinated, afferent nerve fibers.[9,16,46] It has also been turned out that in this way afferent nerve fibers control, besides vascular functions, a variety of local effector systems including the immune system, the respiratory tract and the digestive system (Figure 1). Appreciation of these roles of peptidergic afferent neurons has lit up new aspects in the neural control of tissue functions[16,18] and has even stirred reconsideration of the principal organization of the autonomic nervous system.[52] The present article highlights some of the basic mechanisms of the local effector control by afferent nerve fibers, discusses the relationship of this function to the sensory and afferent activities of the neurons, and addresses some of the questions which have remained open in these respects.

NATO ASI Series, Vol. H 79
Cellular Mechanisms of Sensory Processing
Edited by Laszlo Urban
© Springer-Verlag Berlin Heidelberg 1994

CAPSAICIN AS A PROBE FOR AFFERENT NERVE FUNCTIONS

Our present understanding of the local effector control by afferent nerve fibers goes back to the discovery of N. Jancsó[23] that the afferent nerve fibers responsible for neurogenic inflammation in the skin and eye can pharmacologically be manipulated by capsaicin. Systematic research has confirmed that the afferent neurons being involved in local effector control throughout the body are sensitive to capsaicin, a property which thus has been instrumental in their anatomical, neurochemical and functional investigation.[17] The group of capsaicin-sensitive afferent nerve fibers comprises most of the fine (unmyelinated and thinly myelinated) axons. The excitotoxin capsaicin has two actions on these fibers, both actions being exploited in the neuropharmacological study of sensory nerve mechanisms. Acute administration of low, non-toxic doses of the drug stimulates afferent neurons, whereas systemic administration of high neurotoxic doses of capsaicin causes a long-lasting functional ablation of the neurons sensitive to the drug.[17] The value of capsaicin as a probe for sensory neuron implications lies in the selectivity of its neurotoxic action for fine afferent neurons.

Capsaicin-sensitive afferent neurons supply many somatic and visceral tissues, particularly the arterial vascular system.[18] Neurophysiologically, most of these neurons are nociceptive neurons. The perceived stimuli comprise various modalities ranging from heat, mechanical distortion or trauma to exogenous and endogenous chemicals. Among these chemicals are man-made pollutants such as tobacco smoke, toluene isothiocyanate and hydrogen sulphide, chemicals of bacterial origin such as peptide N-formyl-methionyl-leucyl-phenylalanine and staphylococcal enterotoxin B, antigens provoking allergic reactions, endogenous inflammatory mediators such as histamine, 5-hydroxytryptamine, bradykinin, platelet-activating factor and eicosanoids, gastrointestinal factors such as bile salts, H^+ ions, and hyperosmolarity, and pathological factors such as ischaemia.[17,45] Neurochemically, capsaicin-sensitive afferent neurons are characterized by their expression of biologically active peptides including calcitonin gene-related peptide (CGRP), substance P (SP), somatostatin, dynorphin and vasoactive intestinal polypeptide. These peptides coexist in varying combinations, the pattern of coexistence being characteristic for the different pathways and innervation targets of afferent neurons.[12]

BASIC MECHANISMS OF LOCAL EFFECTOR CONTROL BY AFFERENT NERVES

The basic mechanisms of local effector control by primary afferent nerve fibers are best exemplified by the characteristics of neurogenic inflammation in the skin. CGRP and SP are considered to be the principal neural mediators of the vasodilator and exudative response to afferent nerve stimulation in this tissue. This holds true both for the effects of antidromic electrical stimulation of afferent nerves and for the effects of orthodromic stimulation by, e.g., chemical irritation. The peripheral terminals of peptidergic afferent neurons are well equipped to control local effector systems because the bulk of peptide synthesised in the neuronal somata is transported to the peripheral nerve endings.[4] On excitation, the peptides are released from the varicosities of sensory axon terminals and reach their target receptors by diffusion.[18] CGRP and SP are potent vasodilators in many tissues and SP is, in addition, able to enhance vascular permeability in the skin. The involvement of these peptides in neurogenic inflammatory reactions has been demonstrated by the use of specific peptide antagonists and by immunoneutralization experiments.[18] Afferent nerve axons are thus able to directly control the activity of adjacent effector systems and in this action do not require the participation of autonomic neurons (Figure 1). As in autonomic nerve-effector junctions, morphological specializations of the sensory nerve-effector junctions are lacking except that axon varicosities may come close to the cells which they "innervate". There are obvious morphological and functional analogies between autonomic nerve-effector and sensory nerve-effector communication, similarities which are reflected by the terms "local effector",[16] "afferent-efferent[46,55] and "sensory-motor"[6] functions of fine afferent neurons.

HETEROGENEITY OF AFFERENT NERVES CONTROLLING LOCAL EFFECTOR SYSTEMS

The ability to control adjacent effector systems differentiates fine afferent nerve fibers from thickly myelinated fibers which to our present knowledge do not subserve such a function. Although most, if not all, of these fibers are sensitive to the stimulant and neurotoxic actions of capsaicin,[18] they comprise a heterogeneous group of axons that can be further subdivided on the basis of sensory modality, conduction velocity, stimulation requirements, neurochemical coding and effect on adjacent effector systems.

With regard to the *sensory modality* of the involved fibers it has been shown that cutaneous vasodilatation occurs only when antidromic stimulation of afferent nerve fibers is strong enough to recruit nociceptive afferents.[8,44] Likewise, the fibers which increase vascular permeability in the rat paw skin are connected to polymodal nociceptors[26] but, importantly, not all of the polymodal nociceptor fibers cause protein leakage upon stimulation.[3] The fibers responsible for antidromic vasodilatation and plasma protein extravasation in the rat skin differ from each other

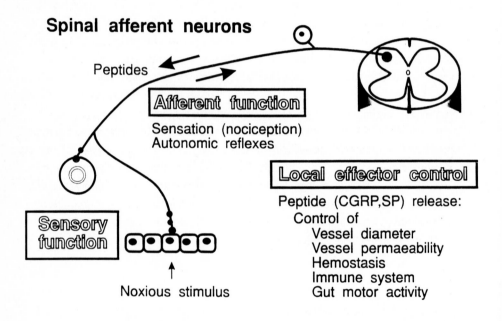

Figure 1. Diagram illustrating the multiple functions of fine afferent neurons. The information perceived by these neurons is transmitted to the central nervous system to produce sensation and initiate autonomic homeostatic reflexes. In addition, peptide transmitters can be released from their peripheral endings to control the function of adjacent effector systems.

with respect to *conduction velocity* and *stimulation requirements*. Whereas only C-fibers are able to augment vascular permeability[22] it is both unmyelinated (C-) fibers[8,39,44] and some thinly myelinated (Aδ-) fibers[22] that can give rise to arteriolar dilatation. The hyperaemic and exudative responses to afferent nerve stimulation are stimulus-dependent but whilst only one or two impulses or a frequency of 0.025 Hz are sufficient to elicit an appreciable increase in cutaneous blood flow,[40,44,56] vascular permeability does not rise unless nerve fibers are stimulated at a frequency of 2 Hz or more.[26,56] These findings demonstrate that the fibers causing vasodilatation are not identical with those increasing vascular permeability. This inference is consistent with a spatial separation of the processes of hyperaemia and plasma protein extravasation. Unlike hyperaemia which occurs by dilatation of arterioles, protein leakage takes place in postcapillary venules whose endothelial cells contract and allow for formation of gaps in the endothelium.[30]

Since there are populations of fine afferent neurons that differ in terms of their *neurochemical coding*, i.e., in the combination of peptide transmitters they contain,[10,12] it has to be inferred that the nerve fibers responsible for local effector control differ in the effect they exert on adjacent tissues according to the peptide mediators which they release and according to the effect these peptides have on the tissues. If so, some polymodal nociceptors may fail to bring about plasma protein extravasation in the skin because they do not contain a mediator that increases vascular permeability.[3] The *heterogeneity of effects* exerted by afferent nerve terminals in different tissues is related to variations in the neurochemical coding of afferent nerve fibers supplying different target tissues[12] and to differences in postjunctional mechanisms such as presence and density of peptide receptors and transduction mechanisms on the effector systems.[18]

LOCAL EFFECTOR CONTROL VERSUS AFFERENT FUNCTION

Afferent nerve fibers monitor their chemical and physical environment and transmit the perceived information to the central nervous system (Figure 1). In face of their additional ability to control local effector functions the question arises as to whether afferent activity and peripheral peptide release operate in parallel or may be activated separately. Evidence is in fact beginning to accumulate that the two functions are not strictly bound to each other and may be differentiated in terms of sensory modality, impulse frequency requirements and neurochemical coding of the respective sensory nerve fibers.

With regard to the *sensory modality* required for induction of afferent activity and peripheral peptide release it would seem that both in visceral[29] and somatic[42] tissues neurogenic vasodilatation and plasma protein extravasation are mediated by a subpopulation of fine afferent nerve fibers that are chemosensitive but insensitive to mechanical stimuli. There is evidence for a similar situation in human skin.[31] The existence of "silent nociceptors" in visceral and somatic tissues[49,53] has added another aspect to this question. These nociceptors are unmyelinated afferent nerve fibers which in normal tissue fail to respond to mechanical and thermal noxious stimuli, although they are responsive to algesic chemicals. It has not yet been determined, however, whether silent nociceptors are involved in the control of local effector systems.

In the skin there is clear evidence that antidromic vasodilatation can be induced by stimulation frequencies of less than 1 Hz,[40,44,56] frequencies that are too low to cause nociception.[14] It would seem, therefore, that there are different *frequency requirements* for activation of the afferent and local effector function of sensory nerve fibers. Differential activation of the two functions will also result from differences in the tissue-specific *neurochemical coding* of different groups of afferents.

INTERACTION BETWEEN SENSORY-AFFERENT ACTIVITY AND PERIPHERAL NEUROPEPTIDE RELEASE

Despite the evidence that the afferent and local effector function of sensory nerve fibers can be activated separately from each other it is clear that with sufficient strengths of stimulation both functions will come into play simultaneously. In other terms, noxious stimulation of afferent nerve fibers will give rise to nociception and nociception-related responses of the organism and at the same time will cause neuropeptide release from the peripheral terminals of the stimulated sensory nerve fibers. Experimental data indicate that the two functions, although they may be activated separately, can interact with each other in a mutual manner. Most importantly, the presence of inflammation leads to *sensitization of nociceptors* including the "waking up" of silent nociceptors, a process in which various non-neurogenic mediators of inflammation such as histamine and prostaglandins play a role.[28,48,49] The protracted stages of neurogenic inflammation in the skin also involve the release of secondary mediators of inflammation from mast cells and leukocytes,[18] mediators which are likely to give rise to sensitization and hyperexcitability of afferent nerve endings. Apart from this indirect sensitising action of sensory neuropeptides, SP has been reported to have a direct conditioning effect on the excitation of afferent nerve terminals by inflammatory mediators.[27] These actions will provide a positive feedback on afferent nerve endings, resulting in hyperalgesia and reinforcement of the inflammatory process.

Another level of interaction refers to the activation of sympathetic and neuroendocrine reflexes which in turn may result in the modulation of the release of neuropeptides from the peripheral terminals of sensory neurons. Noradrenaline and neuropeptide Y, which are released from postganglionic sympathetic neurons, as well as opioid peptides have been found to block the release of peptide mediators and thereby to dampen neurogenic inflammatory reactions.[45]

AXON REFLEX THEORY OF SPREADING FLARE

A peculiar phenomenon pertaining to the local effector control by afferent nerve fibers is the spread of cutaneous hyperaemia (flare) beyond the site at which the skin is stimulated. It has long been known that focal irritation of human skin causes (i) a local reddening and (ii) an area of oedema (the weal) at the site of the stimulus, and (iii) a spread of arteriolar dilatation (the flare) far beyond the point of irritation. The flare component of this "triple response"[34] depends on nerve conduction because it is halted by local anaesthetics and requires an intact sensory innervation because it is abolished by defunctionalization of capsaicin-sensitive afferent neurons.[2,7,11,25]

The classical explanation of the spread of flare[9,16,38,40] holds that this phenomenon results from an axon reflex between collaterals of fine afferent neurons (Figure 2). This term denotes a reflex that takes place entirely within the arborizations of a single nerve axon.[34] When one axon branch is activated by an irritant stimulus, nerve impulses will travel not only centrally but at the branching point will also pass antidromically in the other branches which may happen to come close to some arterioles. If so, the peri-arteriolar branches may release vasoactive peptides and thereby cause arteriolar dilatation.

The axon reflex hypothesis offers an elegant way of explaining the spreading flare but this concept has not yet been proven neurophysiologically and, in fact, has turned out very difficult to test experimentally. Although afferent nerve fibers arborize in the skin, with nerve endings both in the epidermis and along blood vessels, it is not clear whether the epidermal and perivascular branches are collaterals of the same afferent nerve fibers. The axon reflex concept implies that the area of flare is determined by the size of "neurovascular units" made up by the collateral networks (receptive fields) of individual afferent nerve fibers and the area of arterioles innervated by these collateral networks.[15,34] There is in fact a reasonable correlation between the maximum extent of C-fiber receptive fields and the extent of flare in the saphenous area of the lower hind limb of pig, rabbit and rat.[43] Likewise, in the human hand there is a good overlap between C-fiber receptive fields and the size of flare responses.[58] In other body regions, however, discrepancies between the two parameters have been noted.[15] Part of the problem, however, is due to the fact that the flare sizes also depend on the type of stimulus, flare induced by capsaicin being in general larger than that induced by histamine or electrical stimulation.[15,43] The relatively sharp margin of the flare, the inhibition of the spread of flare by local anaesthetics,[11,58] and the apparent failure of the flare to cross the midline of the body[15] (but see also LaMotte et al.[31]) are also consistent with the axon reflex concept. The most serious inconsistency of the axon reflex theory concerns the unexplained delay in the spread of flare which is slower than would be expected if the rate of spread were determined only by conduction delays in unmyelinated nerve fibers.[41]

In view of the delay in the spread of flare both chemical[33,40,41] and electrical coupling between different afferent nerve fibers[3,50] have been considered to participate in the spread of arteriolar flare (Figure 2). The chemical coupling (cascade) theory proposed by Lembeck and Gamse[33] supposes a parallel arrangement of sensory nerve endings in the skin and suggests that the spread of flare is primarily accomplished by a cascade of histamine release from mast cells, activation of sensory nerve endings by histamine, release of neurogenic mediators, followed by further histamine release. In this model, the shape of the flare should be circular and the intensity of vasodilatation should steadily decrease away from the central stimulus. In reality, though, the flare has an irregular shape and a relatively sharp margin, is halted by local anaesthetics[11,58] and does apparently not cross the midline of the body[15] (but see also LaMotte et al.[31]) although it can jump over a strip of skin which has been treated with capsaicin to defunctionalize afferent vasodilator fibers.[56] Taken together, most characteristics of the spreading flare are accounted for by the axon reflex concept but are difficult to reconcile with the cascade theory.[11,15,56,58]

Axon reflex concepts

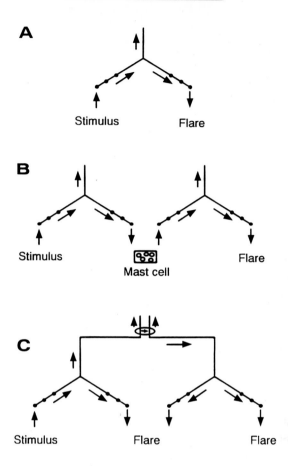

Figure 2. Diagram illustrating 3 different explanations of spreading flare. Panel A depicts the classical axon reflex concept in which a noxious stimulus activates a collateral of an afferent nerve fiber and nerve activity spreads to all other collaterals. Release of vasodilator mediators at their endings evokes arteriolar dilatation. Panel B delineates chemical coupling between collaterals of two different afferent nerve fibers. Coupling is achieved by release of mast cell-derived histamine and other factors that are able to activate adjacent sensory nerve endings and thus allow nerve activity and flare to spread beyond the collateral network of a single afferent nerve fiber. Panel C shows electrical coupling between two afferent nerve fibers, which represents another way by which the flare response may spread beyond the collateral network of a single afferent nerve fiber.

LOCAL AXON REFLEX VERSUS AFFERENT REFLEX REGULATION

Despite its conceptual elegance, the axon reflex theory has not yet solved the enigma of the spreading flare. The lack of solid neurophysiological evidence for the occurrence of axon reflexes advocates caution in extrapolating the axon reflex concept to tissues other than the skin. In the absence of relevant neuroanatomical and neurophysiological data, the conjecture of axon reflexes may be fallacious as is illustrated by the discovery of a role of afferent nerve fibers in gastric mucosal protection.

The intrusion of acid into gastric tissue through a disrupted gastric mucosal barrier causes a prompt increase in gastric mucosal blood flow.[51] The organization of the gastric circulation requires submucosal arterioles to be dilated in order to increase mucosal blood flow, which means that the message of acid influx has to be transmitted over a distance of several hundred micrometers, a distance that separates the surface of the mucosa from submucosal arterioles. The finding that tetrodotoxin and defunctionalization of capsaicin-sensitive nerves inhibit acid-induced hyperaemia in the rat gastric mucosa[21] indicates that communication between the acid-threatened surface mucosa and submucosal arterioles is to a significant extent accomplished by afferent nerve fibers.

It was originally proposed that the acid-induced increase in gastric mucosal blood flow results from an axon reflex between mucosal and submucosal collaterals of afferent neurons.[21,37] The major support for this proposition came from the observation that the CGRP antagonist $CGRP_{8-37}$ attenuated the mucosal hyperaemia caused by acid back-diffusion.[37] Since in the rat stomach CGRP is exclusively contained in afferent nerve endings[13] it appeared as if CGRP released from afferent nerve endings was the local mediator of the vasodilator response to mucosal acid influx. This concept was challenged, though, when it was found that the acid-evoked rise of blood flow relies on intact conduction of nerve activity through afferent/efferent pathways in the splanchnic nerves and the coeliac/superior mesenteric ganglion complex.[19] As these pathways involve ganglionic transmission through nicotinic acetylcholine receptors[19] it is evident that efferent autonomic nerve activity participates in the vasodilator response to acid intrusion. Whilst the precise pathways and mechanisms of acid-induced hyperaemia in the stomach have not yet been worked out it appears conceivable that the acid-induced increase in gastric blood flow is relayed by a peripheral neural circuitry which depends on an excitatory or inhibitory input from efferent nerve fibers in the splanchnic nerves.[18]

PATHOPHYSIOLOGICAL PERSPECTIVES

Recognition of a role of nociceptive afferent nerve fibers in local effector control has revolutionised our understanding of sensory physiology and pharmacology. The pathophysiological significance of this function of afferent neurons can be appreciated if it is seen in context with the stimuli they respond to. These neurons are connected to chemoceptors, chemo-nociceptors and polymodal nociceptors which enable them to detect noxious stimuli that are potentially or actually harmful to the tissue. The overall function of these sensory neurons is to maintain homeostasis, a task in which their afferent and local effector functions cooperate in an efficient manner. The afferent activity of the neurons transmits the perceived information to the central nervous system and initiates both voluntary and autonomic reflexes to maintain homeostasis. The local release of peptide mediators leads to appropriate measures of defence at the very site of stimulation. Hyperaemia and increased vascular permeability facilitate the delivery of macromolecules and leukocytes to the tissue, which will promote resistance of the tissue against further damage and aid the repair of injury. Vasoactive afferent neurons thus represent a system "of first line defence"[32] against trauma, a mechanism that was first embodied by the "nocifensor system" of Lewis.[35,36] The propagation of arteriolar dilatation in the skin (flare) may be considered as a measure to ensure that protective hyperaemia takes place not only in the challenged tissue but also in a "safety margin".[16]

The protective role of local effector control by afferent nerve fibers is portrayed by the ability of afferent nerve stimulation to protect from experimentally imposed damage in the skin,[47] gastrointestinal mucosa[20,57] and other tissues. As a consequence, malfunction or hyperactivity of this neural emergency system is liable to cause homeostatic disorders and inadequate reactions to challenges of homeostasis.

ACKNOWLEDGEMENTS: Research done in the author's laboratory was supported by the Austrian Scientific Research Council (grants P7845 and P9473) and by the Jubiläumsfonds of the Austrian National Bank (grant 4207).

144

REFERENCES

1. BAYLISS, W.M. (1901) On the origin from the spinal cord of the vaso-dilator fibers of the hind-limb, and on the nature of these fibers. *J. Physiol.* **26**, 173-209.
2. BERNSTEIN, J.E., SWIFT, R.M., SOLTANI, K. AND LORINCZ, A.L. (1981) Inhibition of axon reflex vasodilatation by topically applied capsaicin. *J. Invest. Dermatol.* **76**, 394-395.
3. BHARALI, L.A.M. AND LISNEY, S.J.W. (1992) The relationship between unmyelinated afferent type and neurogenic plasma extravasation in normal and reinnervated rat skin. *Neuroscience* **47**, 703-712.
4. BRIMIJOIN, S, LUNDBERG, J.M., BRODIN, E., HÖKFELT, T. AND NILSSON, G. (1980) Axonal transport of substance P in the vagus and sciatic nerves of the guinea pig. *Brain Res.* **191**, 443-457.
5. BRUCE, N.A. (1910) Über die Beziehung der sensiblen Nervenendigungen zum Entzündungsvorgang. *Arch. exp. Pathol. Pharmakol.* **63**, 424-433.
6. BURNSTOCK, G. (1990) Local mechanisms of blood flow control by perivascular nerves and endothelium. *J. Hypertens.* **8**, S95-S106.
7. CARPENTER, S.E. AND LYNN, B. (1981) Vascular and sensory responses of human skin to mild injury after topical treatment with capsaicin. *Br. J. Pharmacol.* **73**, 755-758.
8. CELANDER, O. AND FOLKOW, B (1953) The nature and the distribution of afferent fibers provided with the axon reflex arrangement. *Acta Physiol. Scand.* **29**, 359-370.
9. CHAHL, L.A. (1988) Antidromic vasodilatation and neurogenic inflammation. *Pharmacol. Ther.* **37**, 275-300.
10. COSTA, M., FURNESS, J.B. AND GIBBINS, I.L. (1986) Chemical coding of enteric neurons. *Prog. Brain Res.* **68**, 217-239.
11. FOREMAN, J.C., JORDAN, C.C., OEHME, P. AND RENNER, H. (1983) Structure-activity relationships for some substance P-related peptides that cause weal and flare reactions in human skin. *J. Physiol.* **335**, 449-465.
12. GIBBINS, I.L., FURNESS, J.B. AND COSTA, M. (1987) Pathway-specific patterns of the co-existence of substance P, calcitonin gene-related peptide, cholecystokinin and dynorphin in neurons of the dorsal root ganglia of the guinea-pig. *Cell Tiss. Res.* **248**, 417-437.
13. GREEN, T. AND DOCKRAY, G.J. (1988) Characterization of the peptidergic afferent innervation of the stomach in the rat, mouse, and guinea-pig. *Neuroscience* **25**, 181-193.
14. GYBELS, J., HANDWERKER, H.O. AND VAN HEES, J. (1979) A comparison between the discharges of human nociceptive nerve fibers and the subject's ratings of his sensations. *J. Physiol.* **292**, 193-206.
15. HELME, R.D. AND MCKERNAN, S. (1985) Neurogenic flare responses following topical application of capsaicin in humans. *Ann. Neurol.* **18**, 505-509.
16. HOLZER, P. (1988) Local effector functions of capsaicin-sensitive sensory nerve endings: involvement of tachykinins, calcitonin gene-related peptide and other neuropeptides. *Neuroscience* **24**, 739-768.
17. HOLZER, P. (1991) Capsaicin: cellular targets, mechanisms of action, and selectivity for thin sensory neurons. *Pharmacol. Rev.* **43**, 143-201.

18. HOLZER, P. (1992) Peptidergic sensory neurons in the control of vascular functions: mechanisms and significance in the cutaneous and splanchnic vascular beds. *Rev. Physiol. Biochem. Pharmacol.* **121**, 49-146.

19. HOLZER, P. AND LIPPE, I.T.H. (1992) Gastric mucosal hyperemia due to acid back-diffusion depends on splanchnic nerve activity. *Am. J. Physiol.* 262, G505-G509.

20. HOLZER, P., PABST, M.A., LIPPE, I.T.H., PESKAR, B.M., PESKAR, B.A., LIVINGSTON, E.H. AND GUTH, P.H. (1990) Afferent nerve-mediated protection against deep mucosal damage in the rat stomach. *Gastroenterology* **98**, 838-848.

21. HOLZER, P., LIVINGSTON, E.H. AND GUTH, P.H. (1991) Sensory neurons signal for an increase in rat gastric mucosal blood flow in the face of pending acid injury. *Gastroenterology* **101**, 416-423.

22. JÄNIG, W. AND LISNEY, S.J.W. (1989) Small diameter myelinated afferents produce vasodilatation but not plasma extravasation in rat skin. *J. Physiol.* **415**, 477-486.

23. JANCSÓ, N. (1960) Role of the nerve terminals in the mechanism of inflammatory reactions. *Bull. Millard Fillmore Hosp.* **7**, 53-77.

24. JANCSÓ, N., JANCSÓ-GÁBOR, A. AND SZOLCSÁNYI, J. (1967) Direct evidence for neurogenic inflammation and its prevention by denervation and by pretreatment with capsaicin. *Br. J. Pharmacol.* **31**, 138-151.

25. JANCSÓ, N., JANCSÓ-GÁBOR, A. AND SZOLCSÁNYI, J. (1968) The role of sensory nerve endings in neurogenic inflammation induced in human skin and in the eye and paw of the rat. *Br. J. Pharmacol.* **33**, 32-41.

26. KENINS, P. (1981) Identification of the unmyelinated sensory nerves which evoke plasma extravasation in response to antidromic stimulation. *Neurosci. Lett.* **25**, 137-141.

27. KESSLER, W., KIRCHHOFF, C., REEH, P.W. AND HANDWERKER, H.O. (1992) Excitation of cutaneous afferent nerve endings in vitro by a combination of inflammatory mediators and conditioning effect of substance P. *Exp. Brain Res.* **91**, 467-476.

28. KOCHER, L., ANTON, F., REEH, P.W. AND HANDWERKER, H.O. (1987) The effect of carrageenan-induced inflammation on the sensitivity of unmyelinated skin nociceptors in the rat. *Pain* **29**, 363-373.

29. KOLTZENBURG, M. AND MCMAHON, S.B. (1986) Plasma extravasation in the rat urinary bladder following mechanical, electrical and chemical stimuli: evidence for a new population of chemosensitive primary sensory afferents. *Neurosci. Lett.* **72**, 352-356.

30. KOWALSKI, M.L., SLIWINSKA-KOWALSKA, M. AND KALINER, M.A. (1990) Neurogenic inflammation, vascular permeability, and mast cells. 2. Additional evidence indicating that mast cells are not involved in neurogenic inflammation. *J. Immunol.* **145**, 1214-1221.

31. LAMOTTE, R.H., SHAIN, C.N., SIMONE, D.A. AND TSAI, E.-F.P. (1991) Neurogenic hyperalgesia: psychophysical studies of underlying mechanisms. *J. Neurophysiol.* **66**, 190-211.

32. LEMBECK, F. (1983) Sir Thomas Lewis's nocifensor system, histamine and substance P-containing primary afferent nerves. *Trends Neurosci.* **6**, 106-108.

33. LEMBECK, F. AND GAMSE, R. (1982) Substance P in peripheral sensory

processes. In: *Substance P in the Nervous System.* eds. R. Porter and M. O'Connor. Pitman, London.

34. LEWIS, T. (1927) The Blood Vessels of the Human Skin and Their Responses. Shaw & Sons, London.

35. LEWIS, T. (1937) The nocifensor system of nerves and its reactions. *Br. Med. J.* **I,** 431-435.

36. LEWIS, T. (1937) The nocifensor system of nerves and its reactions. *Br. Med. J.* **I,** 491-497.

37. LI, D-S., RAYBOULD, H.E., QUINTERO, E. AND GUTH, P.H. (1992) Calcitonin gene-related peptide mediates the gastric hyperemic response to acid back-diffusion. *Gastroenterology* **102**, 1124-1128

38. LISNEY, S.J.W. AND BHARALI, L.A.M. (1989) The axon reflex: an outdated idea or a valid hypothesis? *News Physiol. Sci.* **4**, 45-48

39. LOW, A. AND WESTERMAN, R.A. (1989) Neurogenic vasodilation in the rat hairy skin measured using a laser Doppler flowmeter. *Life Sci.* **45**, 49-57.

40. LYNN, B. (1988) Neurogenic inflammation. *Skin Pharmacol.* **1**, 217-224

41. LYNN, B. AND COTSELL, B. (1991) The delay in onset of vasodilator flare in human skin at increasing distances from a localized noxious stimulus. *Microvasc. Res.* **41**, 197-202.

42. LYNN, B. AND COTSELL, B. (1992) Blood flow increases in the skin of the anaesthetized rat that follow antidromic sensory nerve stimulation and strong mechanical stimulation. *Neurosci. Lett.* **137**, 249-252.

43. LYNN, B., COTSELL, B., FAULSTROH, K. AND PIERAU, F.-K. (1993) Flare and C-fiber receptive fields in three mammalian species. *Agents Actions* (in press).

44. MAGERL, W., SZOLCSÁNYI, J., WESTERMAN, R.A. AND HANDWERKER, H.O. (1987) Laser Doppler measurements of skin vasodilation elicited by percutaneous electrical stimulation of nociceptors in humans. *Neurosci. Lett.* **82**, 349-354.

45. MAGGI, C.A. (1991) The pharmacology of the efferent function of sensory nerves. *J. Auton. Pharmacol.* **11**, 173-208.

46. MAGGI, C.A. AND MELI, A. (1988) The sensory-efferent function of capsaicin-sensitive sensory neurons. *Gen. Pharmacol.* **19**, 1-43.

47. MAGGI, C.A., BORSINI, F., SANTICIOLI, P., GEPPETTI, P., ABELLI, L., EVANGELISTA, S., MANZINI, S., THEODORSSON-NORHEIM, E., SOMMA, V., AMENTA, F., BACCIARELLI, C. AND MELI, A. (1987) Cutaneous lesions in capsaicin-pretreated rats. A trophic role of capsaicin-sensitive afferents? *Naunyn-Schmiedeberg's Arch. Pharmacol.* **336**, 538-545.

48. MARTIN, H.A., BASBAUM, A.I., KWIAT, G.C., GOETZL, E.J. AND LEVINE, J.D. (1987) Leukotriene and prostaglandin sensitization of cutaneous high threshold C- and A-delta mechanonociceptors in the hairy skin of rat hindlimbs. *Neuroscience* **22**, 651-659.

49. MCMAHON, S. AND KOLTZENBURG, M. (1990) The changing role of primary afferent neurones in pain. *Pain* **43**, 269-272.

50. MEYER, R.A., RAJA, S.N. AND CAMPBELL, J.N. (1985) Coupling of action potential activity between unmyelinated fibers in the peripheral nerve of monkey. *Science* **227**, 184-187.

51. OATES, P.J. (1990) Gastric blood flow and mucosal defense. In: *Gastric*

Cytoprotection. eds. D. Hollander and A.S. Tarnawski. Plenum, New York.

52. PRECHTL, J.C. AND POWLEY, T.L. (1990) B-afferents: a fundamental division of the nervous system mediating homeostasis? *Behav. Brain Sci.* **13**, 289-331.

53. SCHAIBLE, H.-G. AND SCHMIDT, R.F. (1988) Time course of mechanosensitivity changes in articular afferents during a developing arthritis. *J. Neurophysiol.* **60**, 2180-2195.

54. STRICKER, S. (1876) Untersuchungen über die Gefässwurzeln des Ischiadicus. Sitz-Ber Kaiserl Akad Wiss (Wien) **3**, 173-185.

55. SZOLCSÁNYI, J. (1984) Capsaicin-sensitive chemoceptive neural system with dual sensory-efferent function. In: *Antidromic Vasodilatation and Neurogenic Inflammation.* eds. L.A. Chahl J. Szolcsányi F. Lembeck. Akadémiai Kiadó, Budapest.

56. SZOLCSÁNYI, J. (1988) Antidromic vasodilatation and neurogenic inflammation. *Agents Actions* 23, 4-11.

57. SZOLCSÁNY, J. and BARTHÓ, L. (1981) Impaired defense mechanism to peptic ulcer in the capsaicin-desensitized rat. In: *Gastrointestinal Defense Mechanisms.* eds. G. Mózsik, O. Hänninen and T. Jávor. Pergamon Press and Akadémiai Kiadó, Oxford and Budapest.

58. WÅRDELL, K., NAVER, H.K., NILSSON, G.E. AND WALLIN, B.G. (1993) The cutaneous vascular axon reflex in humans characterized by laser Doppler perfusion imaging. *J. Physiol.* **460**, 185-199.

TRANSMITTERS IN THE SOMATOSENSORY SYSTEM
(SYNAPTOLOGY OF THE SPINAL CORD)

EXITATORY AMINO ACID RECEPTORS IN THE IN VITRO MAMMALIAN SPINAL CORD

Aharon Lev-Tov and M. Pinco
Department of Anatomy, The Hebrew University Medical School
P.O. Box 1172, Jerusalem 91010
ISRAEL

INTRODUCTION

The excitatory synapse between group Ia afferents and α-motoneurons is one of the most frequently used models for central synaptic transmission in mammals. Most of the knowledge regarding this synapse originates from studies of the *in vivo* cat spinal cord preparation (for reviews see Burke,[3] Mendell,[21] Redman[25]). Since spinal neurons *in vivo* are not amenable to manipulations of the external ionic environment, direct studies of neurotransmitters and the nature of their postsynaptic receptors have been carried out on cultured neurons and on mammalian CNS preparations isolated *in vitro* (for reviews see Ascher and Novak,[1] Collingridge and Lester[4], Mayer and Westbrook,[20] Monaghan et al.,[22]). The central dogma regarding the involvement of excitatory amino acid (EAA) receptors in mediation of synaptic excitation in the spinal cord, is that transmission in monosynaptic pathways is mediated primarily by non-N-methyl D-aspartate (non-NMDA) receptors,[6,7,13,27] that the NMDA receptors in these pathways may be activated only as the neurons are substantially depolarised[14], and that interneuronal transmission in polysynaptic pathways is mediated by NMDA receptors.[7,13,14,28] Recent studies from other systems[2,5,9,11,26] and our studies of the neonatal rat spinal cord (see below; see also,[28] for monosynaptic transmission in the embryonic rat spinal cord), have indicated that this concept may not be completely accurate. In this present work, based on recent studies;[15,16,17,24] and on unpublished observations of Lev-Tov and Pinco, we re-evaluate the role of NMDA and non-NMDA receptors in mono- and polysynaptic excitation in the *in vitro* mammalian spinal cord,

NATO ASI Series, Vol. H 79
Cellular Mechanisms of Sensory Processing
Edited by Laszlo Urban
© Springer-Verlag Berlin Heidelberg 1994

and describe the effects and possible mechanisms of action of a different EAA receptor, the L-2-amino-4-phosphonobutyric acid (AP-4) receptor.

NMDA AND NON-NMDA RECEPTOR MEDIATED COMPONENTS OF MONOSYNAPTIC EPSPS

The contribution of NMDA and non-NMDA receptors in the mediation of monosynaptic EPSPs was examined in three different systems: **1**. the synapses between lamina IX axons and α-motoneurons, **2**. the synapses between dorsal root afferents and α-motoneurons, and **3**. the synapses between ventrolateral funiculus (VLF) axons and α-motoneurons. The results are described below:

(1) EAA receptors in monosynaptic transmission between lamina IX axons and α-motoneurons. Excitatory synaptic transmission between lamina IX axons and α-motoneurons was studied in the thin slice preparation of the neonatal rat spinal cord. Motoneurons were visually identified using Nomarski interference optics. Short latency (monosynaptic) EPSCs were induced by extracellular stimulation of unidentified lamina IX axons and recorded using the whole cell patch clamp technique.[15] The stimulated axons could include monosynaptic dorsal root afferents and descending and propriospinal axons, as well as axons of last order polysynaptic excitatory interneurons of various origins. Figure 1A shows the dependence of the peak amplitude of the synaptic currents and of the amplitude of the current measured 20ms following the stimulus artefact on the holding potential. While the fast peak was linearly related to the holding potential (circles and solid linear regression line), the late component (triangles) exhibited a negative slope conductance as is typical for NMDA receptor mediated synaptic currents (see refs.[1,20]). The NMDA and non-NMDA receptor mediated components of these monosynaptic EPSCs could be resolved pharmacologically as shown in Figure 1B. Addition of the NMDA receptor blocker 6-cyano-7-nitroquinoxaline-2,3-dione (CNQX) virtually abolished synaptic currents at holding potential of -60mV. Changing the holding potential to +40mV, revealed a reversed synaptic current which was totally blocked by the NMDA receptor antagonist 3-3 (2 carboxypiperazine-4-yl) propyl-1-phosphonate (CPP).

The use of the thin slice preparation resolved, as mentioned above, dual-component EPSPs, mediated by NMDA and non-NMDA receptor subtypes. However, since spinal neuronal networks as well as dendritic trees of motoneurons

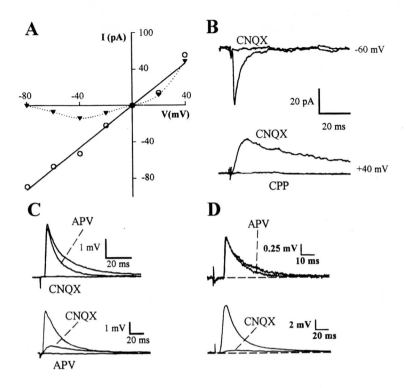

Figure 1. EAA receptors in monosynaptic transmission. A. Dependence of the EPSCs components on the holding potential: EPSCs were generated in α-motoneuron in the thin slice preparation of the neonatal rat by stimulation of lamina IX axon and recorded using the whole-cell patch clamp technique. The EPSC amplitudes were sampled at the peak (circles) and 20 ms after the stimulus artefact (triangles) from 10-sweep computer averaged records at each holding potential.

B. EAA pharmacology of EPSCs in the thin spinal cord slice: Upper set- Superimposed averaged records (11 sweeps each) before, and after bath application of 5µM CNQX. Lower set- Averaged records in the same cell before and after addition of 10µM CPP to the CNQX containing medium. Holding potentials: -60 and +40 mV in the upper and lower sets respectively.

C. EAA pharmacology of monosynaptic EPSPs elicited by dorsal root afferents: Computer averaged monosynaptic EPSPs (26 sweeps each) elicited by stimulation of the segmental dorsal root were shortened by application of 20µM APV and then blocked by 10µm CNQX (upper set). Application of 10µM CNQX to a different motoneuron revealed a CNQX resistant component and then blocked by 20µM APV (lower set, 30 sweep averages).

D. EAA pharmacology of monosynaptic EPSPs elicited by VLF axons. Averaged VLF-induced EPSPs (25 sweep-each) before and after addition of 20µM APV (upper set). VLF-induced EPSPs (25 sweep averages) recorded from a different motoneuron, before and following bath application of 10µM CNQX (lower set). Bathing solutions contained 1mM mephenesin, 5mM strychnine and 10mM bicuculline.

in the thin slice are largely reduced, a more realistic evaluation of the role of NMDA and non-NMDA receptors in monosynaptic transmission, requires the use of in vitro preparations in which motoneurons are intact, neuronal networks are unimpaired and the activated pathways can be identified. The experiments described below therefore, characterised monosynaptic transmission between dorsal root afferents and α-motoneurons in the hemisected and the en-bloc spinal cord preparation of the neonatal rat.

(2) EAA receptors and mono synaptic transmission between dorsal root afferents and α-motoneurons. Activation of dorsal root afferents in the presence of mephenesin, strychnine and bicuculline in the hemisected spinal cord preparation produced monosynaptic EPSPs with a robust NMDA receptor mediated component at resting membrane potential (more negative than -60mV) and normal magnesium concentration (1mM[24]). Figure 1C shows that monosynaptic EPSPs were markedly shortened following application of the NMDA receptor blocker 2-amino-5-phosphonovaleric acid (APV), and were then blocked by addition of CNQX (upper set). Addition of CNQX to a different preparation, revealed an NMDA receptor mediated component, that could reach up to 30% of the peak EPSP amplitude. This component was blocked by bath application of the specific NMDA receptor antagonist APV (lower set).

In order to examine whether the relative contribution of NMDA and non-NMDA receptors to monosynaptic excitation in other monosynaptic connections to α-motoneurons is similar to that described between dorsal root afferents and motoneurons, we characterised EPSPs induced in α-motoneurons by stimulation of ventrolateral funiculus axon in the en-bloc spinal cord preparation of the neonatal rat.

(3) EAA receptors and monosynaptic transmission between VLF axons and α-motoneurons. A different and very potent monosynaptic excitatory connection to α-motoneurons have been recently found by electrical stimulation of ventrolateral funiculus axons in the developing spinal cord of the chick embryo.[12] Stimulation of the surgically peeled ventrolateral funiculus in the neonatal rat spinal cord revealed (after blocking the GABA$_A$ and glycine receptors by bicuculline and strychnine, in the presence of mephenesin) short latency EPSPs. Addition of APV shortened the duration of the VLF induced EPSPs with little effect on their peak amplitudes (Figure 1D, upper set), while addition of CNQX revealed a CNQX resistant component which could be then (similarly to the responses induced by dorsal root stimulation) blocked by APV (Figure 1D, lower set).

Thus, it seems that all the excitatory monosynaptic connection to α-motoneurons described in the present work, are mediated by activation of both NMDA and non-NMDA receptor subtypes. The NMDA component has been shown to have a substantial contribution to monosynaptic excitation at resting potential and normal magnesium concentrations in both the hemisected and the en-bloc preparations. The contribution of the NMDA receptor mediated component can be markedly increased upon depolarization, as has been demonstrated in voltage clamp recordings from motoneurons in the thin slice[15] (see Fig. 1A). Much further increase is expected to occur in dendritic synapses where the local depolarising drive may reach tens of millivolts during normal physiological activities of the spinal cord.

NMDA AND NON-NMDA RECEPTOR MEDIATED COMPONENTS OF POLYSYNAPTIC EPSPS

Polysynaptic EPSPs were generated in motoneurons by activation of non-segmental dorsal roots in the presence of strychnine and bicuculline. These EPSPs were characterised by a prolonged latency and by extreme sensitivity to the stimulation frequency.[24] Addition of CNQX, could either partially (not illustrated) or completely blocked polysynaptic EPSPs (Figure 2, upper set, right panel). At the same time, monosynaptic EPSPs generated in the same motoneuron by stimulation of the segmental dorsal root, revealed a substantial CNQX resistant component of monosynaptic EPSPs (Figure 2, left panel). Complete (Figure 2, lower set, right panel) or partial (not illustrated) block of EPSPs could be also obtained by bath application of APV. The findings that CNQX could completely block polysynaptic transmission, while retaining a CNQX resistant component of monosynaptic EPSPs in the same cell, indicates that unlike previous suggestions[7,13,14,28] the CNQX-induced block of polysynaptic transmission occurred at the interneuronal level. We therefore suggest that interneuronal transmission in polysynaptic pathways between dorsal root afferents and α-motoneurons is mediated by both non-NMDA and NMDA receptors.

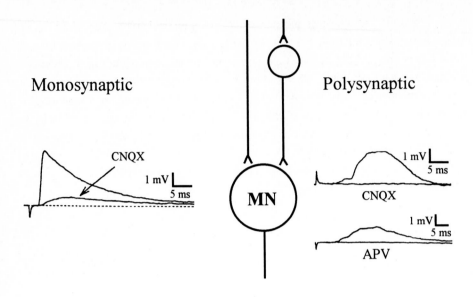

Figure 2 EAA receptors in polysynaptic transmission. Polysynaptic EPSPs (15-sweep averages) elicited in an L5 motoneuron by stimulation of the L4 dorsal root were blocked by 10µM CNQX (upper set, right panel). Monosynaptic EPSPs (15-sweep averages) elicited in the same motoneuron by stimulation of the L5 dorsal root are shown before and in the presence of CNQX (left panel). Polysynaptic EPSPs recorded from another L5 motoneuron (10-sweep averages) are shown before and after administration of 20µM APV (lower set, right panel). Bathing media contained 5mM strychnine and 10mM bicuculline.

AP4 RECEPTORS AND MONOSYNAPTIC EXCITATION

AP4 is a glutamate analogue that has been shown to reduce the excitatory transmission in a number of synaptic systems (for review see Monaghan et al.,[22]). AP4 has also been shown to reduce firing in dorsal horn and Renshaw cells[6,7] and to decrease the stretch reflex *in vivo*[8]. In the *in vitro* mammalian brainstem spinal cord preparation, AP4 has been shown to diminish the inspiratory drive to phrenic motoneurons[18]. In a recent study[24], we have shown that AP4 reduced the monosynaptic EPSPs by a factor of 2-5. We also found that the reduction in EPSP amplitudes was not accompanied by changes in the passive properties of motoneurons, and that AP4 affected equally the NMDA and non-NMDA receptor mediated components of the EPSP. These results taken together with findings that application of AP4 failed to affect the responses to exogeneously applied EAA in phrenic[18] and dorsal horn neurons[6], all suggest that the decrease of EPSP amplitude by AP4 is accounted for by a presynaptic mechanism. This is also supported by the finding that AP4 reduced the amplitude of the EPSCs and increased their coefficient of variation in cultured hippocampal cells[9].

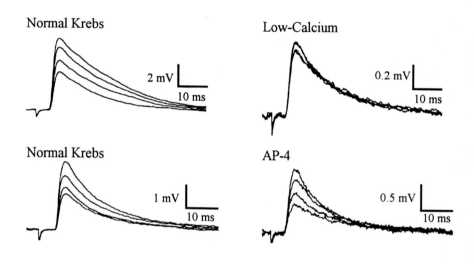

Figure 3. AP4 and monosynaptic transmission. Upper-panel - Computer averaged monosynaptic EPSPs induced by repetitive stimulation of the dorsal root at 1,2, 5 and 10s intervals at normal (Normal Krebs; 20-sweep averages) and 0.8mM Ca^{2+} and 6mM Mg^2 (Low-Ca^{2+}; 40-sweep averages) Krebs saline.
Lower panel - Monosynaptic EPSPs (20sweep averages) induced in a different motoneuron by repetitive stimulation of the dorsal root at 1,2, 5 and 10s intervals, before (Normal Krebs) and in the presence of 75µM L-AP4 (AP-4). All bathing solutions contained 5µM strychnine, 10µM bicuculline and 1mM mephenesin.

The four superimposed traces at the left upper panel of Figure 3 are computer averaged records sampled during repetitive dorsal root activation at 1, 2, 5 and 10s intervals (lower to upper traces respectively; Normal Krebs). The low EPSP amplitudes at shorter intervals reflect a prolonged synaptic depression of presynaptic nature[17], that can be virtually eliminated in low-calcium solutions as the EPSPs are substantially reduced presumably by the decreased calcium influx into afferent terminals and the concomitant reduction in release of transmitter (upper panel, Low-Calcium). Contrary to this, addition of AP-4 to a different preparation, did not alter the frequency dependence of the prolonged synaptic depression despite the substantial decrease in the EPSP amplitude (compare the average records at the respective stimulation intervals before and in the presence of AP4). These findings suggest that if AP4 acts to decrease the release of transmitter, then the mechanism does not involve a decreased release probability from afferent terminals which are invaded by presynaptic action potentials, but rather, might involve either branch point blockade (see ref.[19]) of presynaptic action potentials to afferent terminals, partial depletion in the releasable stores of transmitter, and/or inactivation of presynaptic release sites . In summary, although it seems likely that AP4 acts by a presynaptic mechanism, it is not clear whether the postulated presynaptic receptors act as EAA autoreceptors or involve reduction in EAA re-uptake to presynaptic terminals by AP4 binding to presynaptic EAA uptake-receptors (see ref.[23]) and thereby shunting the membrane of the afferent terminals to incoming afferent volleys.

SUMMARY AND CONCLUSIONS

The studies reviewed above described the involvement of excitatory amino acid receptors in synaptic transmission in the *in vitro* mammalian spinal cord. Both NMDA and non-NMDA receptors were found to play a role in mono- and polysynaptic transmission between dorsal root afferents and α-motoneurons, between VLF axons and α-motoneurons, and between lamina IX axons and α motoneurons. Activation of AP-4 receptors reduced the dorsal root induced monosynaptic EPSPs by a unique presynaptic mechanism involving either branch point block of presynaptic action potentials, depletion of transmitter vesicles and/or inactivation of release sites.

ACKNOWLEDGEMENT: This work was supported by grant No. 363/90 from the Israel Academy for Sciences and Humanities, Jerusalem, Israel to ALT.

REFERENCES

1. ASCHER, P. AND NOWAK, L. (1987) Electrophysiological studies on NMDA receptors. *Trends in Neurosci.* **10**, 284-288.
2. BARRY, M.J. AND O'DONOVAN, M.J. (1987) The effects of excitatory amino acids and their antagonists on the generation of motor activity in the isolated chick spinal cord. *Develop. Brain Res.* **36**, 271-276,
3. BURKE, R.E. (1987) Synaptic efficacy and the control of neuronal input-output relations. Trends in *Neuroscience* **10**, 42-45.
4. COLLINGRIDGE, G.L. AND LESTER R.A.J. (1989) Excitatory amino acid receptors in the vertebrate central nervous system. *Pharmacol. Rev.* **41**, 143-210.
5. DALE, N. AND ROBERTS, A. (1985) Dual component amino acid-mediated synaptic potentials:Excitatory drive for swimming in Xenopus embryos. *J. Physiol.* **384**, 35-59.
6. DAVIS, J.D. AND WATKINS, J.C. (1982) Actions of D and L-forms of 2-amino phosphonovalerate and 2-amino-4-phosphonobutyrate in the cat spinal cord. *Brain Res.* **235**, 378-386.
7. DAVIS, J.D. AND WATKINS, J.C. (1983) Role of excitatory amino acids in mono and polysynaptic excitation in the cat spinal cord. *Exp. Brain Res.* **49**, 280-290.
8. EVANS, R.H., FRANCIS, A.A., JONES, A.W., SMITH, D.A.S. AND WATKINS, J.C. (1982) The effects of series of w-phosphonic a-carboxylic amino-acids on electrically evoked and excitatory amino acid induced responses in isolated spinal cord preparations. *Brit. J. Pharmacol.* **75**, 65-75.
9. FORSYTHE, I.D. AND CLEMENTS, J.D. (1990) Presynaptic glutamate receptors depress excitatory monosynaptic transmission between mouse hippocampal neurons. *J. Physiol.* **429**, 1-16.
10. FORSYTHE, I.D. AND G.L. WESTBROOK, (1988) Slow excitatory postsynaptic currents mediated by N-Methyl-D-Aspartate receptors on cultured mouse central neurons. *J. Physiol.* **396**, 515-533.
11. HESTRIN, S, NICOLL RA, PERKEL DJ, SAH P (1990) Analysis of excitatory synaptic action in pyramidalcells using whole cell recording from rat hippocampal slices. *J. Physiol.* **422**, 203-225.
12. HO, S. AND O'DONOVAN, M.J. (1993) Regionalization and inter-segmental coordination of rhythm generating networks in the spinal cord of the chick embryo. *J. Neurosci.* (in press).

13. JAHR, C.E. AND YOSHIOKA K. (1986) Ia excitation of motoneurons in the in vitro newborn rat spinal cord is selectively antagonized by kynurenate. *J. Physiol.* **370**, 5151-530.
14. JIANG, Z.J., SHEN E. AND DUN, N.J. (1990) Excitatory and inhibitory transmission from dorsal root afferents to neonate rat motoneurons in vitro. *Brain Res.* **235**, 110-118.
15. KONNERTH, A., KELLER B., AND LEV-TOV, A. (1990) Patch clamp analysis of excitatory synapses in mammalian spinal cord slices. *Pflügers Archiv* **417**, 285-290.
16. LEV-TOV, A. AND KONNERTH, A. (1991) Patch clamp studies of synaptic currents in mammalian motoneurons. In: *Plasticity of Motoneuronal Connections*. ed. A. Wernig. Elsevier, Amsterdam.
17. LEV-TOV, A. AND PINCO, M. (1992) In vitro studies of prolonged synaptic depression in the neonatal rat spinal cord. *J. Physiol.* **447**, 149-169.
18. LIU, G., FELDMAN, J.L. AND SMITH, J.C. (1990) Excitatory amino acid-mediated transmission of inhibitory drive to phrenic motoneurons. *J. Neurosci.* **64**, 423-436.
19. LÜSCHER, H-R. RUENZEL, P. AND HENNEMAN, E. (1983) Composite EPSPs in motoneurons of different sizes before and during PTP: Implications for transmission failure and its relief in Ia projections. *J. Neurophysiol.* **49**, 269-289.
20. MAYER, M. L. AND WESTBROOK, G.L. (1987) The physiology of excitatory amino acids in the vertebrate nervous system. *Prog. Neurobiol.* 28: 197-276.
21. MENDELL, L.M. (1984) Modifiability of spinal synapses. *Physiol. Rev.* **64**, 260-324.
22. MONAGHAN, D.T., BRIGES, R.J. AND COTMAN, C.W. (1989) The excitatory amino acids receptors: their classes, pharmacology and distinct properties in the function of the central nervous system. *Ann. Rev..Pharmacol. Toxicol.* **29**, 365-402.
23. MONAGHAN, D.T., MILLS, M.C., CHAMBERLAIN, A.R., AND COTMAN, C.W. (1983) Synthesis of [^{3}H]2-amino-4-phosphonobutyric acid and characterization of its binding to rat brain membranes: a selective ligand for the chloride/calcium dependent class of L-glutamate binding sites. *Brain Res.* **278**, 137-144.
24. PINCO, M. AND LEV-TOV, A. (1993) Characterization and frequency modulation of excitatory amino acid mediated EPSPs in rat spinal motoneurones. *J. Neurophysiol.* (in press).
25. REDMAN, S.J. (1979) Junctional mechanisms at group Ia synapses. *Prog. Neurobiol.* **12**, 33-83.
26. THOMSON, A.M., WEST, D.C, AND LODGE, D.A. (1985) N-methyl aspartate receptor mediated synapse in rat cerebral cortex: a site of action of Ketamine? *Nature.* **313**, 479-481.
27. WALMSLEY, B., AND NICOL, M.J. (1991)The effects of Ca^{2+}, Mg^{2+} and kynurenate on primary afferent synaptic potentials evoked in cat spinal cord neurones in vivo. *J. Physiol.* **433**,409-420.
28. ZISKIND-CONHAIM, L. (1990) NMDA receptors mediate poly and monosynaptic potentials in motoneurons of rat embryos. *J. Neurosci.***10**, 125-135.

MODULATION OF NMDA CURRENTS IN HIPPOCAMPAL NEURONES

Pìotr Bregestovski, Igor Medina and Yezekiel Ben-Ari
INSERM Unite 29
Hopital de Port-Royal
123 Bd de Port-Royal, 75014 Paris
France

INTRODUCTION

Activity of hippocampal neurons is regulated by several types of receptors to neuropeptides, hormones and neurotransmitters.[14,49] Glutamate is the most prominent neurotransmitter of the fast excitatory synapses in hippocampus and other parts of the mammalian brain. Glutamate receptors include ionotropic and metabotropic families[56,60] and the ionotropic ones are divided in two broad classes: N-methyl-D-aspartate (NMDA) and AMPA/kainate.[43] NMDA subtype of the glutamate receptor plays an important role in a number of physiological processes concerning neuronal plasticity (long-term potentiation, model of learning on the cellular level)[5,43] and various physiological disorders such as ischemic cell death and epilepsy.[6,11,51] This subtype is "best characterized of the glutamate receptors and currently the most popular".[4]

The NMDA receptor has a number of fundamental differences from non-NMDA ones which determine its physiological specificity. Thus, the cation selective NMDA-activated ionic channels display high permeability to calcium[34,39] and the receptor itself has several regulatory sites for extracellular and cytoplasmic modulation.[4,5,33]

In this chapter we will describe in short the modulatory properties of NMDA receptors and modulatory interactions between two glutamate receptor subtypes, NMDA and AMPA/kainate, via elevation of intracellular calcium concentration.

Extracellular modulation of the NMDA receptor

Several physiological ways have been described for the modulation of NMDA receptor activity by extracellular factors . (1) Responses to NMDA are potentiated by

NATO ASI Series, Vol. H 79
Cellular Mechanisms of Sensory Processing
Edited by Laszlo Urban
© Springer-Verlag Berlin Heidelberg 1994

micromolar concentrations of glycine at strychnine-insensitive allosteric site.[21] Moreover, glycine may be regarded as NMDA co-agonist as its presence was shown necessary for NMDA channel activation.[16,19,26,30] (2) Physiological concentrations of Mg^{2+} modulate activity of NMDA channels in a voltage-dependent manner.[38,44] (3) NMDA-induced currents are inhibited by protons with an IC_{50} of about pH7.3.[13,53,54] (4) Endogenous polyamines (spermine and spermidine) potentiate NMDA currents by modulating the kinetics of desensitization.[28,46] Thus, polyamine substances known to be present at high concentration in the brain[23] may play regulatory role in the NMDA receptor function. (5) Finally, there is an additional site where divalent cation Zn^{2+} which co-exist in neurons with L-glutamate, inhibits NMDA currents independently of the membrane potential.[45,57,58]

Intracellular modulation of the NMDA receptor

There are several studies which suggest that the NMDA receptor can be modulated from the cytoplasmic side of the membrane through protein kinase-dependent phosphorylation. Thus, phorbol esters, which activate protein kinase C (PKC), increased the activity of NMDA receptor subunits expressed in Xenopus oocytes[24,59] and selectively enhanced the amplitude of NMDA currents in hippocampal[2] and spinal dorsal horn neurons.[17] Stimulation of μ-opioid, metabotropic glutamate and muscarinic receptors, which activate PKC, also caused an elevation of NMDA currents.[1,8,24] PKC potentiates NMDA currents, presumably by reducing the voltage-dependent Mg^{2+} block: a nearly four-fold increase of the apparent dissociation constant for Mg^{2+} block was observed on intracellular application of PKC[9]. Arachidonic acid also potentiates NMDA currents, either by direct binding to the receptor or by interaction with the lipid environment[41]. Nitric oxide reduced NMDA currents and abolished the NMDA-mediated increase in intracellular Ca^{2+}.[36]

Time course of NMDA currents

<u>Synaptic currents</u>

Synaptic responses mediated by NMDA have a prolonged time course relative to the non-NMDA component[12,15,22,58]. The kinetics of excitatory postsynaptic currents (EPSC) is determined by the life-time of the neurotransmitter interaction with the receptor.[31] In cultured hippocampal neurons the authors observed that a brief (100 ms) pulse of glutamate leads to prolonged (>300 ms) activation of NMDA receptors and the decay of NMDA synaptic component is about 100 times longer than the mean open time of NMDA currents.[3,31]

Desensitization

Fast applications of glutamate analogues to the surface of the neuronal membrane with different receptor subtypes show different kinetics of desensitization. With application of quisqualate and AMPA the time course of desensitization is fast, whereas it is slower with NMDA application and the kainate response does not desensitise.[25,40,52,55]

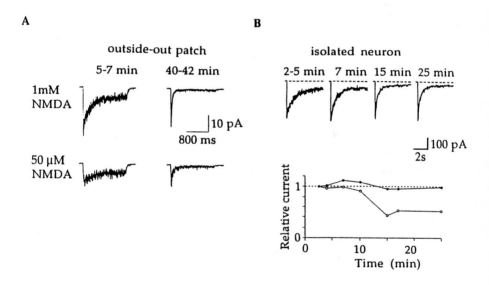

Figure 1. Time-dependent modulation of desensitization kinetics of NMDA- and aspartate-activated currents. A, records of NMDA-gated currents from outside-out patches from mouse neurons soon after the break in and later in the experiment. Time zero was taken as the start of the whole cell recording *(from Sather, et al. 1992)*. B, aspartate-activated responses recorded from isolated hippocampal neurons of the rat at different time of recording (top traces) and time dependence of the mean time constants of the response decay (bottom) *(from Chizhmakov, et al.[10])*.

Desensitization of NMDA receptors can be modulated by several factors. Thus, elevation of glycine concentration decreases desensitization and increases the rate of recovery from desensitization.[40] The authors suggested that this phenomena underlines the potentiating effect of glycine on the NMDA receptor. However, in excised outside-out patches and on acutely isolated neurons, the desensitization was independent of the glycine concentration.[48,50] The speed of desensitization is accelerated with the time of the recording[10,47]; as shown in Figure 1. In the first minutes of dialysis in outside-out patches or isolated neurons the decay of NMDA currents is much slower than after 25-40 min of recording. Recently Lester et al.[32] showed the exsistence of two forms of NMDA receptor desensitization, only one of which depends on the glycine concentration. A glycine-insensitive form increases rapidly during the first minutes of the recording. These results suggest the existence of some intracellular factors which modulate the desensitization of the NMDA receptor.

Recently it was also demonstrated that the desensitization of the NMDA channels depends on the intracellular calcium concentration.[27] The inactivation increased with the elevation of extracellular or intracellular calcium concentrations and it was absent at positive membrane potentials (+40 mV), suggesting that inactivation resulted from transmembrane calcium influx.[27]

Recovery from desensitization

When using low intracellular Ca^{2+} concentrations (7 mM EGTA) the recovery of NMDA currents from desensitization is relatively fast.[47] The time constant of the recovery is single-exponential and does not appear to depend on the duration of the agonist application (Figure 2A). In the whole-cell recording mode in cultured mouse embryonic neurons the time constant of the recovery was about 1 s, while on outside-out patches it was about 0.3 s.

Patch-clamp recordings from cultured pyramidal cells of the rat hippocampus show that in relatively high intracellular Ca^{2+} concentration (50-100 nM) and Mg-ATP (2 mM) the time course of the recovery of NMDA currents evolved in two, clearly distinguished phases (Figure 2 B). The time constant for the first component (τ_1) had a mean value of about 1.0 s, while the time constant for the second component (τ_2) was much slower and varied in different cells from 10 s to 50 s[7]. The time course of the first phase of recovery did not depend markedly on the duration and concentration of conditioning doses of NMDA, similarly to observations of Sather et al.[47] The time constant of the second component depended on the duration of the conditioning NMDA pulses.

All these observations suggest that the behavior of NMDA currents can be modulated from the cytoplasmic side of the membrane.

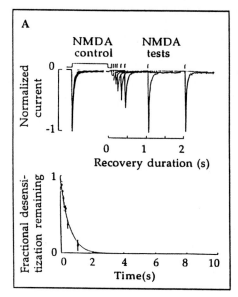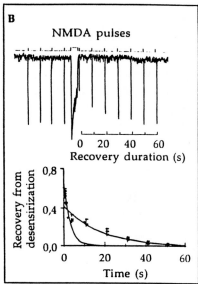

Figure 2. Time course of the recovery of NMDA channels from desensitization. A. Outside-patches from mouse hippocampal neurons. Recording pipette was filled with a solution containing (mM): 84 CsF, 7 CsCl, 7 EGTA, 7 HEPES. Data were fitted by single exponential with a time constant of 0.5 s. Glycine concentration was 10 μM (*modified from W.Sather et al.[47]*).
B. Whole cell recording on cultured rat hippocampal neurons. The recording pipette was filled with a solution containing (mM): 60 K-gluconate, 100 CsCl, 1,1 EGTA, 400 μM CaCl$_2$, 10 HEPES, pH=7.2; pCa=7. Data were fitted by a double exponential with a time constants of 2.5s and 16s respectively. Holding potential: -50 mV. The glycine concentration was 10 μM.

Activation of AMPA receptors by kainate modulates desensitization of NMDA currents via elevation of intracellular Ca^{2+}

There are several observations suggesting modulatory interactions between different receptor systems, i.e. activation of one type of receptors changes properties of the other one. Thus, activation of receptors to acetylcholine[37], μ-opioids[8] or metabotropic (Q$_p$) receptors[1] increase NMDA currents. Short-term potentiation of non-NMDA-induced currents via NMDA receptors was observed in isolated hippocampal neurons.[61] This modulation can arise either at the receptor-channel system or through intracellular second messengers.

Interaction between NMDA and non-NMDA receptor-channel systems may arise from the finding that glutamate receptors could be coupled to a common channel.[13,20] However, more recent results obtained on cultured neurons[18,35] and *Xenopus* oocytes[29] strongly suggest that NMDA and kainate receptors are coupled with separate types of ion channel.

Recently we have shown that application of a long conditioning pulse of kainate (5-10 s) to the surface of cultured pyramidal cells in the rat hippocampus remarkably decreased the amplitude of NMDA test pulses, i.e. the kainate induced desensitization of NMDA receptors (Figure 3). The amplitude of NMDA currents recovered to the control level during 10-30 s after conditioning pulse with single-exponentional kinetics, corresponding to the second (slow) phase of the recovery (see Figure 2B).

Kainate-induced desensitization is not due to a direct activation of the NMDA receptors by kainate.[7] The following observations suggest that recovery of the NMDA current from kainate-induced desensitization is Ca^{2+}-dependent.[7] (1) The simultaneous patch-clamp recording of ionic currents and fluorescent measurement of intracellular Ca^{2+} (Ca_i) with INDO-1[42] show a rise in Ca_i in the presence of kainate, NMDA or due to depolarizing pulses.

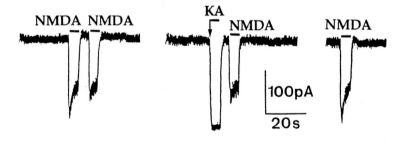

Figure 3. Kainate-induced desensitization of NMDA currents. Note, that a conditioning pulse of kainate decreased the NMDA current similar to that produced by a conditioning pulse of NMDA. Experimental conditions were similar to that described in Fig.2,B.

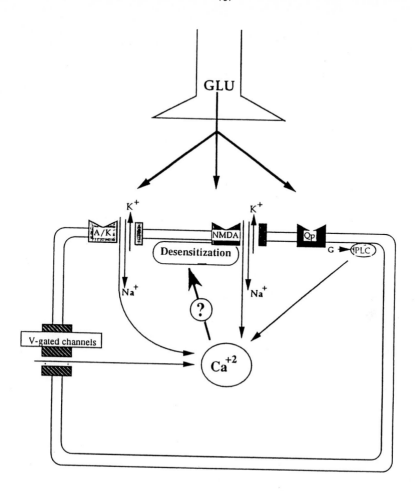

Figure 4. Schematic diagram of the modulation NMDA receptors by intracellular calcium. Transmitter release (Glu) induces activation of three types of glutamate receptors: ionotropic (A/K, NMDA) and metabotropic (Q_p). Stimulation of ionotropic receptors will cause depolarization of neurons and activation of voltage gated calcium channels. Stimulation of Q_p receptors will produce activation of phospholipase C (PLC) and increase in IP_3. These events will induce elevation of intracellular calcium (Ca^{++}) either due to its influx through ionotropic receptor-channel systems and through voltage-operated Ca^{++} channels or by Ca^{2+} release from IP_3-sensitive stores. Elevated Ca^{++} stimulates intermediate systems (to be identified) which induce inactivation of NMDA channels.

(2) Elevation of Ca_i by activation of voltage-dependent Ca^{2+} channels (with depolarising voltage steps) induces desensitization of NMDA currents. Elevation of the extracellular Ca^{2+} concentration to 10 mM enhances the inhibitory effect of

depolarising voltage pulses on NMDA responses. (3) Cadmium (10 µM) prevents development of the desensitization of NMDA currents induced by depolarization but not by kainate. (4) In certain conditions when cells were loaded with the Ca^{2+} chelator BAPTA (15 mM) kainate and conditioning depolarization failed to produce desensitization of NMDA currents.

Thus, the NMDA subtype of the glutamate receptor has several modulatory sites for regulation of its activity under physiological conditions. Amplitude and time course of the NMDA currents are regulated by Ca-dependent intracellular processes as summarized in Figure 4.

REFERENCES

1. ANIKSZTEJN, L., BREGESTOVSKI, P. AND BEN-ARI, Y. (1992) Selective activation of quisqualate metabotropic receptor potentiates NMDA but not AMPA responses. *Eur. J. Pharmacol.* **205**, 327-328.
2. ANIKSZTEJN, L., OTANI, S. AND BEN-ARI, Y. (1992) Quisqualate metabotropic receptor modulate NMDA currents and facilitate induction of long-term potentiation through protein kinase. *Eur. J. Neurosci.* **4**, 500-505.
3. ASCHER, P., BREGESTOVSKI, P. AND NOWAK, L. (1988) N-methyl-D-aspartate-activated channels of mouse central neurones in magnesium-free solutions. *J.Physiol.* **399**, 207-226.
4. ASCHER, P. AND JOHNSON, J.W. (1989) The NMDA receptor, its channel and its modulation by glycine. In: *The NMDA Receptor.* eds J. L. Watkins and G. L. Collingridge. IRL Press.
5. BEN-ARI, Y., ANIKSZTEJN, L. AND BREGESTOVSKI, P. (1992) Protein kinase C modulation of NMDA current: an important link for LTP induction. *Trends Neurosci.* **15**, 333-339.
6. BEN-ARI, Y. AND CHO, M. (1988) Long-lasting modification of the synaptic properties of rat CA3 hippocampal neurones induced by kainic acid. *J. Physiol.* **404**, 365-381.
7. BREGESTOVSKI, P., MEDINA, I AND BEN-ARI, Y. (1993) Calcium-dependent modulation of NMDA currents in cultured hippocampal neurones. In: *Intrac. Channels, Organelles and Cell Function.* Trieste.
8. CHEN, L. AND HUANG, L-Y.M. (1991) Sustained potentiation of NMDA receptor-mediated glutamate responses through activation of protein kinase C by a µ opioid. *Neuron* **7** 319-326.
9. CHEN, L., AND HUANG, L-Y.M. (1992) Protein kinase C reduces Mg^{2+} block of NMDA receptor channels as a mechanism of modulation. *Nature* **356**, 521-523.
10. CHIZHMAKOV, I.V., KISKIN, N.I. AND KRISHTAL, O.A. (1992) Two types of steady-state desensitization of N-methyl-D-aspartate receptor in isolated hippocampal neurones of rat. *J.Physiol.* **448**, 453-472.

11. CHOI, D.W. (1990) Cerebral hypoxia: some new approaches and unanswered questions. *J. Neurosci.* **10**, 2493-2501.
12. CLEMENTS, J.D., LESTER, R.A.J., TONG, G., JAHR, C.E. AND WESTBROOK, G.L. (1992) The time course of glutamate in the synaptic cleft. *Science* **258**, 1498-1501.
13. CULL-CANDY, S. AND USOWICZ, M. (1987) Multiple-conductance channels activated by excitatory amino acids in cerebellar neurons. *Nature* **325**, 525-528.
14. DINGLEDINE, R. (1984) Hippocampus:Synaptic Pharmacology. In: Brain Slices ed. R. Dingledine. Plenum Press New York & London.
15. FORSYTHE, I.D. AND WESTBROOK, G.L. (1988) Slow excitatory postsynaptic currents mediated by N-methyl-D-aspartate receptor on mouse cultured central neurones. *J. Physiol.* **396**, 515-533.
16. FOSTER, A.S., KEMP, J.A. (1989) Glycine maintains excitement. *Nature* **338**, 377-378.
17. GERBER, G., KANGRGA, I., RYU, P.D., LAREW, J. AND RANDIC, M. (1989) Multiple effects of phorbol esters in the rat spinal dorsal horn. *J.Neurosci.* **9**, 3606-3617.
18. HUETTNER, J., BEAN, B. (1988) Block of N-methyl-D-aspartate-activated current by the anticonvulsant MK-801: Selective binding to open channels. *Proc. Natl. Acad. Sci. USA* **85**,1307-1311.
19. HUETTNER, J.E. (1989) Indole-2-carboxylic acid: a competitive antagonist of potentiation by glycine at the NMDA receptor. *Science* **243**, 1611-1613.
20. JAHR, C., STEVENS, C. (1987) Glutamate activated multiple single channel conductances in hippocampal neurones. *Nature* **325**, 522-525.
21. JOHNSON, J.W., ASCHER, P. (1987) Glycine potentiates NMDA response in cultured mouse brain neurones. *Nature* **325**, 529-531.
22. KAUER, J., MALENKA, R.C. AND NICOLL, R.A. (1988) A persistent postsynaptic modification mediates long-term potentiation in the hippocampus. *Neuron* **1**, 911-917.
23. KAWAI, N. (1992) Polyamine toxins as excitatory amino acid receptor ligands. In: *Excitatory Amino Acid Receptors. Design of Agonists and Antagonists* eds. P. Krogsgaard-Larsen and J. J. Hansen. Ellis Horwood New York.
24. KELSO, S.R., NELSON, T.E. AND LEONARD, J.P. (1992) Protein-kinase C-mediated enhancement of NMDA currents by metabotropic glutamate receptors in Xenopus oocytes. *J. Physiol.* **449**, 705-718.
25. KISKIN, N.I., KRISHTAL, O.A AND TSYNDRENKO, A.Y. (1986) Excitatory amino acid receptors in hippocampal neurons: kainate fails to desensitize them. *Neurosci. lett.* **63**, 225230.
26. KLECKNER, N.W. AND DINGLEDINE, R. (1988) Requirement for glycine activation of NMDA receptors expressed in Xenopus oocytes. *Science* **241**, 835-837.
27. LEGENDRE, P., ROSENMUND, C. AND WESTBROOK, G. (1993) Inactivation of NMDA channels in cultured hippocampal neurons by intracellular calcium. *J.Neurosci.* **13**, 674684.
28. LERMA, J. (1992) Spermine regulates N-methyl-D-aspartate receptor desensitization. *Neuron* **8**, 343-352.
29. LERMA, J., KUSHNER, L., SPRAY, D.C., BENNETT, M. AND ZUKIN, S. (1989) mRNA from NCB-20 cells encodes the N-methyl-D-aspartate/phencyclidine

receptor: A Xenopus oocyte expression study. *Proc. Natl. Acad. Sci USA* **86**, 1708-1711.

30. LERMA, J., ZUKIN, S. AND BENNETT, M. (1990) Glycine decreases desensitization of N-methyl-D-aspartate (NMDA) receptors expressed in Xenopus oocytes and is required for NMDA responses. *Proc. Natl. Acad. Sci. USA* **87**, 2354-2358.

31. LESTER, R.A., CLEMENTS, J.D., WESTBROOK, G.L. AND JAHR, C.E. (1990) Channel kinetics determine the time course of NMDA receptor-mediated synaptic currents. *Nature* **346**, 565-567.

32. LESTER, R.A., TONG, G. AND JAHR, C.E. (1993) Interaction between the Glycine and Glutamate binding sites of the NMDA receptors. *J.Neurosci.* **13**, 1088-1096.

33. LODGE, D. (1992) Ligands for NMDA receptor modulatory sites. In: *Excitatory Amino Acid Receptors. Design of Agonists and Antagonists* eds. P. Krogsgaard-Larsen and J. J. Hansen. Ellis Horwood New York.

34. MACDERMOTT, A.B., MAYER, M. WESTBROOK, G.L., SMITH, S.J. AND BARKER, J.L. (1986) NMDA receptor activation increases cytoplasmic calcium concentration in cultured spinal cord neurones. *Nature* **321**, 519-522.

35. MACDONALD, J.F., MILJKOVIC, Z. AND PENNEFATHER, P. (1987) Use-dependent block of excitatory amino acid currents in cultured neurons by ketamine. *J.Neurophysiol.* **58**, 251-266.

36. MANSONI, O.J.J., FINIELS-MARLIER, F., SASSETTI, I., BLOCKAERT, J., PEUCH, C. AND SLADECZEK, F. (1990) The glutamate receptor of the Qp-tupe activates prootein kinase C and is regulated by protein kinase C. *Neurosci. Lett.* **109**, 146-151.

37. MARKRAM, H. AND SEGAL, M. (1992) The inositol 1,4,5-triphosphate pathway mediates cholinergic potentiation of rat hippocampal neuronal responses to NMDA. *J. Physiol.* **447**, 513-533.

38. MAYER, M., WESTBROOK, G.L. AND GUTHRIE, P.B. (1984) Voltage-dependent block by Mg^{2+} of NMDA responses in spinal cord neurones. *Nature* **309**, 261-263.

39. MAYER, M.L., MACDERMOTT, A.B., WESTBROOK, G.L., SMITH, S.J. AND BARKER, J.L. (1987) Agonist- and voltage-gated calcium entry in cultured mouse spinal cord neurons under voltage clamp measured using Arsenazo III. *J. Neurosci.* **7**, 3230-3244.

40. MAYER, M.L., VYKLICKY, L. AND CLEMENTS, J. (1989) Regulation of NMDA receptor desensitization in mouse hippocampal neurones by glycine. *Nature* **338**, 425427.

41. MILLER, B.,, SARANTIS, M., TRAYNELIS, S.F.AND ATTWELL, D. (1992) Potentiation of NMDA receptor currents by arachidonic acid. *Nature* **355**, 722-725.

42. MOLLARD, P., GUERINEAU, N., AUDIN, J. AND DUFY, B. (1989) Measurement of Ca^{2+} transients using simultaneous dual-emission micro-spectrofluorimetry and electrophysiology in individual pituitary cells. *BBRC* **164**, 1045-1052.

43. NICOLL, R.A., MALENKA, R.C. AND KAUER, J.A. (1990) Functional comparison of neurotransmitter receptor subtypes in mammalian central nervous system. *Physiol. Rev.* **70**, 513-565.

44. NOWAK, L., BREGESTOVSKI, P., ASCHER, P., HERBET, A. AND PROCHIANTZ, A. (1984) Magnesium gates glutamate-activated channels in mouse central neurones. *Nature* **307**, 462-465.

45. PETERS, S., KOH, J. AND CHOI, D.W. (1987) Zinc selectively blocks the action of N-methyl-D-aspartate on cortical neurons. *Science* **236**, 589-593.

46. RANSOM, R.W. AND STEC, N.L. (1988) Cooperative modulation of [3H]MK-binding to the N-methyl-D-aspartate receptor ion channel complex by L-glutamate, glycine, and polyamines. *J. Neurochem.* **51**, 830-836.

47. SATHER, W., DIEUDONNE, S., MACDONALD, J.F. AND ASCHER, P. (1992) Activation and desensitization of N-methyl-D-aspartate receptors in nucleated outside-out patches from mouse neurones. *J.Physiol.* **450**, 643-672.

48. SATHER, W., JOHNSON, J.W., HENDERSON, G. AND ASCHER, P. (1990) Glycine-insensitive desensitization of NMDA responses in cultured mouse embryonic neuron. *Neuron* **4**, 725-731.

49. SHEPHERD, G.M. (1974) Hippocampus. In: *Synaptic Organization of the Brain, an Introduction* ed. G. M. Shepherd. University Press Oxford.

50. SHIRASAK, T., NAKAGAWA, T., WAKAMORI, M., TATEISH, N., FUKUDA, A., MURASE, K. AND AKAIKE, N. (1990) Glycine-insensitive desensitization of N-methyl-D-aspartate receptors in acutely isolated mammalian central neurons. *Neurosci. Lett.* **108**, 93-98.

51. SIMON, R.P., SWAN, J.N., GRIFFITHS, T. AND MELDRUM, B.S. (1984) Blockade of N-methyl-D-aspartate receptors may protect against ischemic damage in the brain. *Science* **226,** 850-852.

52. TANG, C.-M., DICHTER, M. AND MORAD, M. (1989) Quisqulate activates a rapidly inactivating high conductance ionic channel in hippocampal neurons. *Science* **243**, 14741477.

53. TANG, C.-M., DICHTER, M. AND MORAD, M. (1990) Modulation of the N-methyl-D-aspartate channel by extracellular H^+. *Proc. Natl. Acad. Sci. USA* **87**, 6445-6449.

54. TRAYNELIS, S.F. AND CULL-CANDY, S.G. (1990) Proton inhibition of N-methyl-D-aspartate receptors in cerebral neurones. *Nature* **345**, 347-350.

55. TRUSSELL, L.O., THIO, L.L., ZORUMSK,I C.F. AND FISCHBACH, G.D. (1988) Rapid desensitization of glutamate receptors in vertebrate central neurons. *Proc. Natl. Acad. Sci. USA* **85**, 4562-4566.

56. WATKINS, J.C., KROGSGAARD-LARSEN, P. AND HONORÉ, T. (1991) Structure-activity relationships in the development of excitatory amino acid receptor agonists and competitive antagonists. *Trends Neurosci.* Special Report 4-12.

57. WEISS, J.H., KOH, J.-Y., CHRISTINE, C.W. AND CHOI, D. (1989) Zinc and LTP. *Nature* **338**, 212.

58. WESTBROOK, G.L. AND MAYER, M.L. (1987) Micromolar concentration of Zn^{++} antagonize NMDA and GABA responses on hippocampal neurones. *Nature* **328**, 640643.

59. YAMAZAKI, M., MORI, H., ARAKI, K., MORI, K.J. AND MISHINA, M. (1992) Cloning, expression and modulation of a mouse NMDA receptor subunit. *FEBS Lett.* **300**, 39-45.

60. YOUNG, A.B. AND FAGG, G.E. (1991) Excitatory amino acid receptors in the brain: membrane binding and receptor autographic approaches. *Trends Neurosci.* Special Report 18-24.
61. ZILBERTER, Y.I., UTESHEV, VV., SOKOLOVA, S.N., MOTIN, L.G. AND EREMJAN, H.H. (1990) Potentiation of glutamate-activated currents in isolated hippocampal neurons. *Neuron* **5**, 597-602.

EXCITATORY AMINO ACID RECEPTORS IN THE SPINAL CORD

David Lodge and Ann Bond
Lilly Research Centre Limited
Erl Wood Manor, Windlesham
SURREY GU20 6PH
United Kingdom

INTRODUCTION

The spinal cord of the cat was until the mid-1970s the major preparation used for the developing pharmacology of glutamate receptors. The pioneering studies of Curtis and Watkins[1] in the early 1960s laid the groundwork for the subsequent mushrooming of knowledge in this area. They showed that endogenous dicarboxylic amino acids such as L-glutamate and L-aspartate were ubiquitous excitants of central neurons, although some small differences in sensitivity between the two agonists on dorsal and ventral horn neurons were noted. A few years later, studies with structurally constrained amino acids from exogenous sources, quisqualate and kainate along with synthetic N-methyl-D-aspartate (NMDA) revealed populations of cells preferentially activated by one or more of these analogues.[2,3] Other analogues, such as D-alpha-amino-adipate, glutamate-diethyl ester (GDEE), γ-D-glutamyl-amino-methyl-sulphonate (GAMS) and the pyrrolidone, HA-966, showed differential effects on the above agonists.[4,5,6] This led to the subdivision of glutamate receptors into NMDA, quisqualate and kainate subtypes which mediated the fast synaptic or ionotropic responses to L-glutamate. It was soon obvious, however, that L-glutamate and some of its analogues, had additional longer term actions which included effects on second messenger systems such as phospholipases and cyclases.[7,8,9] Quisqualate was one such analogue acting as an agonist for these metabotropic responses. Hence for the nomenclature of ionotropic receptors, the term "quisqualate", was dropped in favour of AMPA (α-amino-3-hydroxy-5-methylisoxazole-4-propionate), a more selective agonist for this site.[10]

NATO ASI Series, Vol. H 79
Cellular Mechanisms of Sensory Processing
Edited by Laszlo Urban
© Springer-Verlag Berlin Heidelberg 1994

Although the terms, NMDA, AMPA, kainate and metabotropic are commonly accepted for glutamate receptors, the known number of genes coding for ionotropic receptor subunits is in double figures and that for metabotropic receptors is not far behind. Clearly the nomenclature issue will have to be faced in the near future. For this paper, however, the traditional terminology will be used.

PHARMACOLOGY OF NMDA RECEPTORS

There has been surprisingly little advance in the agonist pharmacology for NMDA receptors. Three compounds L-α-2S,3R,4S-(carboxycyclopropyl) glycine,[11] cis-methano-glutamate[12] and (tetrazol-5-yl)glycine,[13] have been discovered as more potent and selective ligands for the NMDA receptor than NMDA itself. It is an interesting reflection on natural product chemistry that no highly potent or selective NMDA receptor ligands (agonist or antagonist) have been discovered in either plants or invertebrates other than L-aspartate and L-glutamate themselves: the invertebrate nervous system has few if any NMDA receptors.

The situation with synthetic NMDA antagonists is, however, very different. From the weak and rather non-selective compounds, medicinal chemists have developed competitive NMDA antagonists with binding values in the nanomolar range. The greatest advance was the discovery that replacement of the ω-carboxylic acid group of pentanoic and heptanoic acids with a phosphonate produced potent and selective antagonists.[14] Inclusion of piperidines, piperazines, decahydro-isoquinolines or double bonds in the carbon chain backbone has led to further increases in potency.[15]

Beside the NMDA recognition site, there are several other sites on the NMDA receptor-channel complex which can be pharmacologically manipulated.[16] These include the ion channel itself:

Divalent cations produce a partial and voltage-dependent block of the channel.[17,18] It should, however, be noted that NMDA is a potent excitant of otherwise quiescent neurons in the spinal cord and so depolarization by some other means is not a prerequisite for functional channel activation even in the presence of normal extracellular levels of magnesium.

Compounds such as ketamine, phencyclidine, cyclazocine, dextrorphan and MK-801 all produce a voltage- and use-dependent block of the NMDA channel.[16,19,20] The common behavioral effects of this group of compounds include psychotomimetic activity, analgesia and anticonvulsant activity as well as neuroprotection in various ischaemia and trauma models and are likely due to their NMDA antagonist profile.

Other sites of physiological and pharmacological importance on the NMDA receptor complex include the "glycine site". Discovered almost serendipidously by Johnson and Ascher[21] who showed that activation at this site was necessary for the full effects of NMDA receptor occupancy to be realised. In many studies of the intact CNS, addition of exogenous glycine was found to give only small potentiations of the responses to NMDA whereas antagonists of glycine were able to block its activation.[16,22,23] The activity of HA-966, one of the older established NMDA antagonists, is mediated via the glycine site where it acts as a weak partial agonist. Such results suggest that this site is almost fully activated *in vivo*. Development of more potent and selective glycine-site antagonists and careful experimentation with glycine-free media on isolated systems have shown that co-activation at this site is necessary for NMDA channel opening.[23] Whether glycine is co-released with L-glutamate or whether the ambient extracellular glycine contributes to NMDA receptor-mediated synaptic potentials is still an open question.

Polyamines, zinc, tricyclic antidepressants, alcohol and many other compounds are reported to interact more-or-less specifically with the NMDA receptor-channel complex.[16]

Although there are two genes, nmdaR1 and nmdaR2 with various splice variants[24], there is no clear heterogeneity of NMDA receptor pharmacology well established. The cloned receptors appear to express sites for NMDA, glycine, divalent cations and PCP-like compounds.

With respect to their role in physiology, it has been clear from the earliest studies that NMDA receptors are involved in synaptic processing of spinal afferent information.[4,6] The NMDA receptor component comes into greater prominence with stimuli of higher amplitude and frequency.[25] Polysynaptic reflexes and nociceptive responses of motoneurons are particularly susceptible to NMDA antagonists.[26,27] Activation of conductance changes via the NMDA receptor are, however, intrinsically slower than at AMPA receptors and this may probably accounts for the slow rise time of the EPSPs. NMDA receptors also contribute to neuronal plasticity in the spinal cord,[25,27] as is better established in other areas of the CNS. The use of NMDA antagonists both to ameliorate the symptoms of chronic pain and to prevent the development of hyperexcitable states of nociceptive spinal neurons remains inter alia a distinct therapeutic possibility for this group of drugs.

PHARMACOLOGY OF NON-NMDA RECEPTORS

From the earlier observations on spinal neurons, some pharmacological separation of responses to kainate from those to quisqualate/AMPA were observed with antagonists such as GDEE and GAMS (see above). Displacement of kainate and AMPA by these antagonists was, however, not observed in binding studies. The development of more potent and selective antagonists for these agonists was therefore essential if any advances in non-NMDA pharmacology were to be made. The discovery of such properties within the quinoxalinediones by Honore's group[28] has thus been invaluable. 6,7-Dinitro- (DNQX) and 6-cyano-7-nitro- (CNQX) quinoxaline-2,3-diones are commonly used now for distinguishing non-NMDA receptors but they do suffer from some non-specificity to the glycine site of the NMDA complex, which is absent from 6-nitro-7-sulphamoylbenzo(f) compound (NBQX)[29,30] Furthermore NBQX has an approximately 30-fold greater affinity for AMPA over kainate binding whereas, for DNQX and CNQX, the difference is 3-5-fold.[29]

The ability of even NBQX to select between AMPA and kainate responses of central neurons has, however, been variable. In most cases responses to both agonists applied to the somatic region, e.g. of spinal neurons, are reduced in parallel. This is also the case for spinal neurons,[28,30] suggesting that both AMPA and kainate act on pharmacologically similar receptors. Responses to AMPA are generally rapidly desensitising whereas those to kainate desensitise only marginally. In the presence of desensitised response to AMPA the response to kainate is occluded, suggesting that both agonists share the same receptor.[31]

In other preparations, however, where AMPA and kainate are administered to other than the soma, NBQX preferentially reduces responses to AMPA. Thus, on rat cortical wedges, there is a 30-fold preference for AMPA over kainate responses, suggesting separate receptors mediating the effects of these two agonists.[29,30] This difference is less marked on hemisected rat spinal cords where the kainate dose-response curve shows two phases, a lower part which is resistant to NBQX and an upper part which is sensitive.[32] This was interpreted as showing that at low concentrations kainate acts on NBQX-resistant kainate receptor and at higher concentrations acts on NBQX-sensitive AMPA receptors. Which tissue elements contribute to these responses is at present unknown. Unmyelinated afferent C fibers, however, are uniquely sensitive to kainate rather than AMPA and the potency of NBQX on such responses is similar to that on kainate responses in the cortical wedges (RH Evans personal comm.). Interestingly several barbiturates, of which methoxexitone was the most potent and selective, and the divalent cation, nickel, had the opposite effect, i.e. preferentially antagonising responses to kainate.[32,33]

In addition to competitive antagonists, some 2,3-benzodiazepines, e.g. GYKI52466, are also selective non-NMDA antagonists. They were first described as central muscle relaxants reducing spinal reflexes by a postsynaptic mechanism.[34] Subsequently, GYKI52466 was shown to reduce selectively responses to AMPA rather than those to kainate and NMDA on cortical wedges and AMPA and kainate rather than NMDA on spinal neurons *in vivo*,[35] a pattern of activity similar to that described above for NBQX. But in drug combination experiments it is quite clear that NBQX and GYKI52466 act synergistically rather than additively (AJ Palmer unpublished results), suggesting that they act at different sites on the AMPA receptor complex. No use-dependency has been noticed and hence these compound are likely to act allosterically rather than as channel blockers.

On the other hand, certain polyamine-containing invertebrate toxins such as philanthotoxin from the Egyptian Digger Wasp do block AMPA and kainate responses on spinal neurons *in vivo* in a use-dependent manner consistent with a channel blocking action as suggested at the glutamate receptor on insect muscle.[16,36] In other *in vitro* preparations, however, the selectivity between non-NMDA and NMDA responses is variable and so such toxins must be used with caution as pharmacological tools.[37]

Cyclothiazide and related compounds have recently been shown to reduce the desensitisation of responses to AMPA.[38,39] We found that, on spinal neurons in vivo, cyclothiazide given locally or intravenously (2-5mg/kg) selectively enhanced responses to AMPA and kainate more-or-less equally but not those to NMDA.[40] On cortical wedges, cyclothiazide potentiated AMPA but had little effect on responses to either kainate or NMDA.[41]

Interestingly in both preparations, AMPA antagonism by 2,3-benzodiazepines such as GYKI52466 was almost completely reversed by cyclothiazide whereas inhibition by NBQX was only marginally reduced.[40,41] Such results are very reminiscent of the glycine reversal of HA-966 but not of that by competitive NMDA antagonists and they are consistent with the notion that cyclothiazide and the 2,3-benzodiazepines are acting at the same site.

Since AMPA receptors are thought to be responsible for fast monosynaptic EPSPs and since both responses to AMPA and the synaptic event have a short duration of action due to desensitisation, cyclothiazide would be expected to prolong monosynaptic EPSPs in the spinal cord as has been demonstrated for EPSPs between hippocampal neurons in culture.[38]

In summary, non-NMDA receptor subtypes which are AMPA- or kainate-preferring can be distinguished pharmacologically. Which of the cloned receptor subunits (*gluR1-7, kai1-2*) combine to give such produce such heterogeneity is as yet unknown. Cyclothiazide does, however, enhance currents in Xenopus oocytes expressing *gluR1/2* subunits (L. Simmonds personal comm.) and AMPA is the more potent agonist at *gluR1-4* whereas kainate is more potent at *gluR5-7* and *kai1-2*.

PHARMACOLOGY OF METABOTROPIC GLUTAMATE RECEPTORS

The first described agonists at metabotropic receptors[7,8,9] as measured by a G-protein-coupled increase in phosphatidyl inositol (PI) hydrolysis were L-glutamate, quisqualate and ibotenate but these compounds also activate ionotropic receptors. Aminocyclopentane-dicarboxylic acid (ACPD) also has a similar mixed metabotropic/ionotropic pharmacology but the separation into the four enantiomers showed that 1S,3R-ACPD is the active constituent increasing phospholipase C and decreasing adenylyl cyclase activity.[9] 1S,3R-ACPD has thus become the drug of choice for investigating metabotropic receptors, but see comments below. The L-isomers of two 2-(carboxycyclopropyl)glycines (L-CCG-I and L-CCG-II) are also agonists at the PI coupled metabotropic receptor. Phenyl-glycine (PG) derivatives have proved useful for characterising and differentiating various effects of 1S,3R-ACPD. 4-Carboxy-PG and 3-hydroxy-4-carboxy-PG have a partial agonist profile on PI hydrolysis whereas a-methyl-4-carboxy-PG shows a pure antagonist profile[43] and 3,5-dihydroxy-PG is an agonist.[44]

In electrophysiological tests in non-spinal tissue,[9,45] 1S,3R-ACPD enhances postsynaptic responses to ionotropic agonists and reduces N-type calcium currents and reduces potassium currents. Interestingly low frequency synaptic responses, the predominant effect of 1S,3R-ACPD appears to be a reduction of excitatory synaptic events and this is likely to be due to the reduction in presynaptic calcium currents. By contrast, high frequency stimulation is in part mediated by metabotropic glutamate receptors since 1S,3R-ACPD potentiates such events and the above PG derivatives reduce long term potentiation and nociceptive responses in the thalamus, effects which may be related to reduction of potassium conductances.

On dissociated spinal neurons, 1S,3R-ACPD potentiates the action of AMPA, kainate and NMDA[46]. We have also found *in vivo* that these three agonist are potentiated more or less equally but also that the actions of glycine and GABA are

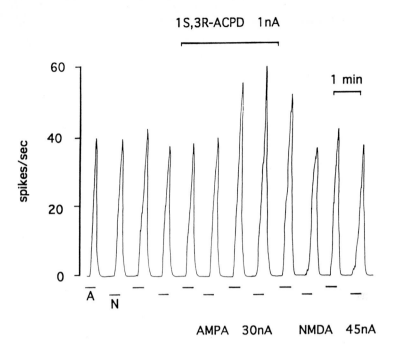

Fig. 1. Effect of 1S,3R-ACPD on responses of a spinal neuron in a pentobarbitone-anaesthetised rat to electrophoretic ejection of AMPA and NMDA for the times and currents indicated. 1nA ejection of 1S,3R-ACPD slowly and reversibly increased the responses to both agonists. Ordinate: spikes/sec. Abscissae: time in min.

also potentiated by similar concentrations of 1S,3R-ACPD (A Bond & D Logde unpublished observation). Such effects are consistent with a decrease in potassium conductance. The time-course of such effects of 1S,3R-ACPD are slower than that of ionotropic agonists such as NMDA and AMPA and are consistent with mediation via second messenger systems. Reflex synaptic potentials between dorsal and ventral roots of neonatal rats are reduced by 1S,3R-ACPD, an effect which is partially antagonised by a-methyl-4-carboxy-PG but not by 4-carboxy-PG.[47] The former antagonist also reduces the similar synaptic depressant effects of L-2-amino-4-phosphonobutyrate (L-AP4).

These results suggest that the metabotropic receptor involved in this response is different from that mediating PI hydrolysis. It seems more likely that the effects are mediated via inhibition of adenylyl cyclase, a common mechanism for presynaptic modulation via reduction of calcium entry.

The nature of metabotropic receptors[48] mediating these effects are unknown. It seems less likely that the PI-linked mGluRs1 & 5 are involved than the negatively cyclase-coupled mGluRs 2-4 & 6. In fact, mGluR4 & 6 are the most probable candidates for the action of L-AP4, although the likelihood of more as yet unknown metabotropic receptors remains.

CONCLUSIONS

There have been considerable developments during the last five years with regard to the molecular biology of glutamate receptors. The pharmacology of the cloned and expressed glutamate receptors, both ionotropic and metabotropic, is emerging rapidly. The medicinal chemistry of non-NMDA ionotropic and metabotropic receptor ligands is proceeding at a similar breath-taking pace. The physiological pharmacology of information processing mediated by glutamate receptors within the spinal cord is still in its infancy but it is reasonable to assume that non-NMDA and NMDA ionotropic receptors mediate synaptic events which have time courses in the order of 10s of msec, 100s of msec and seconds respectively.

REFERENCES

1. CURTIS, D.R. AND WATKINS, J.C. (1963)   Acidic amino acids with strong excitatory actions on mammalian neurons. *J. Physiol.* **166**, 1-14.
2. CURTIS, D.R. AND JOHNSTON, G.A.R. (1974) Amino acid transmitters in the mammalian central nervous system. *Ergebn. Physiol.* **69**,97-188.
3. MCLENNAN, H. (1983) Receptors for excitatory amino acids in the mammalian central nervous system. *Prog. Neurobiol.* **20**,251-271.
4. DAVIES, J. AND WATKINS, J.C. (1979) Selective antagonism of amino acid-induced and synaptic excitation in the cat spinal cord. *J. Physiol.* **297**, 621-636.

5. MCLENNAN, H. AND LODGE, D. (1979) The antagonism of amino acid-induced excitation of spinal neurons in the cat. *Brain Res.* **169**, 83-90.
6. WATKINS, J.C. AND EVANS, R.H. (1981) Excitatory amino acid transmitters. *Ann. Rev. Pharmacol Toxicol.* **21**, 165-204.
7. SLADECZEK, F.A.J., RECASENS, M. AND BOCKAERT, J. (1988) A new mechanism for glutamate receptor action: phosphoinositide hydrolysis. *Trends Pharmacol. Sci.* **11**, 545-549.
8. BASKYS, A. (1992) Metabotropic receptors and 'slow' excitatory actions of glutamate agonists in the hippocampus. *Trends Neurosci.* **15**, 92-96.
9. SCHOEPP, D.D. AND CONN, P.J. (1993) Metabotropic receptors in brain function and pathology. *Trends Pharmacol. Sci.* **14**,13-25.
10. KROGSGAARD-LARSEN, P.. HONORE, T., HANSEN, J.J., CURTIS, D.R. AND LODGE, D. (1980) New class of glutamate agonist structurally related to ibotenic acid. *Nature* **284**, 64-66.
11. SHINOZAKI, H., ISHIDA, K., SHIMAMOTO, K. AND OHFUNE, Y. (1989) A conformationally restricted analogue of L-glutamate, the threo-folded form of L-a-(carboxycyclopropyl)glycine activates the NMDA-type receptor more markedly than NMDA in the isolated rat spinal cord. *Brain Res.* **480**, 355-359.
12. LANTHORN, T.H., HOOD, W.F., WATSON, G.B., COMPTON, R.P., RADER, R.K., GAONI, Y. AND MONAHAN, J.B. (1990) cis-2,4-Methano-glutamate is a potent and selective N-methyl-D-aspartate receptor agonist. *Eur. J. Pharmacol.* **182**, 397-404.
13. SCHOEPP, D.D., SMITH, C.L., LODGE, D., MILLAR, J.D., LEANDER, J.D., SACAAN, A.I. AND LUNN, W.H.W. (1991) D,L-(Tetrazol-5-yl) glycine: a novel and highly potent NMDA receptor agonist. *Eur. J. Pharmacol.* **203**, 237-243.
14. EVANS, R.H., FRANCIS ,A.A., JONES, A.W., SMITH, D.A.S. AND WATKINS, J.C. (1982) The effects of a series of w-phosphonic a-carboxylic amino acids on electrically evoked and excitant amino acid-induced responses in isolated spinal cord preparations. *Brit. J. Pharmacol.* **75**, 65-75.
15. ORNSTEIN, P.L., SCHOEPP, D.D., FULLER, R.W., LEANDER, J.D. AND LODGE, D. (1992) The discovery and development of competitive NMDA antagonists as therapeutic agents. In: *Drug Research Related to Neuroactive Amino Acids,* Alfred Benzon Symposium 32. eds. A. Schousboe, N.H. Diemer and H. Kofod. Copenhagen: Munksgaard.
16. LODGE, D. and JOHNSON, K.M. (1990) Noncompetitive excitatory amino acid antagonists. *Trends Pharmacol. Sci.* **11**, 81-86.
17. AULT, B., EVANS, R.H., FRANCIS, A.A., OAKES, D.J. and WATKINS, J.C. (1980) Selective depression of excitatory amino acid induced depolarizations by magnesium ions in isolated spinal cord preparations. *J. Physiol.* **307**, 413-428.
18. NOWAK, L., BREGESTOVSKI, P., ASCHER, P., HERBET, A. AND PROCHIANTZ, A. (1984) Magnesium gates glutamate-activated channels in mouse central neurons. *Nature* **307**, 462-466.
19. ANIS, N.A., BERRY, S.C., BURTON, N.R. AND LODGE, D. (1983) The dissociative anaesthetics, ketamine and phencyclidine, selectively reduce excitation of central mammalian neurons by N-methylaspartate. *Brit. J. Pharmacol.* **79**, 565-575.

20 MACDONALD, J.F., NOWAK, L.M. (1990) Mechanisms of blockade of excitatory amino acid receptor channels. *Trends Pharmacol. Sci.* **11**, 167-172.

21. JOHNSON, J.W.AND ASCHER, P. (1987) Glycine potentiates the NMDA response in cultured mouse brain neurons. *Nature* **325**, 529-531.

22.. FLETCHER EJ, LODGE D, Glycine reverses antagonism of N-methyl-D-aspartate (NMDA) by 1-hydroxy-3-pyrrolidone-2 (HA-966) but not be D-2-amino-5-phosphonovalerate (D-AP5). *Eur. J. Pharmacol.* **151**, 161-162.

23. KEMP, J.A., LEESON, P.D. (1993) The glycine site of the NMDA receptor - five years on. *Trends Pharmaco. Sci.* **14**, 20-25.

24. SOMMER, B. AND SEEBURG, P.H. (1992) Glutamate receptor channels: novel properties and new clones. *Trends Pharmacol. Sci.* **13**, 291-296.

25. DAVIES, S.N. AND LODGE, D. (1987) Evidence of involvement of N-methylaspartate receptors in 'wind up' of class 2 neurons in the dorsal horn of the rat. *Brain Res.* **424**, 402-406.

26. LODGE, D. AND ANIS, N.A. (1984) Effects of ketamine and three other short acting anaesthetics on spinal reflexes and inhibition in the cat. *Brit. J. Anaesth.* **56**, 1143-1151.

27. HEADLEY, P.M. AND GRILLNER, S. (1990) Excitatory amino acids and synaptic transmission: the evidence for physiological function. *Trends Pharmacol. Sci.* **11**, 205-211.

28. HONORE, T., DAVIES, S.N., DREJER, J., FLETCHER, E.J., JACOBSEN, P. AND LODGE, D. NIESEN FE (1988) Quinoxalinediones: Potent and competitive non-N-methyl-D-aspartate glutamate receptor antagonists. *Science* **241**, 701-703.

29. SHEARDOWN, M.J., NIELSEN, E.O., HANSEN, A.J., JACOBSEN, P. AND HONORE, T. (1990) 2,3-Dihdroxy-6-nitro-7-suphamoylbenzo [f]quinoxaline: a neuro-protectant in cerebral ischaemia. *Science* **247**, 571-574.

30. LODGE, D., JONES, M.G. AND PALMER, A.J. (1990) Excitatory amino acids: new tools for old stories. *Can. J. Physiol. Pharmacol.* **69**, 1123-1128.

31. PATNEAU, D.K. AND MAYER, M.L. (1991) Kinetic analysis of interactions between kainate and AMPA: evidence for activation of a single receptor in mouse hippocampal neurons. *Neuron* **6**, 785-798.

32. ZEMANL, S. AND LODGE, D., (1992) Pharmacological characterisation of non-NMDA subtypes of glutamate receptor in the neonatal hemisected rat spinal cord. *Eur. J. Pharmacol.* **106**, 367-372.

33. PALMER, A.J., ZEMAN, S. AND LODGE, D. (1992) Methohexitone and nickel are selctive antagonistsof kainate on rat cortical slices. *Mol. Neuropharmacol.* **2**, 43-45.

34. TARNAWA, I.S., FARKAS, P., BERSENYI, P., PATAKI, A. AND ANDRASI, F. (1989) Electrophysiological studies with a 2,3-benzodiazepine muscle relaxant: GYKI52466. *Eur. J. Pharmacol.* **167**, 193-199.

35. LODGE, D., JONES, M.G., PALMER, A.J. AND ZEMAN, S. (1992) Electrophysiology of glutamate receptors. In: *Drug Research Related to Neuroactive Amino Acids.* Alfred Benzon Symposium 32. eds. A. Schousboe, N.H. Diemer, H. Kofod. Copenhagen: Munksgaard.

36. JONES, M.G. AND LODGE, D. (1991) Comparison of some arthropod toxins and toxin fragments as antagonists of excitatory amino acid-induced excitation of rat spinal neurons. *Eur. J. Pharmacol.* **106**, 367-372.

37. SCOTT, R.H., SUTTON, K.G. AND DOLPHIN, A.C. (1993) Interactions of polyamines with neuronal ion channels. *Trends Pharmacol. Sci.* **16**, 153-160.

38. PATNEAU, D.K., VYKLICKY, L, JR. AND MAYER, M.L. (1992) Cyclothiazide modulates excitatory synaptic transmission and AMPA/kainate receptor desensitisation in hippocampal cultures. *Soc. Neurosci. Abst.* **18**, 115.

39. YAMADA, K.A. (1992) Thiazide diuretics reversibly block postsynaptic glutamate receptor desensitisation in rat hippocamapl neurons. *Soc. Neurosci. Abst.* **18**, 757

40. LODGE, D., BOND, A. AND PALMER, A.J. (1993) Interaction between cyclothiazide and 2,3-benzodiazepines on non-N-methyl-D-aspartate receptors in rat neocortex in vitro and spinal cord in vivo. *Brit. J. Pharmacol.* (in press).

41. PALMER, A.J. AND LODGE, D. (1993) Cyclothiazide reverses AMPA receptor antagonism of the 2,3-benzodiazepine, GYKI53655. *Eur. J. Pharmacol.* **244**, 193-194.

42. SHINOZAKI, H. AND ISHIDA, M. (1991) Recent advances in the study of glutamate agonists. *Asia Pacif. J. Pharmacol.* **6**, 293-316.

43. PORTER, R.H.P., ROBERTS, P.J., JANE, D.E., SUNTER, D.C. AND WATKINS, J.C. (1993) Phenylglycine derivatives as competitive antagonists at glutamate metabotropic receptors (mGluRs) *Brit. J. Pharmacol.* (in press).

44. ITO, I., KOHDA, A., TANABE, S., HIROSE, E., HAYASHI, M., MITSUNGA, S. AND SUGIYAMA, H. (1992) 3,5-Dihydroxyphenylglycine: a potent agonist of metabotropic glutamate receptors. *NeuroReport* **3**, 1013-1016.

45. MILLER, R.J. (1991) Metabotropic excitatory amino acid receptors reveal their true colours. *Trends Pharmacol. Sci.* **12**, 365-368.

46. BLEAKMAN, D., RUSIN, K.I., CHARD, P.S., GLAUM, S.R. AND MILLER, R.J. (1992) Metabotropic glutamate receptors potentiate ionotropic glutamate responses in the rat dorsal horn. *Mol. Pharmacol.* **42**, 192-196.

47. POOK, P.C.-K., BIRSE, E.F., JANE, D.E., JONES, A.W., JONES, P.L.S.T.J., MEWETT, K.N., SUNTER, D.C., UDVARHELYI, P.M., WHARTON, B. AND WATKINS, J.C. (1993) Differential actions of the metabotropic glutamate receptor antagonists 4C-PG and aM4C-PG at L-AP4-like receptors in neonatal rat spinal cord. *Brit. J. Pharmacol. Proc.* (in press).

48. TANABE, Y., MASU, T., ISHII, T., SHIGEMOTO, R. AND NAKANISHI, S. (1992) A family of metabotropic receptors. *Neuron* **8**, 169-179.

EXCITATORY AMINO ACID RELEASE IN DORSAL ROOT GANGLION CULTURES

Fang Liu, Ksenija Jeftinija and Srdija Jeftinija
Department of Veterinary Anatomy and Neuroscience Program
Iowa State University, Ames, Iowa 50011
USA

INTRODUCTION

The mechanisms underlying chemical transmission at $A\delta$ and C fiber synapses in the dorsal horn are not resolved. A great deal of interest has been directed towards excitatory amino acids (EAA) , L-aspartate (Asp) and L-glutamate (Glu), as sensory neurotransmitters in the spinal cord. Chemical[10] and immunocytochemical studies have shown that 15-30% of rat dorsal root ganglion (DRG) neurons were immunoreactive to Glu.[2] Furthermore, Asp- and Glu-like immunoreactivity are contained in 15% and 8.2% of unmyelinated and 4% and 2.3% of myelinated dorsal root (DR) axons, respectively.[22,23] Electrophysiological studies provided the evidence that EAA depolarise spinal neurons and excitatory postsynaptic potentials (EPSP), evoked by primary afferent stimulation, are blocked by EAA antagonists.[10,14,21] More recent evidence suggests a role for EAAs in pain transmission as nociceptive stimulation produces a significant increase in the apparent release of Asp and Glu in the dorsal spinal cord of awake rats.[15] The presence of EAAs in neurons and glia intrinsic to the spinal dorsal horn as well as descending spinal projections could be responsible for release of EAA in the dorsal horn area in response to DR stimulation. In light of that uncertainty, the specific objective of the present study was to determine whether EAAs are released specifically from primary afferent neurons. We used high K^+ and chemical irritants capsaicin[17,19] and bradykinin[6,8,16] to evoke EAA release from organotypic DRG cultures which offer several advantages over *in vivo* and *in vitro* slice preparations.

NATO ASI Series, Vol. H 79
Cellular Mechanisms of Sensory Processing
Edited by Laszlo Urban
© Springer-Verlag Berlin Heidelberg 1994

METHODS

Experiments were performed on organotypic Petri dish cultures of dorsal root ganglions (DRG) from Sprague-Dawley rats. Organotypic DRG cultures were prepared according to methods described by Gähwiler[9] with some modifications.[11] Following anesthesia with ether or decapitation, the spinal cord with DRG from 1 to 8 days old rats was rapidly removed and washed in cold (4°C) oxygenated Gey's balanced salt solution (GBSS; Gibbco) modified by the addition of 2.0% glucose. Culturing was carried out on glass coverslips. DRGs were cleaned of connective tissue and stored in the modified GBSS for 1 hour at 4°C. Isolated explants were placed on a glass coverslip completely covered with chicken plasma coagulated with thrombin. The coverslips bearing the explants were placed into 35mm Petri dishes and incubated in a humid 5% CO_2 atmosphere at 36°C. The culture medium contained 25% horse serum, 25% Earls Balanced Salt Solution, and 50% Basal Medium Eagles with glucose (6.4mg/ml).

DRG explants cultured for 1 to 2 weeks were then mounted into a perfusion chamber. The coverslip bearing 2-3 DRG cultures was placed into recesses of a 50µl plexiglas chamber. Ringer solution (in mM: NaCl 127, KCl 1.9, KH_2PO_4 1.2, $CaCl_2$ 2.4, $MgSO_4$ 1.3, $NaHCO_3$ 26, glucose 10, pH=7.4, 31±1°C) was perfused at a rate of 200 µl/min. After equilibration 200µl perfusate samples were taken at one min intervals for determination of basal concentrations of amino acids. Following this control period, the cultures were exposed for a 1-2 min period to potassium (50mM), capsaicin and bradykinin (for details see Jeftinija et al., 1991).[11]

In some experiments neurite cultures were prepared from established DRG cultures (4-6 day old cultures): the DRG explant was removed (leaving the neurites only) 4-6 hours prior to the release experiments.

Glia cultures were prepared by removing DRGs from established cultures (4 to 5 days old cultures) and allowing only glial elements to grow for an additional 72 hours.

Amino acid content in the samples of bathing solution were determined by high-performance liquid chromatography (HPLC) with fluorescence detection. The amounts of L-Glu and L-Asp were expressed in nMols. Basal rates of EAA released were determined as the mean of the EAA content in 3 samples collected just prior to stimulation with potassium, capsaicin or bradykinin. All data are presented as the mean values±S.E.M. Groups were compared using Student's t-test.

RESULTS

Excitatory amino acids are released from cultured sensory neurons in response to chemical stimulation

High potassium, capsaicin and bradykinin were used to stimulate DRG cultures. Exposure of DRG cultures to Ringer's buffer containing 3.6mM KCl results in a resting or basal release of Glu (58.3±7.9nM/1min; n=28) and Asp (33.4±3.9nM/min; n=28). When the extracellular concentration of KCl was increased to 50mM, the release of Asp and Glu was increased significantly to 166±17% and 155±12% of the control concentration, respectively (n=6; Figure 1A).

Application of capsaicin, a selective excitant of nociceptive primary afferent neurons, in concentrations of 1 to 10µM, produced an increase in the concentrations of Asp and Glu (Figure 1). The peak concentrations of Asp and Glu significantly increased to 204±11% (P<0.01) and 165±15% (P<0.01) of basal concentrations respectively, in response to a 1min exposure to 10µM capsaicin. When cultures were exposed to the vehicle alone no increase in concentrations of Asp and Glu was observed (n=6).

The recently introduced capsaicin antagonist capsazepine[20] was tested in our model in order to establish the role of capsaicin receptors. Capsazepine (10µM) blocked the release of EAAs evoked by 3µM capsaicin (Figure 1B). On the other hand capsazepine did not affect the release of EAAs evoked by high potassium (Figure 1B).

Tetrodotoxin (10µM) did not affect the release of Asp and Glu evoked by capsaicin or high potassium. Furthermore, when cultures were superfused with a sodium-free solution for over 30 min, brief application of capsaicin still resulted in an increase in the release of EAAs.

To test the requirement of calcium in the effects of capsaicin cultures were preincubated for 15 min or longer in a solution containing 0.2mM Ca²⁺, 1mM EGTA and 2.5 mM Mg. Capsaicin was applied for the same period as in control experiments and tissues were washed in a low Ca, EGTA solution. Under these conditions capsaicin (10µM) and high potassium failed to induce an increase in the release of EAAs (Figure 1C).

Ruthenium red (1µM) when applied for 4 min prior to the application of 10µM capsaicin completely abolished capsaicin-evoked release of EAAs (Figure 1D). This effect of ruthenium red was selective against capsaicin, because high potassium-evoked EAA-release was not affected (Figure 1D).

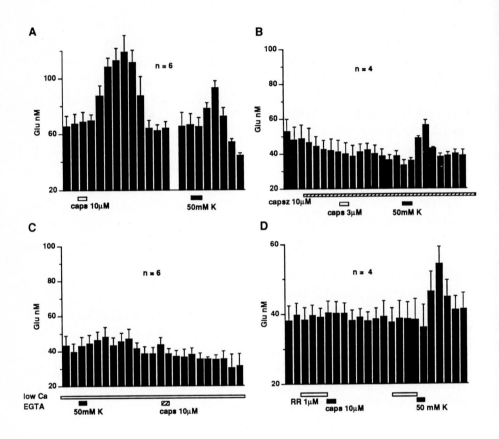

Figure 1. A. Time course of changes in the concentration of glutamate following exposure of the culture to capsaicin (10μM) and 50mM potassium. Each bar represents the concentration of glutamate in 200μl of 1 min sample.
B. Bath application of capsazepine abolished the effect of capsaicin and was without effect on potassium-evoked release of glutamate.
C. Time course and magnitude of the increase in the concentration of glutamate induced by high potassium and capsaicin in culture perfused for 30 min in low Ca^{2+} EGTA solution.
D. Ruthenium red (RR, 1μM) applied for four min prior to application of capsaicin on DRG cultures abolished the effect of capsaicin but was without effect on potassium-induced increase in the concentration of glutamate.

Release of excitatory amino acids from neurites

The basal release of glutamate and aspartate from neurites was 55±12 nM (n=5) and 14±2 nM respectively. Addition of 10µM capsaicin for one min caused a 210±20% increase in the release of glutamate and a 250±24% increase in the release of aspartate. High potassium produced approximately a 150% increase in the release of glutamate and aspartate. This stimulatory effect of high potassium and capsaicin on neurite cultures was abolished in low Ca-EGTA solution (n=6).

The concentration of the amino acid serine did not change in response to high potassium or capsaicin (n=18).

Glia as source of excitatory amino acids

Using primary glial cultures from DRG we demonstrated that bradykinin releases Glu and Asp by mobilising calcium from internal stores.

The basal release of glutamate and aspartate from glial cultures was 26±2nM and 6±1nM respectively. Addition of bradykinin caused a dose-dependent increase in the release of glutamate and aspartate. Ten nM bradykinin caused greater than nine-fold increase in the release of glutamate to 239±41nM and a five-fold increase in the release of aspartate to 30±4nM (Figure 2a,b). A second application of bradykinin similarly caused EAA release, although the magnitude of this response was attenuated compared to the first bradykinin response. This action is receptor-mediated since the B_2 receptor antagonist (D-Arg[0], Hyp[3], ß-Thi[5,8], D-Phe[7])-bradykinin (5uM) reversibly blocked the stimulatory action of bradykinin (Figure 2c). Bradykinin did not significantly affect the release of serine from glial cultures. The basal level of serine was 14±2nM compared to 16±2 in the presence of bradykinin (n=13; P>0.5). These data demonstrate that bradykinin potently causes release of glutamate and aspartate from glia.

The removal of external calcium from the bathing medium did not prevent bradykinin from stimulating the release of EAAs from glial cultures (Figure 2d). However, a second application of bradykinin in 0.2mM Ca/1mM EGTA saline solution failed to stimulate EAA release (Figure 2d). These data suggest that bradykinin mobilised calcium from intracellular stores. To test this hypothesis, we incubated glial cultures for 30 minutes in 50µM BAPTA-AM [5,5'-dimethyl-1,2-bis(2-aminophenoxy)ethane-N,N,N',N'-tetraacetic-acid acetoxymethyl ester]. This membrane permeant calcium chelator blocked the stimulatory action of bradykinin on EAA release (Figure 2e). Furthermore thapsigargin, the Ca-ATPase inhibitor [18], blocked the BK induced release of EAAs (n=8). As a critical test of the "calcium hypothesis" we exposed cultures to the Ca^{2+} ionophore ionomycin for 2 minutes in calcium-containing saline. Addition of ionomycin (1μM) stimulated the release of both Glu (Figure 2f) and Asp from cultured glia. Subsequent addition of bradykinin (10nM) stimulated the release of EAAs (Figure 2f). Ionomycin was ineffective to

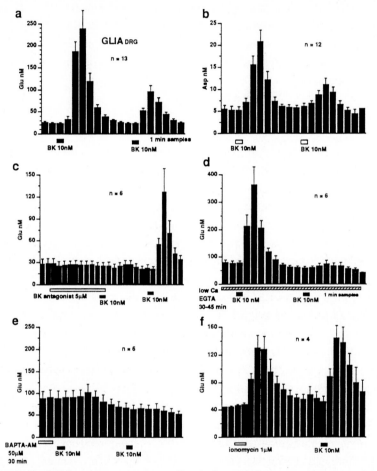

Figure 2. Bradykinin causes a receptor-mediated release of glutamate and aspartate from glia. Addition of bradykinin (10nM) caused a 9-fold elevation of glutamate (a), and a 6-fold elevation of aspartate release (b). Second application of bradykinin resulted in increase of EAA release. The B2 receptor antagonist (D-Arg[0], Hyp[3], ß-Thi[5,8], D-Phe[7])-bradykinin (5μM) reversibly blocked stimulatory effect of bradykinin (c). Removal of extracellular calcium did not prevent the stimulatory effect of bradykinin, however, abolished the effect of successive application of bradykinin (d). BAPTA-AM, a membrane permeant calcium chelator, blocked the stimulatory action of bradykinin on glutamate release (e). Addition of ionomycin stimulated the release of glutamate from cultured Schwann cells and subsequent addition of bradykinin stimulated the release of glutamate (f).

stimulate EAA release when calcium was omitted from the bathing medium (n=4). These data demonstrate that calcium is necessary for stimulating the release of EAAs from glial cultures. The specific mechanism of EAA release from glial cultures is unclear. Glial cultures were free of immunoreactivity for the synaptic proteins synaptophysin and synaptotagmin while axons of DRG explants (separate cultures; data not shown) were immunopositive for these synaptic proteins. Thus, proteins characteristic of neuronal transmitter release apparatus are absent in the glia.

DISCUSSION

The present results demonstrate that aspartate and glutamate are released into the bathing medium following depolarization of cultured sensory neurons with either high K^+ or capsaicin. The basal concentrations of neither amino acid changed if the same stimuli were used on cultures consisting of glial elements only. These data suggest that activation of capsaicin-sensitive C-fibers may result in the release of Asp and Glu. These results are consistent with the previous findings that electrical or chemical stimulation of sensory neurons increased the concentration of EAAs in spinal cord perfusate *in vitro*[12] and in extracellular fluid of the dorsal spinal cord *in vivo*.[15] While the origin of the EAA pools was unknown in previous work, the results of the present study directly demonstrate the ability of the primary afferent fibers to release Asp and Glu and suggest that part of the EAA released *in vivo* may have originated from sensory neuronal input to the spinal cord.

Our findings, establishing a relationship between effective concentrations of capsaicin and release of EAAs are in agreement with previous studies.[13] Ten µM capsaicin was reported to evoke maximal EAA-release and a decreased response was evident with repeated application,[13] therefore we did not use higher concentrations of capsaicin than 10µM.

Using primary glial cultures from DRG we demonstrated that bradykinin released calcium from internal stores which in turn stimulated the release of the EAAs glutamate and aspartate.

The specific mechanism of EAA release from glial cultures is unclear. Glial cultures were free of immunoreactivity for synaptic proteins while axons of DRG cultures (separate cultures) were immunoreactive for these synaptic proteins. The regulated release of glutamate and aspartate from glia may be a widespread property. Since many neurotransmitters utilized by the nervous system, can mobilise calcium in glia (for review see Barres[1]), it is possible that neurons have in addition to their fast neuron-to-neuron synaptic interactions, a calcium mobilising action on neighboring glia[5] which in turn leads to the release of other neurotransmitters.

The specific roles for release of EAA from glial cells remains to be elucidated. However, elevations of external glutamate and aspartate are likely to modulate neuronal properties including excitability and synaptic transmission. Given the important role of glutamate in the induction of long-term potentiation, it is important to determine whether glia would regulate synaptic plasticity, learning and memory, and whether excessive glutamate release from glia leads to neurodegenerative disorders (for review see Choi[3]).

ACKNOWLEDGEMENT: We thank Drs A. Fox and L. Urban for helpful comments on the manuscript. This work was supported by National Institute of Health Grant NS 27751.

REFERENCES

1. BARRES, B.A., (1991) New roles for glia. *J. Neurosci.* **11**, 3685-3694.
2. BATTAGLIA, G. AND RUSTIONI, A., (1988) Co-existence of glutamate and substance P in dorsal root ganglion neurons of the rat and monkey, *J. Comp. Neurol.*, **277**, 302-312.
3. CHOI, D.W. (1988) Glutamate neurotoxicity and diseases of the nervous system. Neuron **1**, 623-634.
4. CHRISTENSEN, B.N. AND PERL, E.R. (1970) Spinal neurons specifically excited by noxious or thermal stimuli: marginal zone of the dorsal horn. *J. Neurophysiol.* **33**, 293-307.
5. DANI, J.W., CHERNJEVSKY, A. AND SMITH, S J. (1992) Neuronal activity triggers calcium waves in hippocampal astrocyte networks. *Neuron* **8**, 429-440.
6. DRAY, A., PATEL, I.A., PERKINS, M.N. AND RUEFF, A. (1992) Bradykinin-induced activation of nociceptors: receptor and mechanistic studies on the neonatal reat spinal cord-tail preparation *in vitro*. *Br. J. Pharmacol.* **107**, 1129-1134.
7. DUGGAN, A.W. AND JOHNSTON, G.A.R. (1970) Glutamate and related amino acids in cat spinal roots, dorsal root ganglion, and peripheral nerves. *J. Neurochem.* **17**, 1205-1208.

8. DUNN, P.M. AND RANG, H.P. (1990) Bradykinin-induced depolarisation of primary afferent nerve terminals in the neonatal rat spinal cord in vitro. *Br. J. Pharmacol.* **100**, 656-660.

9. GÄHWILER, B.H. (1981) Organotypic monolayer cultures of nervous tissue. *J. Neurosci. Methods* **4**, 329-342.

10. JEFTINIJA, S. (1989) Excitatory transmission in the dorsal horn is in part mediated through APV-sensitive NMDA receptors. *Neurosci. Lett.* **96**, 191-196.

11. JEFTINIJA, S., JEFTINIJA, K., LIU, F., SKILLING, S. R., SMULLIN, D. H. AND LARSON, A. A. (1991) Excitatory amino acids are released from rat primary afferent neurons *in vitro. Neurosci. Lett.* **125**, 191-194.

12. KAWAGOE, R., ONODERA, K. AND TAKEUCHI, A. (1986) The release of endogenous glutamate from the newborn rat spinal cord induced by dorsal root stimulation and substance *P. Biomed. Res.* **7**, 253-259.

13. MARSH, S.J., STANSFELD, C.E., BROWN, D.A., DAVEY, R. AND MCCARTHY, D. (1987) The mechanism of action of capsaicin on sensory C-type neurons and their axons *in vitro, Neuroscience* **23**, 275-289.

14. SALT, T.E. AND HILL, R.G. (1983) Neurotransmitter candidates of somatosensory primary afferent fibers. *Neuroscience* **10**, 1083-1103.

15. SKILLING, S.R., SMULLIN, D. H. AND LARSON, A.A. (1988) Extracellular amino acid concentrations in the dorsal spinal cord of freely moving rats following veratridine and nociceptive stimulation. *J. Neurochem.* **51,** 127-132.

16. STERANKA, L.R., MANNING, D.C., DEHAAS, J.R., CONNOR, R.J., VAVREK, J. M., STEWART, S. AND SNYDER, S.H. (1988) Bradykinin as a pain mediator: Receptors are localized to sensory neurones, and antagonists have analgesic actions. *Proc. Natl. Acad. Sci. U.S.A.* **85**, 3245-3249.

17. SZOLCSANYI, J. (1984) Capsaicin: hot new pharmacological tool. *Trends Neurosci.* **4**, 495-497.

18. THASTRUP, O., CULLEN, P.J., DROBAK, B.K., HANLEY, M.R. AND DAWSON, A.P. (1990) Thapsigargin, a tumor promoter, discharges intracellular Ca2+ stores by specific inhibition of the endoplasmic reticulum Ca2+-ATPase. *Proc. Natl. Acad. Sci. USA* **87**, 2466-2470.

19. URBAN, L. AND DRAY, A. (1992) Synaptic activation of dorsal horn neurons by selective C-fibre excitation with capsaicin in the mouse spinal cord in vitro. *Neuroscience* **47**, 693-702.

20. URBAN, L. AND DRAY, A. (1991) Capsazepine, a novel capsaicin antagonist, selectively antagonises the effects of capsaicin in the mouse spinal cord in vitro. *Neurosci. Lett.*, **134, 9-11.**

21. WATKINS, J.C. AND EVANS, R.H. (1981) Excitatory amino acid transmitters. *Annu. Rev. Pharmacol. Toxicol.* **21**, 165-204.

22. WESTLUND, K.N., MCNEILL, D.L. AND COGGESHALL, R.E. (1989) Glutamate-immunoreactive axons in normal rat dorsal roots. *Neurosci. Lett.* **96**, 13-17.

23. WESTLUND, K.N., MCNEILL, D.L., PATTERSON, J.T. AND COGGESHALL, R.E. (1989) Aspartate immunoreactive axons in normal rat L_4 dorsal roots. *Brain Res.* **489**, 347-351.

THE INVOLVEMENT OF EXCITATORY AMINO ACIDS AND THEIR RECEPTORS IN THE SPINAL PROCESSING OF NOCICEPTIVE INPUT FROM THE NORMAL AND INFLAMED KNEE JOINT IN THE RAT

Hans-Georg Schaible, Volker Neugebauer, Thomas Lücke
Physiologisches Institut, Universität Würzburg
Röntgenring 9, D-8700 Würzburg
F.R.G.

INTRODUCTION

Several studies have shown that excitatory amino acids such as L-glutamate are involved in the processing of nociceptive information in the dorsal and ventral horn of the spinal cord. Since it has become clear that excitatory amino acids activate different types of receptors on postsynaptic neurons efforts are made to identify the importance of these receptor types for the different aspects of nociceptive processing, namely (1) the mediation of nociceptive information under normal conditions and (2) the development of hyperexcitability of neurons which is seen in pathophysiological states such as injury or inflammation of the tissue and nerve lesions. Briefly, glutamate receptor subtypes include the ionotropic NMDA receptor (activated by the specific agonist N-methyl-D-aspartate), the ionotropic non-NMDA receptors (activated by the agonists alpha-amino-3-hydroxy-5-methyl-4-isoxazolepropionic acid, AMPA, and kainate), and the metabotropic receptor activated by trans-(±)-1-amino-(1S,3R)-cyclopentane dicarboxylic acid (t-ACPD). [8,16,17,29,30,43] The NMDA receptor has gained considerable interest since it is a "conditional" receptor[10] that is blocked by Mg^{2+} ions unless the depolarization of the neuron is sufficient to remove the block.[28,29,38] When opened, NMDA receptors allow the entry of Ca^{2+} into the neuron.[4,39] It is thought that these characteristics qualify the NMDA receptor to play a key role in processes of neuronal plasticity.

In studies of nociception most attention has been directed towards the NMDA receptors. In awake animals the intrathecal application of NMDA caused

NATO ASI Series, Vol. H 79
Cellular Mechanisms of Sensory Processing
Edited by Laszlo Urban
© Springer-Verlag Berlin Heidelberg 1994

nociceptive behavior.[2,5,40] Furthermore the development of hyperalgesia in the course of neuropathies,[11,26,27,51,62,] ischemia,[54,52] formalin-induced tissue damage,[7,31] heat injury[6] and carrageenan- or Freund's complete adjuvant-induced subcutaneous inflammation of the foot[42] is attenuated or prevented by intraperitoneal and/or intrathecal application of NMDA antagonists suggesting a role of NMDA receptors in these conditions. The non-NMDA antagonist 6-cyano-7-nitroquinoxaline-2,3-dione (CNQX) had antinociceptive effects in the hot plate, tail flick and formalin tests in one study[33] but not in the formalin test in another one.[7] Thermal hyperalgesia in neuropathic rats could be reduced by pre-injury treatment with CNQX but not by application of CNQX at day 3 after nerve ligation. [26]

Electrophysiological studies *in vitro* have shown the involvement of NMDA and non-NMDA receptors in the responses of spinal cord neurons evoked by electrical stimulation of dorsal roots[18,24,25,32,49,63] or by application of capsaicin to dorsal roots[32,60]. Indications for different roles of NMDA and non-NMDA receptors in the nociceptive processing have come in particular from studies which showed that non-selective antagonists reduce the responses of spinal cord neurons to electrical stimulation of A and C fibers in peripheral nerves whilst NMDA antagonists reduce only or preferentially the "wind up" phenomenon, i.e. the increase of the responses to repetitive C-fiber stimulation.[12,13,18,24,59] The involvement of NMDA receptors in the processing of natural noxious stimuli is not settled. NMDA receptors seem to be involved in the neuronal discharges in pathological conditions such as inflammation,[42,44] ischemia,[54] application of mustard oil,[61] injection of formalin into the paw[20] and intradermal injections of capsaicin.[14] On the other hand NMDA antagonists also reduced the responses of spinal cord neurons to noxious mechanical stimuli under normal conditions[9,21] suggesting that the role of NMDA receptors is not necessarily restricted to pathophysiological states. There are less electrophysiological studies on the importance of non-NMDA receptors. The non-NMDA receptor antagonist CNQX reduced the responses of spinothalamic neurons in the monkey to innocuous and noxious stimulation of the skin and to the intradermal injection of capsaicin and CNQX reduced the generation of hyperexcitability following the injection of capsaicin.[14]

Spinal cord neurons with joint input show pronounced hyperexcitability during the development of inflammation in the joint.[15,36,37,45,48] There is already some evidence that excitatory amino acids and their receptors are involved in the neuronal activity during joint inflammation. In a model of acute arthritis CNQX and NMDA antagonists reduced or delayed the intraspinal release of glutamate and aspartate in the awake rat[56] that is usually associated with development of arthritis.[55,57] Spinal cord neurons with joint input in the cat[44] and spinothalamic neurons with joint input in the monkey[15] were activated by excitatory amino acids and the activity of neurons in the spinal cord with input from the inflamed knee was reduced by NMDA antagonists.[44] In the present experiments the involvement of NMDA and non-NMDA receptors in the processing of afferent input from the knee joint was further addressed in the anesthetized rat using microionophoresis of antagonists and agonists close to the neurons. Firstly, we examined whether the application of NMDA and/or non-NMDA antagonists would interfere with the responses of spinal neurons to innocuous and noxious mechanical stimuli applied to the normal knee joint. Secondly, we investigated whether the application of non-NMDA and/or NMDA antagonists would influence the development of hyperexcitability of the neurons with joint input which is usually seen in the course of an acute inflammation. Part of the data have been published elsewhere.[34,35]

METHODS

Anesthesia and dissection. All experiments were performed on male Wistar rats (220-360g) anesthetized by an initial intraperitoneal injection of 75-125 mg/kg sodium thiopentone (Trapanal, BYK Ltd) and further i.p. injections as required for deep anesthesia. The depth of anesthesia was assessed by regularly testing the corneal blink and hind paw withdrawal reflexes which had to be absent and, after insertion of the cannula in the carotid artery, by measurement of the mean arterial blood pressure (it was usually stable between 100-120 mmHg during surgery and recordings). Spontaneous respiration was assisted by blowing a gentle jet of oxygen towards the opening of the tracheal cannula. The body temperature was kept at 37-39°C using a homeothermic blanket system.

Induction of experimental inflammation. In part of the experiments an experimental inflammation was induced in the left knee joint whilst a neuron was recorded. A small needle was inserted into the joint cavity through the patellar ligament. First about 0.06 ml kaolin (4%) were slowly injected and after removal of the needle the knee joint was flexed and extended for 15 min. Thereafter 0.06 ml carrageenan (2%) were injected using the same approach and the joint was flexed and extended for 5 min. The development of inflammation was documented by measuring the circumference of the leg in the knee region. Details of this experimental inflammation are described elsewhere.[45,46,47,48]

Recording from neurons with joint input. After a laminectomy (segments L1-L6), dorsal horn neurons were recorded extracellularly in the segments L2-L3 using glass insulated carbon filaments. Neurons were identified that responded to pressure applied across the knee joint but not to stimulation of the skin overlying the knee. The source of the afferent inputs of the neurons (skin, deep tissue, joint) and the threshold for excitation (innocuous or noxious intensity) were determined and the size of the receptive fields in the deep tissue and in the skin were mapped. Each neuron was characterised as either a nociceptive specific (NS) neuron or a wide dynamic range (WDR) neuron taking into account all inputs.

Ionophoretic application of agonists and antagonists. For ionophoretic application of compounds close to the recorded neuron a five-barrel glass microelectrode was bent near the tip and glued to the recording electrode by using a u.v. bonded adhesive. The array of ionophoresis electrodes had a tip diameter of 5-8 µm. The barrels were filled with the following solutions: ketamine (50 mM in 150 mM NaCl, pH4.8) or DL-2-amino-5-phosphonovalerate (AP5, 50 mM in 150 mM NaCl, pH9.4), 6-cyano-7-nitroquinoxaline-2,3-dione (CNQX, 1 mM in 150 mM NaCl, pH 9.4), N-methyl-D-aspartate (NMDA, 50 mM in 150 mM NaCl, pH 8.17), and (RS)-alpha-amino-3-hydroxy-5-methyl-4-isoxazolepropionic acid (AMPA, 10 mM in 200 mM NaCl, pH 7.5). One barrel was filled with NaCl (1M) and used for automatic current balancing. In all barrels containing compounds retaining currents were used (10-20 nA) to prevent drug leakage. Ketamine was ejected with positive (cationic) current, AP5, CNQX, NMDA, and AMPA with negative (anionic) current.

Stimulation For stimulation of the deep tissue with innocuous intensity holding pressure was applied manually across the knee and a clip was used at the ankle joint and paw (applying a force of 110 g/mm^2, corresponding to holding pressure). For stimulation with noxious intensity strong compression was applied manually to the knee (felt painful when applied to the experimenter) and a clip was used at the ankle joint and paw (applying a force of 595 g/mm^2). To measure reproducibility of the two intensities of the stimuli applied to the knee the experimenter compressed a small balloon connected to a pressure gauge whilst the reading from the scale was done by another person. In this test the application of the pressure stimuli at the two intensities was found fairly reproducible (variation of 10% or less of the mean in each session) within one experiment and also between the different experiments. For innocuous stimulation of the skin brush stimuli were applied to the hind limbs using a soft-haired artist's brush. Noxious cutaneous pinch was applied to a skin fold using a pair of blunt, non-serrated forceps. All stimuli were applied for 15s.

Quantification of results The responses to pressure stimuli were calculated by subtracting the ongoing activity in the preceding 15 s (if present) from the total activity during the stimulus. To assess effects of a drug at least 3-4 responses to mechanical stimuli were averaged prior to drug application and set to 100%. A significant effect of the drug was assumed if the response during drug application differed from the mean of the pre drug period by±2 standard deviations. Ongoing activity was counted per minute in a period of 10 minutes before drug application and the average was set to 100%. The impulses per minute during and after drug application were expressed as percentage of the control and a significant effect was assumed if the values reached a level lower or higher than the mean±2 standard deviations of the pre drug value. To evaluate changes of the responses of a neuron by the acute arthritis the mean of the responses to each stimulus in the control period was set to 100% and the values after induction of inflammation were expressed as percentage of the mean. For the comparison of the responses to noxious pressure in the control period to those obtained at every hour after kaolin the t-test for unpaired samples was used for each neuron.

RESULTS

Nociceptive processing from the normal joint

In the segments L2-L3 twenty-seven neurons were studied that could be driven by pressure applied across the knee joint. They were located in the superficial (330-440 mm; n=6) and deep (570-1230 mm; n=21) dorsal horn. Seven cells were NS neurons and 20 were WDR neurons. Sixteen of these neurons had also receptive fields in the ankle joint. Cutaneous receptive fields were present in 11 neurons but they were not located at the knee (and ankle). Nine neurons showed ongoing activity (< 1Hz).

All neurons tested were affected by the agonists AMPA and NMDA and the vast majority of them was also affected by the non-NMDA and NMDA antagonists. Figure 1 shows the protocol used and a typical result. The neuron displayed is a WDR neuron that was recorded at depth of 729 mm. The receptive field was located in the knee joint and in the adjacent thigh and lower leg. We applied pressure to the knee joint (these responses are shown in Figure 1A) and we administered ionophoretically the specific agonists AMPA and NMDA (these responses are displayed in Figure 1B). After having established the baseline of the responses in the control period either the non-NMDA antagonist CNQX or the NMDA antagonist

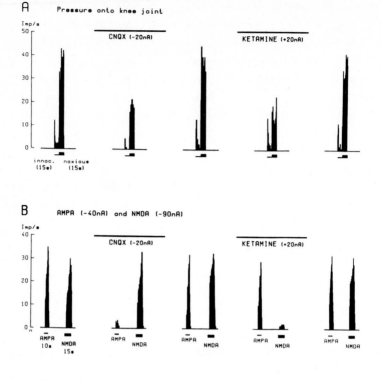

Figure 1. Effects of the ionophorectic administration of the non-NMDA antagonist 6-cyano-7-nitroquinoxaline-2,3-dione (CNQX) and the NMDA antagonist ketamine on the responses of a wide dynamic range neuron to innocuous (innoc.) and noxious pressure applied to the knee (A) and on the responses to AMPA and NMDA (B). The duration of the mechanical stimuli and the administration of NMDA was 15s, the duration of the application of AMPA 10s.

ketamine was administered ionophoretically and the mechanical and chemical stimuli were repeated. CNQX (ejected with -20 nA) selectively reduced the responses to AMPA (left side in Figure 1B) and during partial blockade of the non-NMDA receptor the responses to innocuous and noxious pressure were decreased (Figure 1A). The selective blockade of the NMDA receptor by ketamine (right side in Figure 1B) also reduced the response to noxious pressure but not the response to innocuous pressure (Figure 1A). The neurons' responses showed full recovery after switching off the ejection of the antagonists.

Table I. DIFFERENTIAL EFFECTS OF THE NON-NMDA ANTAGONIST AND THE NMDA ANTAGONISTS AP5 AND KETAMINE ON THE RESPONSES EVOKED BY STIMULATION OF THE NORMAL JOINT

	Responses to AMPA	Responses to NMDA	Responses to innocuous pressure	Responses to noxious pressure
CNQX	reduced (to 0-55%)	not reduced	reduced in 17/19 WDR cells (to 0-34%)	reduced in 17/19 WDR cells 7/7 NS cells (to 10-57%)
AP5 and ketamine	not reduced	reduced (to 0-38%)	reduced in 1/17 WDR cells (to 71%)	reduced in 17/17 WDR cells 5/5 NS cells (to 21-58%)

Table I summarises the results obtained in a sample of 27 neurons with ejection of the antagonists at 20 nA. (1) With ejections at 20 nA the antagonists selectively suppressed either the responses to AMPA or to NMDA. (2) The responses to noxious pressure applied to the knee were reduced by both CNQX and the NMDA antagonists AP5 and ketamine. NS and WDR neurons were similarly affected. (3) The responses of WDR neurons to innocuous pressure applied to the knee joint were reduced by CNQX but not by the NMDA antagonists AP5 and ketamine except in one case. Ejection of ketamine and AP5 at higher currents (50 and 75 nA) was used in 7 neurons and the responses to innocuous pressure were still not affected but in 4/7 neurons the responses to noxious pressure were further reduced. (4) When pressure was applied to the ankle CNQX reduced the effects to innocuous and noxious pressure while the NMDA antagonists reduced only the responses to noxious pressure. (5) The effects of the antagonists were similar in neurons of the superficial and deep dorsal horn. (6) Ongoing discharges were reduced in 5/9 WDR neurons by AP5/ketamine and in 6/9 WDR neurons by CNQX. Thus in our hands the responses to noxious pressure involved non-NMDA and

NMDA receptor activation whilst the responses to innocuous pressure seemed to be mediated predominantly or exclusively by non-NMDA receptors.

NOCICEPTIVE PROCESSING DURING DEVELOPMENT OF INFLAMMATION

In the course of an experimental inflammation in the joint spinal cord neurons with input from the inflamed joint become hyperexcitable. Typical changes in the neurons consist of (1) increased responses to firm mechanical stimuli applied to the inflamed joint, (2) increased responses to innocuous mechanical stimuli in WDR neurons and a lowering of threshold in NS neurons such that they are activated by innocuous stimuli, (3) increased responsiveness to mechanical stimuli applied to areas adjacent to and remote from the inflamed joint (lower limb, ankle region and paw) including expansion of the total receptive field in some neurons and (4) increase or induction of ongoing discharges in some neurons.[36,37,45,48] In the present experiments we assessed whether the application of NMDA or non-NMDA antagonists would influence the changes in responsiveness usually seen during development of inflammation. In each experiment one neuron with input from the knee was identified and recorded continuously in a control period and during development of acute inflammation. During induction of inflammation and also in several periods in the first 90 minutes after injection of kaolin either the NMDA antagonists ketamine or AP5 or the non-NMDA antagonist CNQX were ionophoretically administered. Care was taken to choose doses of the antagonists which were selective for one of the receptor agonists by testing the antagonists against the agonists NMDA and AMPA. In some neurons the intravenous injetion of ketamine was used.

Control experiments. Figure 2A shows the typical time course of the development of hyperexcitability in a dorsal horn NS neuron with afferent inputs from the knee, adjacent thigh and lower leg (recorded at a depth of 880 mm). In the control period neurons showed stable responses to noxious pressure applied to the knee (dots) but did not respond to innocuous pressure (crosses). The responses to noxious pressure were reduced during the ionophoretic administration of CNQX and AP5 (see boxes). The intraarticular injections of kaolin and then of carrageenan led to an increase in the responses to noxious pressure and to the appearance of responses to innocuous pressure applied to the knee (Figure 2A) and to an expansion of the total receptive field since the neuron became also activated by innocuous and noxious pressure applied to the ankle and paw when the inflammation developed in the knee (not shown). These changes were mainly noted within the first and second hour after injection of kaolin.

After development of hyperexcitability CNQX and then AP5 were administered ionophoretically. Both antagonists reduced the responses to innocuous and noxious pressure applied to the knee joint. This point will be further addressed in the next section. Here it should be noted that the ionophoretic application of the antagonists in the control period (in order to test the effects on the responses to innocuous and noxious pressure applied to the normal joint) had no influence on the development of hyperexcitability since the time course of the neuronal changes was the same in neurons in rats in which no pharmacology was studied.

Figure 3 summarises the inflammation-evoked changes of the responses to noxious pressure applied to the knee. The dots show 6 neurons tested in 6 control animals. Each dot displays the responses of one neuron (mean±SD). The left graph shows the responses in the control period (normalised to 100%), the second graph shows the responses at about 2 hours after injection of kaolin and the right graph displays the responses at about 4 hours after injection of kaolin. In the 6 control animals the responses of the neurons to noxious pressure applied to the knee were consistently enhanced 2 hours after kaolin (significantly different from control with $p < 0.0005-0.00005$ in each neuron, t-test).

Administration of NMDA antagonists or CNQX during and post induction of inflammation. The ionophoretic administration of ketamine or AP5 or the ionophoretic administration of CNQX during the injections of kaolin and carrageenan and during several periods post induction (up to 103 minutes post kaolin) prevented the development of hyperexcitability although the circumference of the leg in the knee region showed an increase similar to that seen in control animals (arthritic, non-treated). Figure 2B shows the responses to innocuous and noxious pressure applied to the knee in a NS neuron with afferent input from the knee joint, adjacent thigh and lower leg (recorded at a depth of 1122mm). The NMDA antagonist ketamine was ionophoretically applied during the injections of kaolin and carrageenan and also in 3 periods within the 73 min after kaolin (indicated by the boxes). During application of ketamine and in the intervals between the applications there was no increase of the responses to noxious pressure as usually seen in control rats. Figure 2C shows an experiment in which CNQX was used (WDR neuron with afferent inputs from knee, thigh and lower leg, recorded at a depth of 953mm). Again the responses to innocuous and noxious pressure applied to the knee did not show an increase during CNQX. In both neurons in Figure 2B and 2C, however, the responses to pressure showed a pronounced increase about 1 hour after termination of the administration of ketamine or CNQX and the neurons also showed the other phenomena of

Pressure knee joint

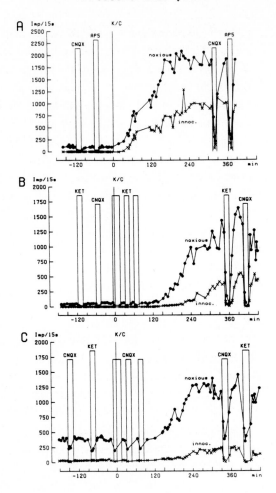

Figure 2. Development of hyperexcitability in 3 spinal cord neurons with input from the knee joint. The graphs show the responses to innocuous pressure (crosses) and to noxious pressure (dots) applied to the knee obtained in extracellular long term recordings. At the time point "0 min" an experimental inflammation was induced by injections of kaolin and carrageenan (at about 20 min post kaolin) into the knee joint. During the time indicated by the boxes the non-NMDA antagonist CNQX (-20nA) or the NMDA antagonists ketamine (+20 nA) or AP5 (-20 nA) were administered ionophoretically. A. Control experiment on a NS neuron located a at depth of 880 mm. No antagonist applied during induction of inflammation. B. Recordings from a NS neuron at a depth of 1122 mm. Ionophoretic application of ketamine during injection of kaolin and in 3 subsequent periods. C. Recording from a WDR neuron at a depth of 953 mm. Ionophoretic administration of CNQX during the injections of kaolin and in 3 subsequent periods.

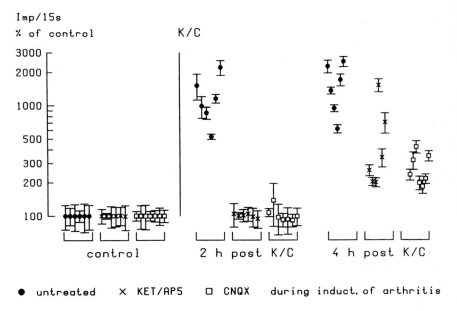

Figure 3. Summary of the responses of dorsal horn neurons to noxious pressure applied to the knee in different experimental groups of rats. The left graph shows the responses in the control period (120-205 minutes), the middle graphs shows the responses at 2 hours after the injection of kaolin (90-150 min post kaolin) and the right graph the responses at 4 hours after kaolin (210-270 min post kaolin). Each symbol shows the responses of one neuron (mean ± SD). All values are expressed as percentage of control (mean response in the control period). The dots show the responses of the 6 neurons in untreated control rats. The crosses display 6 neurons of 6 experiments in which the NMDA antagonists AP5 or ketamine were administered ionophoretically during induction of inflammation (see experimental protocol in Figure 2B). The squares show the responses of 7 neurons in 7 rats in which the non-NMDA antagonist was ionophoretically administered during induction of inflammation (see experimental protocol in Figure 2C).

hyperexcitability usually seen in control animals. When the antagonists were tested in the hyperexcitable state the responses of the neurons to innocuous and noxious pressure were reduced by the NMDA antagonists and by CNQX. This was different to the normal situation in that the application of NMDA antagonists in the control period only reduced the responses to noxious pressure (see Section I).

The prevention of hyperexcitability by the antagonists is summarised in Figure 3. The crosses show the neurons in rats in which ketamine (n=4 neurons) and AP5 (n=2 neurons) were ionophoretically administered during the injections of kaolin and carrageenan and in the subsequent 73-100 minutes. The responses to noxious pressure were not significantly different from controls at 2 hours post kaolin ($0.05 < p < 0.5$, t-test). Later, within 3-4 hours after kaolin the responses showed a gradual enhancement (different from control with $p < 0.05 - 0.00005$ three hours after kaolin). It should be noted, however, that in 4 of the 6 neurons the increase in the responses did not reach the level usually seen in control rats. Similar results were seen when ketamine was applied in bolus injections of 2 mg/kg, a dose that selectively suppresses NMDA receptors.[3,44] Similar as the NMDA antagonists, CNQX delayed the increase of the responses to noxious pressure applied to the knee (neurons displayed by squares). In the second hour after kaolin the responses to noxious pressure were not different from control ($0.05 < p < 0.5$, t-test) but increases of the responses developed 50-90 min after the last application of CNQX. Three hours after kaolin the difference from control was significant in 5 of 6 neurons ($p < 0.0005 - 0.00005$) and at 4 hours it was significant in all neurons tested. Similar results were obtained for noxious pressure applied to the ankle. In 4 of these 6 neurons the effects of CNQX on the responses to the agonists were tested. The responses to AMPA were reduced (to 5, 7, 16 and 30 % of control) whereas the responses to NMDA were not changed.

Effects of the NMDA antagonists and CNQX on the size of the receptive fields.
In 13 of 22 neurons the receptive field showed an expansion to the ipsilateral ankle and/or the paw during development of inflammation in the knee. In 20 of these neurons and in another 6 neurons sampled in these animals 4.5-9.5 h post kaolin the effects of the antagonists on the receptive fields were tested. Figure 4 shows an example. This NS neuron was recorded at a depth of 1080 mm in the segment L2. Initially it had a high threshold receptive field in the knee and in the deep tissue in adjacent areas (Figure 4A). At 5 hours after kaolin the receptive field included also the ankle and the paw and the mechanical threshold was reduced (Figure 4B). The ionophoretic application of ketamine (+20 nA for 13 min, 342 min post kaolin) caused a shrinkage of the receptive field and an increase of threshold in the areas adjacent to the knee (Figure 4C) and this effect was reversible (Figure 4D). The ionophoretic application of CNQX (-20 nA for 14 min, 380 min post kaolin) also led to a reduction of the receptive field to the initial size and to an increase in mechanical threshold (Figure 4E). These effects were also reversible (Figure 4F).

Receptive field of NS neuron

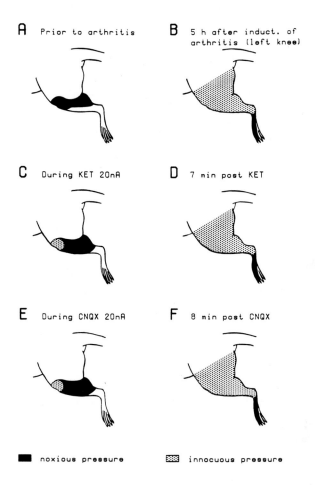

A Prior to arthritis

B 5 h after induct. of arthritis (left knee)

C During KET 20nA

D 7 min post KET

E During CNQX 20nA

F 8 min post CNQX

■ noxious pressure   ▨ innocuous pressure

Figure 4. Effects of ketamine and CNQX on the size of the receptive field of a hyperexcitable NS neuron recorded at a depth of 1080 mm in the segment L2. A. Size of the receptive field in the control period prior to inflammation. B. Size of the receptive field during inflammation (5 hours post kaolin). C. Reduction of the size of the expanded receptive field by the ionophoretic application of ketamine (+20 nA) and, D., recovery from the effect of ketamine. E. Reduction of the size of the expanded receptive field by the ionophoretic application of CNQX (-20 nA) and, F. Recovery from the effect of CNQX. The black areas indicate a high threshold, the shaded areas a low threshold for mechanical stimuli. The receptive field of this neuron was located in the deep tissue only.

The ionophoretic application of CNQX (294-603 minutes post kaolin) led to a reduction in the size of the receptive fields in 10 of 15 neurons. Similar results were found in 11 of 15 neurons when AP5 and ketamine were applied ionophoretically (275-582 min post kaolin). The intravenous injection of ketamine was most effective, reducing the size of the receptive fields in 11 of 13 neurons. Selecting the results obtained in the sample of those 13 neurons which were monitored during inflammation and showed an enlargement of the receptive field in the course of inflammation 12 neurons exhibited a reduction of the size of the receptive field during the application of the antagonists. In the pre-inflammatory control period a reduction of the receptive field size of the neurons was only exceptionally seen. Following intravenous ketamine 1 of 10 neurons and during ionophoretic application of ketamine and CNQX 1 of 12 neurons exhibited a reduction of the receptive field size.

DISCUSSION

Role of excitatory amino acids, NMDA and non-NMDA receptors in the signalling of nociceptive information from the normal joint

This study shows two important aspects of the spinal processing of sensory information from the normal joint. Firstly, the NMDA and non-NMDA antagonists had differential effects on the responses to innocuous and noxious pressure applied to the knee and the ankle suggesting that the processing of noxious input from the joint involves NMDA and non-NMDA receptors whilst innocuous stimuli such as holding pressure activate mainly non-NMDA receptors. A similar conclusion was recently made for the processing of cutaneous stimuli in spinothalamic neurons in monkeys in which the spinal cord was perfused with non-NMDA and NMDA antagonists using dialysis fibers.[14] Since biophysical studies indicate that NMDA receptors are particularly activated when the Mg^{2+} block is removed by marked depolarization of the neuron[29,38] the weaker sensory inflow during application of innocuous stimulation may not be sufficient to activate the NMDA receptor whereas the strong afferent inflow during noxious pressure may activate both receptor types. It should be noted, however, that the threshold for activation of NMDA receptors has not been exactly determined in these experiments, i.e. it has not been examined whether the mechanical stimulus has to be painful in order to activate NMDA receptors or whether firm yet not frankly noxious pressure might be sufficient.

The second point is that the NMDA receptor does not seem to be only active in pathophysiological conditions such as inflammation in which the neurons are hyperexcitable. The application of noxious stimuli to the normal tissue seems to activate NMDA receptors as well. It could be argued that the laminectomy and the searching stimuli may have induced hyperexcitability in these neurons and that it is virtually impossible to study nociception under "normal" conditions. Although this possibility cannot be entirely ruled out we do not assume for several reasons that this complication is severe in the present study. (1) Numerous neurons in the present experiments appeared as NS neurons whereas our previous studies and also this new one have clearly demonstrated that inflammation-evoked afferent input from the deep tissue leads to definite changes in the spinal neurons with deep input such that NS neurons show changes of threshold and appear as WDR neurons[19,36,37,48] (see, however, Hylden et al.[22]). (2) Some of the neurons were studied prior to arthritis and during development of inflammation. All of these neurons showed dramatic changes of the response properties in the course of inflammation in the knee suggesting that surgery-induced hyperexcitability was weak if at all present. (3) In the state of hyperexcitability NMDA antagonists typically reduced the responses to noxious as well as to innocuous mechanical stimuli such as holding pressure. We assume, therefore, that the involvement of NMDA receptors in the mediation of innocuous mechanical stimuli may be a characteristic feature of hyperexcitability, at least in the sample of neurons studied in these experiments.

Role of excitatory amino acids, NMDA and non-NMDA receptors in the hyperexcitability during inflammation

The typical development of hyperexcitability could be prevented as long as NMDA antagonists or CNQX were applied during the injections of kaolin and carrageenan and in subsequent periods. Since the development of hyperexcitability could be totally prevented with either a NMDA or a non-NMDA antagonist, it must be concluded that both the NMDA and non-NMDA receptors must be activated in order to render the neuron hyperexcitable. This conclusion seems to be valid since (1) at least in some experiments we could demonstrate the specificity of the antagonists by testing them against the agonists and (2) the development of inflammation in the injected knee was not impaired by the application of the antagonists judged from the increase of the circumference of the knee region.

At this time it is a matter of speculation why the coactivation of both NMDA and non-NMDA receptors is necessary to produce hyperexcitability. The NMDA receptor is different from the non-NMDA receptors in several aspects. The NMDA receptor allows strong influxes of Ca^{2+} upon activation and the channel is blocked by Mg^{2+} unless the neuron is sufficiently depolarised.[29] It may be, therefore, that the influx of calcium is an important factor contributing to the change of excitability. If the activation of the NMDA receptor and the processes triggered by receptor activation are regarded as the essential step involved in the generation of hyperexcitability the phenomena of hyperexcitability should not occur when NMDA antagonists are applied. If the NMDA receptor, on the other hand, is activated by depolarization which is mediated by non-NMDA receptors the prevention of hyperexcitability by CNQX may be due to the missing activation of NMDA receptors as a consequence of the initiating step.

Once the hyperexcitability was established the inflammation-induced increases of the responses to mechanical stimuli and the expansion of the receptive fields were reduced by both the NMDA antagonists and CNQX. The continuous observation of the neurons during development of inflammation and during the application of the antagonists at later stages showed that the inflammation-evoked changes of the responses and the expansion of the receptive fields were almost reversed. A reduction of the size of receptive fields was also seen in dorsal horn neurons in rats with Freund's complete adjuvant-induced inflammation of the paw after intravenous application of the NMDA antagonist MK-801.[42] Similar to our study, the NMDA antagonist had no obvious effect on the receptive fields of dorsal horn neurons in normal animals. In the hyperexcitable state the effects of CNQX were similar to those of the NMDA antagonists. These data demonstrate that the maintenance of inflammation-evoked hyperexcitability is at least in part dependent on continuous activation of non-NMDA and NMDA receptors. In this respect there might be a difference to the long term potentiation in the hippocampus where NMDA receptors are only required for induction of the potentiation but not for its maintenance.[23,58]

An important contribution of NMDA receptors to the generation and maintenance of hyperalgesia in "pathophysiological states" has been suggested in several behavioral experiments using different models of tissue and/or nerve injury (see Introduction). The effectiveness of intrathecal application of the antagonists in some behavioral experiments and the demonstration of the presence and the functional aspects of non-NMDA and NMDA receptors in the spinal cord by electrophysiological *in vitro* experiments (see Introduction) and in further *in vivo* experiments[1,41,50,53] may allow the conclusion that the development of hyperalgesia in "pathophysiological conditions" is at least in part a process that is based on the activation of non-NMDA and NMDA receptors in spinal cord neurons. The results from the present electrophysiological experiments and those from others[14,42] may support this conclusion by directly demonstrating the involvement of non-NMDA and NMDA receptors in the generation of hyperexcitability in spinal neurons in the course of pathophysiological conditions. In this context it should also be mentioned that in most studies the hyperalgesia or hyperexcitability were induced by stimuli which cause immediately considerable discharge rates in afferent fibres (formalin, capsaicin, mustard oil) and thus a strong afferent barrage during the initial event which may lead to excessive depolarization of the spinal cord neurons. Our study shows that a gradually developing inflammation is sufficient to involve NMDA receptors in the generation of hyperexcitability. The activity in the spinal cord neurons during the injections was usually less than that elicited by noxious compression of the knee.

REFERENCES

1. AANONSEN, L.M., LEI, S. AND WILCOX, G.L. (1990) Excitatory amino acid receptors and nociceptive neurotransmission in rat spinal cord. *Pain* **41**, 309-321.
2. AANONSEN, L.M. AND WILCOX, G.L. (1986) Phencyclidine selectively blocks a spinal action of N-methyl-D-aspartate in mice. *Neurosci. Lett.* **67**, 191-197.
3. ANIS, N.A., BERRY, S.C., BURTON, N.R. AND LODGE, D. (1983) The dissociative anaesthetics, ketamine and phencyclidine, selectively reduce excitation of central mammalian neurones by N-methyl-aspartate. *Br. J. Pharmacol.* **79**, 565-575.
4. BÜHRLE, C.P. AND SONNHOF, U. (1983) The ionic mechanism of the excitatory action of L-glutamate upon the membranes of motoneurones of the frog. *Pflügers Arch.* **396**, 154-162.
5. CAHUSAC, P.M.B., EVANS, R.H., HILL, R.G., RODRIQUEZ, R.E. AND SMITH, D.A.S. (1984) The behavioural effects of an N-methyl-D-aspartate receptor antagonist following application to the lumbar spinal cord of conscious rats. *Neuropharmacology* **23**, 719-724.
6. CODERRE, T.J. AND MELZACK, R. (1991) Central neural mediators of secondary hyperalgesia following heat injury in rats: neuropeptides and excitatory amino acids. *Neurosci. Lett.* **131**, 71-74.
7. CODERRE, T.J. AND MELZACK, R. (1992) Contribution of excitatory amino acids to central sensitization and persistent nociception after formalin-induced tissue injury. *J. Neurosci.* **12**, 3665-3670.
8. COLLINGRIDGE, G.L. AND LESTER, R.A.J. (1989) Excitatory amino acid

receptors in the vertebrate central nervous system. *Pharmacol. Rev.* **41**, 143-210.

9. CONSEILLER, C., BENOIST, J.M., HAMANN, F., MAILLARD, M.C. AND BESSON, J.-M. (1972) Effects of ketamine (CI 581) on cell responses to cutaneous stimulations in laminae IV and V in the cat's dorsal horn. *Eur. J. Pharmacol.* **18**, 346-352.

10. COTMAN, C.W., MONAGHAN, D.T. AND GANONG, A.H. (1988) Excitatory amino acid neurotransmission: NMDA receptors and Hebb-type synaptic plasticity. *Annu. Rev. Neurosci.* **11**, 61-80.

11. DAVAR, G., HAMA A., DEYKIN, A., VOS, B. AND MACIEWICZ, R. (1991) MK-801 blocks the development of thermal hyperalgesia in a rat model of experimental painful neuropathy. *Brain Res.* **553**, 327-330.

12. DAVIES, S.N. AND LODGE, D. (1987) Evidence for involvement of N-methylaspartate receptors in `wind-up` of class 2 neurones in the dorsal horn of the rat. *Brain Res.* **424**, 402-406.

13. DICKENSON, A.H. AND SULLIVAN, A.F. (1990) Differential effects of excitatory amino acid antagonists on dorsal horn nociceptive neurones in the rat. *Brain Res.* **506**, 31-39.

14. DOUGHERTY, P.M., PALECEK, J., PALECKOVA, V., SORKIN, L.S. AND WILLIS, W.D. (1992a) The role of NMDA and non-NMDA excitatory amino acid receptors in the excitation of primate spinothalamic tract neurons by mechanical, chemical, thermal, and electrical stimuli. *J. Neurosci.* **12**, 3025-3041.

15. DOUGHERTY, P.M., SLUKA, K.A., SORKIN, L.S., WESTLUND, K.N. AND WILLIS, W.D. (1992b) Neural changes in acute arthritis in monkeys. I. Parallel enhancement of responses of spinothalamic tract neurons to mechanical stimulation and excitatory amino acids. *Brain Res. Rev.* **17**, 1-13.

16. FAROOQUI, A.A. AND HORROCKS, L.A. (1991) Excitatory amino acid receptors, neural membrane phospholipid metabolism and neurological disorders. *Brain Res. Rev.* **16**, 171-191.

17. FOSTER, A.C. AND FAGG, G.E. (1984) Acidic amino acid binding sites in mammalian neuronal membranes: their characteristics and relationship to synaptic receptors. *Brain Res. Rev.* **7**, 103-164.

18. GERBER, G. AND RANDIC, M. (1989) Participation of excitatory amino acid receptors in the slow excitatory synaptic transmission in the rat spinal dorsal horn in vitro. *Neurosci. Lett.* **106**, 220-228.

19. GRUBB, B.D., STILLER, R.U. AND SCHAIBLE, H.-G. (1993) Dynamic changes in the receptive field properties of spinal cord neurons with ankle input in rats with chronic unilateral inflammation in the ankle region. *Exp. Brain Res.* **92**, 441-452.

20. HALEY, J.E., SULLIVAN, A.F. AND DICKENSON, A.H. (1990) Evidence for spinal N-methyl-D-aspartate receptor involvement in prolonged chemical nociception in the rat. *Brain Res.* **518**, 218226.

21. HEADLEY, P.M., PARSONS, C.G. AND WEST,, D.C. (1987) The role of N-methylaspartate receptors in mediating responses of rat and cat spinal neurons to defined sensory stimuli. *J. Physiol.* **385**, 169-188.

22. HYLDEN, J.L.K., NAHIN, R.L., TRAUB, R.J. AND DUBNER, R. (1989) Expansion of receptive fields of spinal lamina I projection neurons in rats with

unilateral adjuvant-induced inflammation: the contribution of dorsal horn mechanisms. *Pain* **37**, 229-243.

23. IZUMI, Y., CLIFFORD, D.B. AND ZORUMSKI, C.F. (1991) 2-amino-3-phosphonopropionate blocks the induction and maintenance of long-term potentiation in rat hippocampal sices. *Neurosci. Lett.* **122**, 187-190.

24. JEFTINJIA, S. (1989) Excitatory transmission in the dorsal horn is in part mediated through APV-sensitive NMDA receptors. *Neurosci. Lett.* 96, 191-196.

25. KING, A.E., THOMPSON, S.W.N., URBAN, L. AND WOOLF, C.J. (1988) An intracellular analysis of amino acid induced excitations of deep dorsal horn neurones in the rat spinal cord slice. *Neurosci. Lett.* **89**, 286-292.

26. MAO, J., PRICE, D.D., HAYES, R.L., LU, J. AND MAYER D.L. (1992) Differential roles of NMDA and non-NMDA receptor activation in induction and maintenance of thermal hyperalgesia in rats with painful peripheral mononeuropathy. *Brain Res.* **598**, 271-278.

27. MAO, J., PRICE, D.D., MAYER, D.J., LU, J. AND HAYES, R.L. (1992) Intrathecal MK-801 and local nerve anesthesia synergistically reduce nociceptive behaviors in rats with experimental peripheral mononeuropathy. *Brain Res.* **576**, 254-262.

28. MAYER, M.L., WESTBROOK, G.L. AND GUTHRIE, P.B. (1984) Voltage-dependent block by Mg^{2+} of NMDA responses in spinal cord neurones. *Nature* **309**, 261-263.

29. MAYER, M.L. AND WESTBROOK, G.L. (1987) Permeation and block of N-methyl-D-aspartic acid receptor channels by divalent cations in mouse cultured central neurones. *J. Physiol.* **394**, 501-527.

30. MONAGHAN, D.T., BRIDGES, R.J. AND COTMAN, C.W. (1989) The excitatory amino acid receptors: their classes, pharmacology, and distinct properties in the function of the central nervous system. *Annu. Rev. Pharmacol. Toxicol.* **29**, 365-402.

31. MURRAY, C.W., COWAN, A. AND LARSON, A.A. (1991) Neurokinin and NMDA antagonists (but not a kainic acid antagonist) are antinociceptive in the mouse formalin model. *Pain* **44**, 179-185.

32. NAGY, I., MAGGI, C.A., DRAY, A., WOOLF, C.J. AND URBAN, L. (1993) The role of neurokinin and N-methyl-D-aspartate receptors in synaptic transmission from capsaicin-sensitive primary afferents in the rat spinal cord in vitro. *Neuroscience* **52**, 1029-1037.

33. NÄSSTRÖM, J., KARLSSON, U. AND POST, C. (1992) Antinociceptive actions of different classes of excitatory amino acid receptor antagonists in mice. *Eur. J. Pharmacol.* **212**, 21-29.

34. NEUGEBAUER, V., LÜCKE, T. AND SCHAIBLE, H.-G. (1993a) Differential effects of N-methyl-D-aspartate (NMDA) and non-NMDA receptor antagonists on the responses of rat spinal neurons with joint input. *Neurosci. Lett.,* (in press).

35. NEUGEBAUER, V., LÜCKE, T. AND SCHAIBLE, H.-G. (1993b) N-methyl-D-aspartate (NMDA) and non-NMDA receptor antagonists block the hyperexcitability of dorsal horn neurons during development of acute arthritis in rat`s knee joint. (submitted).

36. NEUGEBAUER, V. AND SCHAIBLE, H.-G. (1988) Peripheral and spinal components of the sensitization of spinal neurons during an acute

arthritis. *Agents Actions* **25**, 234-236.

37. NEUGEBAUER, V. AND SCHAIBLE, H.-G. (1990) Evidence for a central component in the sensitization of spinal neurons with joint input during development of acute arthritis in cat's knee. *J. Neurophysiol.* **64**, 299-311.

38. NOWAK, L., BREGESTOVSKI, P., ASCHER, P., HERBET, A. AND PROCHI-ANTZ, A. (1984) Magnesium gates glutamate-activated channels in mouse central neurones. *Nature* **307**, 462-465.

39. PUMAIN, R. AND HEINEMANN, U. (1985) Stimulus- and amino acid-induced calcium and potassium changes in the rat neocortex. *J. Neurophysiol.* **53**, 1-16.

40. RAIGORODSKY, G. AND URCA, G. (1987) Intrathecal N-methyl-D-aspartate (NMDA) activates both nociceptive and antinociceptive systems. *Brain Res.* **422**, 158-162.

41. RAIGORODSKY, G. AND URCA, G. (1990) Involvement of N-methyl-D-aspartate receptors in nociception and motor control in the spinal cord of the mouse: behavioral, pharmacological and electrophysiological evidence. *Neuroscience* **36**, 601-610.

42. REN, K., HYLDEN, J.L.K., WILLIAMS, G.M., RUDA, M.A. AND DUBNER, R. (1992) The effects of a non-competitive NMDA receptor antagonist, MK-801, on behavioral hyperalgesia and dorsal horn neuronal activity in rats with unilateral inflammation. *Pain* **50**, 331-334.

43. ROBINSON, M.B. AND COYLE, J.T. (1987) Glutamate and related acidic excitatory neurotransmitters: from basic science to clinical application. *FASEB J.* **1**, 446-455.

44. SCHAIBLE, H.-G., GRUBB, B.D., NEUGEBAUER, V. AND OPPMANN, M. (1991a) The effects of NMDA antagonists on neuronal activity in cat spinal cord evoked by acute inflammation in the knee joint. *Eur. J. Neurosci.* **3**, 981-991.

45. SCHAIBLE, H.-G., NEUGEBAUER, V., CERVERO, F. AND SCHMIDT, R.F. (1991b) Changes in tonic descending inhibition of spinal neurons with articular input during the development of acute arthritis in the cat. *J. Neurophysiol.* **66**, 1021-1032.

46. SCHAIBLE, H.-G. AND SCHMIDT, R.F. (1985) Effects of an experimental arthritis on the sensory properties of fine articular afferent units. *J. Neurophysiol.* **54**, 1109-1122.

47. SCHAIBLE, H.-G. AND SCHMIDT, R.F. (1988) Time course of mechanosensitivity changes in articular afferents during a developing experimental arthritis. *J. Neurophysiol.* **60**, 2180-2195.

48. SCHAIBLE, H.-G., SCHMIDT, R.F. AND WILLIS, W.D. (1987) Enhancement of the responses of ascending tract cells in the cat spinal cord by acute inflammation of the knee joint. *Exp. Brain Res.* **66**, 489-499.

49. SCHNEIDER, S.P. AND PERL, E.R. (1988) Comparison of primary afferent and glutamate excitation of neurons in the mammalian spinal dorsal horn. *J. Neurosci.* **8**, 2062-2073.

50. SCHOUENBORG, J. AND SJÖLUND, B. (1986) First-order nociceptive synapses in rat dorsal horn are blocked by an amino acid antagonist. *Brain Res.* **397**, 394-398.

51. SELTZER, Z., COHN, S., GINZBURG, R. AND BEILIN, B.Z. (1991) Modulation of neuropathic pain behavior in rats by spinal disinhibition and NMDA

receptor blockade of injury discharge. *Pain* **45**, 69-75.

52. SHER, G.D., CARTMELL, S.M., GELGOR, L. AND MITCHELL, D. (1992) Role of N-methyl-D-aspartate and opiate receptors in nociception during and after ischaemia in rats. *Pain* **49**, 241-248.

53. SHER, G.D. AND MITCHELL, D. (1990a) Intrathecal N-methyl-D-aspartate induces hyperexcitability in rat dorsal horn convergent neurones. *Neurosci. Lett.* **119**, 199-202.

54. SHER, G.D. AND MITCHELL, D. (1990b) N-methyl-D-aspartate receptors mediate responses of rat dorsal horn neurones to hindlimb ischaemia. *Brain Res.* **522**, 55-62.

55. SLUKA, K.A. AND WESTLUND, K.N. (1992) An experimental arthritis in rats: dorsal horn aspartate and glutamate increases. *Neurosci. Lett.* **145**, 141-144.

56. SLUKA, K.A. AND WESTLUND, K.N. (1993) An experimental arthritis model in rats: the effects of NMDA and non-NMDA antagonists on aspartate and glutamate release in the dorsal horn. *Neurosci. Lett.* **149,** 99-102.

57. SORKIN, L.S., WESTLUND, K.N., SLUKA, K.A., DOUGHERTY, P.M. AND WILLIS, W.D. (1992) Neural changes in acute arthritis in monkeys. IV. Time-course of amino acid release into the lumbar dorsal horn. *Brain Res. Rev.* **17**, 39-50.

58. TEYLER, T.J. AND DISCENNA, P. (1987) Long-term potentiation. *Annu. Rev. Neurosci.* **10**, 131-161.

59. THOMPSON, S.W.N., KING, A.E. AND WOOLF, C.J. (1990) Activity-dependent changes in rat ventral horn neurons in vitro; summation of prolonged afferent evoked postsynaptic depolarizations produce a D-2-amino-5-phosphonovaleric acid sensitive windup. *Eur. J. Neurosci.* **2**, 638-649.

60. URBAN, L. AND DRAY, A. (1992) Synaptic activation of dorsal horn neurons by selective C-fibre excitation with capsaicin in the mouse spinal cord in vitro. *Neuroscience* **47**, 693-702.

61. WOOLF, C.J. AND THOMPSON, S.W.N. (1991) The induction and maintenance of central sensitization is dependent on N-methyl-D-aspartic acid receptor activation; implications for the treatment of post-injury pain hypersensitivity states. *Pain* **44**, 293-299.

62. YAMAMOTO, T. AND YAKSH, T.L. (1992) Studies on the spinal interaction of morphine and the NMDA antagonist MK-801 on the hyperesthesia observed in a rat model of sciatic mononeuropathy. *Neurosci. Lett.* **135**, 67-70.

63. YOSHIMURA, M. AND JESSELL, T.M. (1990) Amino acid-mediated EPSPs at primary afferent synapses with substantia gelatinosa neurons in the rat spinal cord. *J. Physiol.* **430**, 315-335.

TACHYKININ RECEPTORS AND THEIR ANTAGONISTS

Carlo Alberto Maggi and Alessandro Lecci
Department of Pharmacology, A. Menarini Pharmaceuticals
Via Sette Santi 3, 50131, Florence
Italy

INTRODUCTION

Tachykinins (TKs) are a family of peptides which share the common C-terminal sequence Phe-Xaa-Gly-Leu-MetNH$_2$. Three peptides of this family, substance P (SP), neurokinin A (NKA) and neurokinin B (NKB) (Table I), have an established role as neurotransmitters in mammals. SP and NKA are produced through the expression of the same gene, preprotachykinin I (PPT I) while the PPT II gene encodes NKB.[23,24] Two N-terminally extended forms of NKA, neuropeptide K and neuropeptide γ are also produced from the PPT I gene, but their status of neurotransmitters is not yet firmly established.

TKs are widely distributed into the central and peripheral nervous system. At the peripheral level, a major source of TKs is represented by the peripheral endings of capsaicin-sensitive primary afferent neurons: the neuronal bodies of these elements, which express the PPT I gene, are located in dorsal root ganglia and TKs synthesised at this level are transported in both central and peripheral directions. Both the PPT I and PPT II gene are expressed, with discrete differences in localization, in the mammalian central nervous system and spinal cord.[1,17,22]

Since the original discovery that SP is concentrated in the dorsal half of the spinal cord[31], the proposal has been advanced that TKs may be important mediators for signalling noxious events from the periphery to the central nervous system. This basic concept has received strong experimental support in the past 20 years. The use of specific antisera enabled to demonstrate that a subpopulation of

NATO ASI Series, Vol. H 79
Cellular Mechanisms of Sensory Processing
Edited by Laszlo Urban
© Springer-Verlag Berlin Heidelberg 1994

primary afferent neurons located in dorsal root ganglia contain SP[19]. Since then, immunohistochemical techniques have been used to document the distribution and pattern of innervation of these primary afferent neurons at various peripheral targets (in both the somatic and visceral domains) and, at spinal cord level, in the dorsal grey matter where sensory input is processed. The development of the first generation of SP antagonist, at the beginning of the '80s (see rev. by Maggi et al.,[34]) provided pharmacological tools to demonstrate the role of SP as a neurotransmitter, especially in the peripheral nervous system. The topic became more complicated following the discovery, in the mid '80s, of the existence of NKA and NKB, and the demonstration of their status of neurotransmitters in mammals.

Table I. AMINO ACID SEQUENCES OF MAMMALIAN TACHYKININS HAVING AN ESTABLISHED STATUS OF NEUROTRANSMITTERS

SP	H-Arg-Pro-Lys-Pro-Gln-Gln-<u>Phe</u>-Phe-<u>Gly-Leu-Met-NH2</u>
NKA	H-His-Lys-Thr-Asp-Ser-<u>Phe</u>-Val-<u>Gly-Leu-Met-NH2</u>
NKB	H-Asp-Met-His-Asp-Phe-<u>Phe</u>-Val-<u>Gly-Leu-Met-NH2</u>

SP = substance P; NKA = neurokinin A (also known as substance K, neuromedin L or neurokinin a); NKB = neurokinin B (also known as neurokinin b or neuromedin K). The common C-terminal sequence is underlined.

The biological actions of mammalian TKs which are encoded by their common C-terminal sequence (underlined in Table I) are mediated by three distinct receptors, termed NK-1, NK-2 and NK-3.[34] Amongst mammalian TKs, SP, NKA and NKB possess higher affinity for the NK-1, NK-2 and NK-3 receptor, respectively. The existence of distinct TK receptors has been originally suggested by pharmacological and radioligand binding experiments showing different rank order of potencies of natural TKs or their fragments in different systems.[30,46] This concept, further supported by data obtained with synthetic receptor-selective agonists and antagonists (see below), has been more recently enriched by the isolation and cloning of TK receptors from mammalian tissues: the three receptors belong to the superfamily of rhodopsin-like G-protein coupled receptors (see rev. by Nakanishi[39]). Stimulation of phosphoinositide turnover is currently held as the major second messenger system activated by the three TK receptors.[16]

TACHYKININ RECEPTOR ANTAGONISTS

The widespread distribution and variety of biological actions of TKs have attracted much interest to the development of TK receptor antagonists. Such molecules are important not only to establish the physiological role of peptides of this family, but also for their possible use in the treatment of a variety of human diseases.

The first generation of TK receptor antagonists has been developed at the beginning of the '80s by insertion of D-Trp residues in the sequence of SP. Such antagonists (the prototype of which is Spantide) have been instrumental to define the status of transmitters of TK peptides, particularly in the peripheral nervous system (e.g. in the gut).[26] These antagonists suffer from a number of drawbacks (Table II) which have limited their usefulness as tools in neuroscience research.

The best known of these drawbacks is the neurotoxic effect produced by Spantide or other D-Trp-containing analogues after direct administration into the CNS or spinal cord. Although Spantide has been successfully used to implicate TKs in certain physiological events at spinal cord level,[41] its neurotoxic effect, apparently linked to induction of vasoconstriction and ischemia,[12] has prevented a full characterization of the biological roles of TKs at the central level.

Important limitations of the first generation of TK receptor antagonist are their low potency and poor ability to discriminate between NK-1 and NK-2 receptors[5]. Since SP and NKA are co-expressed by and co-released from the same neurons, especially from nociceptive primary afferent neurons, the availability of receptor selective antagonists is necessary to exactly define the relative biological roles of different peptides of this family. Owing to the limitations of Spantide and its congeners, several groups have attempted to get more potent and selective peptide TK antagonists which represent the second generation of TK receptor antagonists (Table III).

Table II. FIRST GENERATION OF TK RECEPTOR ANTAGONISTS AND DRAWBACKS

<u>Examples :</u>
[D-Pro^2, D-Trp^{7,9}] substance P
[D-Arg^1, D-Trp^{7,9}, Leu^{11}] substance P (Spantide I)
<u>Drawbacks :</u>
Low potency
Neurotoxicity
Local anesthetic activity
Mast cells degranulation
Partial agonism
Blockade of bombesin receptors
Blockade of endothelin receptors
Poor discrimination between NK-1 and NK-2 receptors

The third generation of tachykinin receptor antagonists comprises ligands of nonpeptide nature. The first example to be described in this category is the quinuclidine derivative CP 96,345[47] which possesses nM affinity for NK-1 receptors. Another important example of non peptide NK-1 receptor antagonists is RP 67,580[13]. A radioiodinated derivative of CP 96,345 has been also developed which will enable to study the distribution of NK-1 receptors in further depth.[7]

The first potent and selective non-peptide antagonist for NK-2 receptor, SR 48,968 has also been recently described[10]. This compound possesses nM affinity at NK-2 receptors and is 1,000-10,000 more potent at NK-2 than NK-1 or NK-3 receptors.

To date no clear example of potent and selective antagonists for tachykinin NK-3 receptor has been reported.

Table III. SECOND GENERATION OF PEPTIDE TK RECEPTOR ANTAGONISTS

NK-1 receptor selective

L668,169 : cyclo(Gln,D-Trp,(NMe)Phe(R)Gly[ANC-2]Leu,Met)$_2$
Spantide II : [D-NicLys^1,3-Pal^3,D-Cl$_2$Phe^5, Asn^6,D-Trp^{7,9}, Nle^{11}] SP
GR 82,334 : [D-Pro^9 [spiro-g-lactam]Leu^{10}, Trp^{11}]physalaemin (1-11)
FR113,680 : Ac-Thr-DTrp(CHO)-Phe-NMeBzl
FK 888 : (2-(N-Me)indolil-CO-Hyp-NAl-NMeBzl

NK-2 receptor selective

L659,877 : cyclo (Gln-Trp-Phe-Gly-Leu-Met)
MEN10,207 : [Tyr^5,D-Trp^{6,8,9}, Arg^{10}] NKA(4-10)
MEN 10,376 : [Tyr^5, D-Trp^{6,8,9}, Lys^{10}] NKA (4-10)
R396 : Ac-Leu-Asp-Gln-Trp-Phe-GlyNH$_2$
MDL 29,913 : cyclo[Leu-Y(CH$_2$NCH$_3$)-Leu-Gln-Trp-Phe-Gly]
MEN 10,573 : cyclo(LeuY[CH$_2$NH]Asp(OBzl)-Gln-Trp-Phe-bAla)
MEN 10,612 : cyclo(LeuY[CH$_2$NH]Cha-Gln-Trp-Phe-bAla)

HETEROGENEITY OF TACHYKININ NK-1 AND NK-2 RECEPTOR : SPECIES DIFFERENCES VERSUS RECEPTOR SUBTYPES

The introduction of second and third generation of NK-1 and NK-2 receptor antagonists has led to the recognition of a remarkable pharmacological heterogeneity for both receptor types.

For the NK-1 receptor, a species-related difference in the potency of competitive receptor antagonists has been disclosed following the introduction of CP 96,345 and RP 67,580 : CP 96,345 is about 100 times more potent at human, guinea-pig rabbit and bovine than at rat or mouse NK-1 receptor.[15,43] In contrast, RP 67,580 is more potent at rat or mouse NK-1 receptor than at human or guinea-pig NK-1 receptor.[13] These differences in the potency of competitive receptor antagonists have been shown to be linked to species-related amino acid variations in the sequence of transmembrane segments of the NK-1 receptor. Fong et al. (1992) compared the ability of CP 96,345 and RP 67,580 in binding to human or rat NK-1 expressed in COS cells : CP 96,345 has a higher affinity for the human NK-1 receptor (IC_{50} 0.5 nM) than for rat NK-1 receptor (IC_{50} = 35 nM), while the binding affinity of RP 67,580 for the rat NK-1 receptor (IC_{50} = 4 nM) is 5-fold higher than for human NK-1 receptor (IC_{50} 20 nM).[11] However, when a double mutant of the human NK-1 receptor was prepared in which Val-116 and Ile-290 were substituted by the rat homologs Leu and Ser, the binding affinity of both antagonists was similar to that observed for the wild type rat NK-1 receptor.[11]

The introduction of potent and selective antagonists led to the recognition of the pharmacological heterogeneity of NK-2 receptor. Some antagonists, like MEN 10,207 or its close analogue, MEN 10,376 (Table III and IV), recognise with high affinity the NK-2 receptor in e.g. rabbit smooth muscles and are much more potent than at NK-2 receptor in hamster smooth muscles; other antagonists such as R 396 or L 659,877 (Tables III and IV) show the converse picture of affinities for NK-2 receptor expressed in these species.[32,50]

The second criterion for recognition of species-related variation in the pharmacology of NK-2 receptor originates from the use of the pseudopeptide derivative of NKA(4-10), MDL 28,564.[3,42] MDL 28,564 acts as a full agonist at e.g. rabbit NK-2 receptor, while being ineffective as agonist but active as antagonist at e.g. hamster NK-2 receptor. Combining the two criteria, two broad categories of NK-2 are recognised : a) NK-2A receptors, characterised by high affinity for MEN 10,207 and MEN 10,376, at which MDL 28,564 act as a full agonist, and NK-2B receptor characterised by high affinity for R 396 (in hamster only) and L 659,877 and the lack of agonist activity of MDL 28,564 (for review Maggi et al.,[34]). Rabbit, human, guinea-pig and bovine NK-2 receptor fall in the first category while rat and hamster NK-2 receptor fall in the second category. These species-related differences have been mainly established for NK-2 receptor -mediated smooth muscle contraction.

At the present time, only one form of the NK-1 or NK-2 receptor has been detected in the genoma of the various species examined. Thus, the above mentioned differences in the pharmacology of NK-1 and NK-2 receptor may simply reflect the existence of species-related differences but not that of true receptor subtypes (for review see Gerard et al.,[14]). In addition to this species-related difference, NK-1 receptor subtypes could exist, however : Petitet et al.[44] presented evidence supporting the idea that a novel 'septide-sensitive' tachykinin receptor could exist in the guinea-pig ileum. Maggi et al.[33] showed that CP 96,345 has a very high affinity for the septide-sensitive receptor in the ileum, about 10 fold higher than that for the 'classical' NK-1 receptor. Similar findings were obtained by Meini et al.[35] in the rat isolated urinary bladder, with the only exception that, owing to the above mentioned species-related differences RP 67,580 was more potent than CP 96,345.

Table IV. AFFINITIES (PKB VALUES AND 95 % CONFIDENCE LIMITS) OF VARIOUS TK RECEPTOR ANTAGONISTS SELECTIVE FOR NK-1 OR NK-2 RECEPTORS

Antagonist	NK-1 receptor GPI	NK-2 receptor RPA	HT	NK-3 receptor RPV
L 668,169	6.44 (6.1 - 6.7)	inactive *	6.16 (5.8 - 6.4)	inactive *
Spantide II	7.08 (6.8 - 7.3)	5.43 (5.2-5.6)	6.00 (5.8-6.2)	inactive *
GR 82,334	7.59 (7.2 - 8.0)	5.10 (4.9 - 5.3)	inactive *	inactive *
FR 113,680	6.61 (6.3 - 6.9)	5.37 (5.2 -5.5)	5.21 (4.9 - 5.5)	inactive *
(±)CP 96,345	8.11 (7.9 - 8.3)	inactive *	inactive *	inactive *
RP 67,580	7.37 (6.9 - 7.9)	inactive **	inactive **	inactive **
MEN 10,207	5.52 (5.3 - 5.8)	7.89 (7.7 - 8.1)	5.94 (5.7 - 6.2)	4.90 (4.7-5.1)
MEN 10,376	5.66 (5.4 - 5.9)	8.08 (7.8 - 8.3)	5.64 (5.5 - 5.8)	inactive *
L 659,877	5.60 (5.2 - 5.9)	6.72 (6.5 - 7.0)	7.92 (7.8 - 8.0)	5.40 (5.1-5.7)
R 396	inactive *	5.42 (5.2 - 5.6)	7.63 (7.3 - 7.9)	inactive *
MDL 29,913	5.37 (5.2 - 5.6)	7.77 (7.6 - 7.9)	8.65 (8.4 - 8.8)	inactive *
MEN 10,573	6.37 (5.9 - 6.5)	7.31 (7.2 - 7.4)	8.66 (8.5 - 8.8)	inactive **
MEN 10,612	6.09 (5.7 - 6.3)	7.41 (7.3 - 7.7)	9.06 (8.9 - 9.2)	inactive **
SR 48,968	inactive ***	9.60 (9.4 - 9.8)	8.50 (8.3 - 8.6)	inactive **

GPI = guinea-pig ileum; RPA = endothelium-denuded rabbit pulmonary artery; HT = hamster trachea; RPV = rat portal vein

Thus the septide-sensitive receptor could be an NK-1 receptor subtype. Kage et al.[71] reported the existence of two forms of NK-1 receptor in rat submaxillary glands, which apparently differ in the length of their C-termini. Whether these two forms of NK-1 receptor have any bearing to the proposed 'septide-sensitive' receptor remains to be established.

For the NK-2 receptor pharmacological evidence for intra-species heterogeneity has been presented as well[2,40,53] : it is at present unclear if these cases of intra-species heterogeneity of the NK-2 receptor accommodate the above mentioned criteria used to define NK-2A and NK-2B receptors.

The affinities of the various antagonists was assessed against substance P methylester as an agonist at NK-1 receptors in the GPI, against neurokinin A as an agonist at NK-2 receptors in the RPA and HT, and against neurokinin B as an agonist at NK-3 receptors in the RPV. * inactive at 10 µM, ** inactive at 1-3 µM.

TACHYKININ RECEPTOR ANTAGONISTS, SENSORY TRANSMISSION TO THE SPINAL CORD AND PAIN

The introduction of receptor selective TK receptor antagonists of second and third generation, has enabled to assess the exact relative role of TKs, and of NK-1 and NK-2 receptors in various responses which are of physiological or pathophysiological relevance.[34] With special reference to the topic of this book, firm evidence has been obtained, by the use of receptor selective antagonists of both peptide and non-peptide nature, for a role of TKs as afferent transmitters/modulators of both nociceptive and non-nociceptive information from the periphery to the spinal cord.

Neurophysiological evidence has been presented to indicate that CP 96,345 blocks the excitatory response of nociceptive, SP-responsive dorsal horn neurons to peripheral nociceptive stimulation in cat[8,45] and monkey spinal cord.[9] Evidence for analgesic action of NK-1 receptor antagonists CP 96,345 and RP 67,580 in various behavioural models of nociception for small rodents has been reported;[4,13,27,37,51] however, the interpretation of data on the analgesic activity of CP 96,345 in rat or mice models of nociception is complicated by unspecified effects unrelated to NK-1 receptor blockade.[36]

While the above mentioned studies provide strong support to the general idea that SP[31] or, anyway, TKs act indeed as primary afferent transmitters through NK-1 receptor, less information is available about the role of NK-2 receptors. Nagy et al.[38] showed that the depolarising response recorded in rat dorsal horn neurons produced by application of capsaicin to dorsal root ganglion involves activation of glutamate and NK-2 receptor, but not NK-1 receptor. Likewise, the ventral root potential produced by single shock stimulation at C-fiber strength of the ipsilateral dorsal root in the rat spinal cord *in vitro* is inhibited by an NK-2 but not an NK-1 receptor antagonist, while with train stimulation the contribution of NK-1 receptor to the overall response becomes evident[49,52,53] used a rat model in which the facilitation of a spinal nociceptive flexor reflex is produced by conditioning stimulation of cutaneous or gastrocnemius nerve. Doses of NK-1 and NK-2 receptor antagonists were used which selectively block, after intrathecal administration, the facilitatory effect on the flexor reflex produced by exogenously administered SP or NKA : from these studies, evidence for an involvement of both NK-1 and NK-2 receptors in the facilitation produced by conditioning stimulation was provided; furthermore evidence was obtained that NK-2 receptors selectively mediate the facilitation produced by gastrocnemius but not cutaneous conditioning nerve stimulation.[52,53] These studies suggest that, depending upon different peripheral targets of innervation, different types of TK receptors play a role in processing of nociceptive input to the spinal cord.

Knowledge on the role of TKs and TK receptor in primary afferent transmission is beginning to accumulate also for visceral reflex pathways: thus, Hill et al.[18] showed that the exercise pressor reflex, which is the reflex cardiovascular and ventilatory response evoked by static muscular contraction through group III and IV afferent fibers in the skeletal muscle, is attenuated by intrathecal administration of NK-1 but not NK-2 receptor antagonists in cats. Lecci et al.[28,29] investigated a panel of NK-1 and NK-2 receptor selective antagonists for producing blockade of micturition-related reflexes after intrathecal administration in rats: the outcome of these studies was that, in normal rats, NK-1 receptor antagonist of both peptide and nonpeptide nature block the chemonociceptive vesico-vesical reflex activated by topical application of capsaicin onto the rat urinary bladder and modulate the distension-activated micturition reflex, while NK-2 receptor antagonists are ineffective.[28,29] Furthermore, the effect of NK-1 receptor blockade and capsaicin pretreatment on the distension-induced micturition reflex, which are qualitatively and quantitatively similar, is non-additive indicating that the functional integrity of capsaicin -sensitive primary afferents is required for this effect to occur.[29]

Overall, a rapidly growing body of evidence is available to indicate a major role of TKs as primary afferent transmitters from the periphery to the spinal cord and their participation to pain-producing mechanisms. The recent availability of potent and selective antagonists for NK-1 and NK-2 receptors provides a solid ground for physiological and behavioural studies in this field. On the other hand, two areas are still awaiting for development of new pharmacological tools : first, no potent and selective antagonist for NK-3 receptor is at present available; NK-3 receptors and their preferred endogenous ligand, NKB are both present in the dorsal half of the spinal cord[17] and putatively take part to sensory input processing. Second, N-terminal fragments of SP, like SP(1-7), which do not interact with NK-1, NK-2 and NK-3 receptors produce behavioural effects suggestive of an interaction with pain-producing mechanisms at spinal cord level[25,48] and interact in a complex manner with excitatory amino acids.[6] Since a high affinity specific receptor for SP(1-7) has been described in mouse spinal cord[20] it is possible that the N- and C-terminal ends of the SP molecule exert different actions on nociceptive input via distinct mechanisms.

Much work is still needed to fully elucidate the biological role of different TKs and different TK receptors in processing of sensory information in both normal and pathological-like conditions. Beside of its pharmacological and physiological relevance this line of research is expected to provide a better understanding of mechanisms of pain generation and, possibly, to new therapeutic strategies for pain control.

ACKNOWLEDGEMENTS: I wish to thank my co-workers at Menarini Pharmaceuticals, especially Drs. S. Meini and R. Patacchini for their active participation to research on tachykinin receptors and role of tachykinins in physiological responses and Prof. A. Giachetti for encouragement and support.

REFERENCES

1. ARAI, H. AND EMSON, P.C. (1986) Regional distribution of neuropeptide K and other tachykinins (neurokinin A, neurokinin B and substance P) in rat central nervous system. *Brain Res.* **399**, 240-249.
2. BRUNELLESCHI, S., CENI, E., FANTOZZI, R. AND MAGGI, C.A. (1992) Evidence for tachykinin NK-2B-like receptors in guinea-pig alveolar macrophages. *Life Sci - Pharmacology Lett.* **51**, PL177-PL181.
3. BUCK, S.H., HARBESON, S.L., HASSMANN, III C.F., SHATZER, S.A., ROUISSI, N., NANTEL, F. AND VAN GIERSBERGEN, P.L.M. (1990) [Leu^{9}Y(CH$_2$NH$_2$)Leu^{10}]-neurokinin A(4-10) (MDL 28,564) distinguishes tissue tachykinin peptide NK-2 receptors. *Life Sci - Pharmacology Lett.* **47**, PL37-PL41.
4. BIRCH, P.J., HARRISON, S.M., HAYES, A.G., ROGERS, H. AND TYERS, M.B. (1992) The nonpeptide NK-1 receptor antagonist, (±)CP 96,345, produces antinociceptive and antioedema effects in the rat. *Br. J. Pharmacol.* **105**, 508-510.
5. BUCK, S.H. AND SHATZER, S.A. (1988) Agonist and antagonist binding to tachykinin peptide NK-2 receptor. *Life Sci.* **42**, 2701 -2708.
6. BUDAI, D., WILCOX, G.L. AND LARSON, A.A. (1992) Modulation of NMDA and AMPA responses of spinal nociceptive neurons by a N-terminals fragment of Substance P. *Eur. J. Pharmacol.* **216**, 441-444.
7. CASCIERI, M.A., BER, E., FONG, T.M., SADOWSKI, S., BANSAL, A., SWAIN, C., SEWARD, E., FRANCES, B., BURNS, D. AND STRADER, C.D. (1992) Characterization of the binding of a apotent, selective radioiodinated antagonist to the human neurokinin-1 receptor. *Mol. Pharmacol.* **42**, 458-463.
8. DE KONINCK, Y. AND HENRY, J.L. (1991) Substance P-mediated slow excitatory postsynaptic potential elicited in dorsal horn neurons in vivo by noxious stimulation. *Proc. Natl. Acad. Sci. USA* **88**, 11344-11348.
9. DOUGHERTY PM, PALECECK J, PALECKOVA V, SORKIN LS, WILLIS WD (1993) The role of NMDA, non-NMDA and NK-1 receptors in the excitation of spinothalamic tract neurons in anaesthetized monkeys. *J. Physiol.* **459**, 209P.
10. EMONDS ALT, X., VILAIN, P., GOULAOUIC, P., PROIETTO, V., VAN BROECK, D., ADVENIER, C., NALINE, E., NELIAT, G., L.E. FUR, G. AND BRELIERE, J.C. (1992) A potent and selective nonpeptide antagonist of the neurokinin A (NK-2) receptor. *Life Sci. - Pharmacology Lett.* **50**, PL101-106.
11. FONG, T.M., YU, H. AND STRADER, C.D. (1992) Molecular basis for the species selectivity of the NK-1 receptor antagonists CP 96,345 and RP 67,580. *J. Biol. Chemistry* **267**, 25668-25671.
12. FREEDMAN. J., POST, C., KAHRSTROM, J., HOKFELT, T., OHLEN, A., MOLLENHOLT, P., OWMAN, C., ALARI, L. AND HOKFELT, T. (1988)

Vasoconstrictor effects in spinal cord of the substance P antagonist [D-Arg^1, D-Trp^{7,9}, Leu^{11}]-substance P (spantide) and somatostatin and interaction with thyrotropin releasing hormone. *Neuroscience* **27**, 267-278.

13. GARRET, C., CARRUETTE, A., FARDIN, V., MOUSSAOUI, S., PEYRONEL, J.F., BLANCHARD, J.C. AND LADURON, P.M. (1991) Pharmacological properties of a potent and selective nonpeptide substance P antagonist. *Proc. Natl. Acad. Sci. USA* **88**, 10208-10211.

14. GERARD, N.P., BAO, L., XIAO-PING, H. AND GERARD, C. (1993) Molecular aspects of the tachykinin receptors, *Regul. Peptides* **43**, 21-35.

15. GITTER, B.D., WATERS, D.C., BRUNS, R.F., MASON, N.R., NIXON, J.A. AND HOWBERT, J.J. (1991) Species differences in affinities of nonpeptide antagonists for substance P receptors. *Eur. J. Pharmacol.* **197**, 237-238.

16. GUARD, S. AND WATSON, S.P. (1991) Tachykinin receptor types: classification and mebrane signalling mechanisms. *Neurochem. Int.* **18**, 149-165.

17. HELKE, C.J., KRAUSE, J.E., MANTYH, P.W., COUTURE, R. AND BANNON, M.J. (1990) Diversity in mammalian tachykinin peptidergic neurons : multiple peptides, receptors and regulatory mechanisms. *FASEB J.* **4**, 1606-1615.

18. HILL, J.M., PICKAR, J.G. AND KAUFMAN, M.P. (1992) Attenuation of reflex pressor and ventilatory responses to static contraction by an NK-1 receptor antagonist. *J. Appl. Physiol.* **73**, 1389-1395.

19. HOKFELT, T., KELLERTH, J.O., NILSSON, G. AND PERNOW, B. (1975) Experimental immunohistochemical studies on the localization and distribution of substance P in cat primary sensory neurons. *Brain Res.* **100**, 235-252.

20. IGWE, O.J., SUN, X. AND LARSON, A.A. (1990) Specific binding of substance P aminoterminal heptapeptide SP(1-7) to mouse brain and spinal cord membranes. *J. Neurosci.* **10**, 3653-3663.

21. KAGE, R., LEEMAN, S.E. AND BOYD, N.D. (1993) Biochemical characterization of two different forms of the substance P receptor in rat submaxillary glands, *J. Neurochemistry* **60**, 347-351.

22. KANAZAWA, I., OGAWA, T., KIMURA, S. AND MUNEKATA, E. (1984) Regional distribution of substance P, neurokinin A and neurokinin B in rat central nervous system. *Neurosci. Res.* **2**, 111-120.

23. KOTANI, H., HOSHIMARU, M., NAWA, H., AND NAKANISHI, S. (1986) Structure and gene organization of bovine neuromedin K precursor. *Proc. Natl. Acad. Sci. USA* **83**, 7074 - 7078.

24. KRAUSE, J.E., CHIRGWIN, J.M., CARTER, M.S., XU, Z.S. AND HERSHEY, A.D. (1987) Three rat preprotachykinin mRNAs encode the neuropeptides substance P and neurokinin A. *Proc. Natl. Acad. Sci. USA* **84**, 881-885.

25. LARSON, A.A. AND SUN, X. (1992) Aminoterminus of substance P potentiates kainic acid-induced activity in the mouse spinal cord. *J. Neurosci.* **12**, 4905-4910.

26. LEANDER, S., HAKANSON, R., ROSELL, S., FOLKERS, K., SUNDLER, F. AND TORNQVIST, K. (1981) A specific substance P antagonist blocks smooth

muscle contractions induced by noncholinergic nonadrenergic nerve stimulation. *Nature* **294**, 467-469.

27. LECCI, A., GIULIANI, S., PATACCHINI, R., VITI, G. AND MAGGI, C.A. (1991) Role of NK-1 tachykinin receptors in thermonociception : effect of (±)CP 96,345, a nonpeptide substance P antagonist on the hot plate test in mice. *Neurosci. Lett.* **129**, 299-302.

28. LECCI, A., GIULIANI, S. AND MAGGI, C.A. (1992) Effect of the NK-1 receptor antagonist GR 82,334 on reflexly-induced bladder contractions. *Life Sci. - Pharmacology Lett.* **51**, PL277-PL280.

29. LECCI, A, GIULIANI S., GARRET, C. AND MAGGI, C.A. (1993) Evidence for a role of tachykinins as sensory transmitters in the activation of micturition reflex. *Neuroscience* (in press).

30. LEE, C.M., IVERSEN, L.L., HANLEY, M.R. AND SANDBERG, B.E.B. (1982) The possible existence of multiple receptors for substance P. *Naunyn Schmied Arch. Pharmacol.* **318**, 281-288.

31. LEMBECK, F. (1953) Zur Frage der zentralen Ubertragung afferenter Impulse III Mitteilung. Das Vorkommen und die Bedeutung der Substanz P in den dorsalen Wurzeln des Ruckenmarks. *Arch. Exp. Path. Pharmakol.* **219**, 197-213.

32. MAGGI, C.A., PATACCHINI, R., GIULIANI, S., ROVERO, P., DION, S., REGOLI, D., GIACHETTI, A. AND MELI, A. (1990) Competitive antagonists discriminate between NK-2 tachykinin receptor subtypes. *Br. J. Pharmacol.* **100**, 588-592.

33. MAGGI, C.A., PATACCHINI, R., MEINI, S. AND GIULIANI, S (1993) Evidence for the presence of a septide-sensitive tachykinin receptor in the circular muscle of the guinea-pig ileum. *Eur. J. Pharmacol.* (in press).

34. MAGGI, C.A., PATACCHINI, R., ROVERO, P., AND GIACHETTI, A. (1993) Tachykinin receptors and receptor antagonists. *J. Autonom. Pharmacol.* **13**, 1-70.

35. MEINI, S., PATACCHINI, R. AND MAGGI, C.A. (1993) Tachykinin NK-1 receptor subtypes in the rat urinary bladder *Br. J. Pharmacol.* (in press).

36. NAGAHISA, A., ASAI, R., KANA,I Y., MURASE, A., TSUCHIYA-NAKAGAKI, M., NAKAGAKI, T., SHIEH, T.C. AND TANIGUCHI, K. (1992b) Nonspecific activity of (±)CP 96,345 in models of pain and inflammation. *Br. J. Pharmacol.* **107**, 273-275.

37. NAGAHISA, A., KANAI, Y., SUGA, O., TANIGUCHI, K., TSUCHIYA, M., LOWE, III J.A. AND HESS, H.J. (1992a) Antinflammatory and analgesic activity of a nonpeptide substance P receptor antagonist. *Eur. J. Pharmacol.* **217**, 191-195.

38. NAGY, I., MAGGI, C.A., DRAY, A., WOOLF, C.J. AND URBAN, L. (1993) The role of neurokinin and NMDA receptors in synaptic transmission from capsaicin-sensitive primary afferents in the rat spinal cord in vitro. *Neuroscience* **52**, 1029-1037.

39. NAKANISHI, S. (1991) Mammalian tachykinin receptors. *Annu. Rev. Neuroscience* **14**, 123 - 136

40. NIMMO, A., CARSTAIRS, J.R., MAGGI, C.A. AND MORRISON, J.F.B. (1992) Evidence for the co-existence of multiple NK-2 tachykinin receptor subtypes in rat bladder. *Neuropeptides* **22**, 48.

41. OTSUKA, M. AND YANAGISAWA, M. (1988) Effect of a tachykinin antagonist on a nociceptive reflex in the isolated spinal cord-tail preparation of the newborn rat. *J. Physiol.* **395**, 255-270.

42. PATACCHINI, R., ASTOLFI, M., QUARTARA, L., ROVERO, P., GIACHETTI, A., AND MAGGI, C.A. (1991) Further evidence for the existence of NK-2 tachykinin receptor subtypes. *Br. J. Pharmacol.* **104**, 91-96.

43. PATACCHINI, R., SANTICIOLI, P., ASTOLFI, M., ROVERO, P., VITI, G. AND MAGGI, C.A. (1992) Activity of peptide and non-peptide antagonists at peripheral NK-1 tachykinin receptors. *Eur. J. Pharmacol.* **215**, 93-98.

44. PETITET, F., SAFFROY, M., TORRENS, Y., LAVIELLE, S., CHASSAING, G. LOEUILLET, D., GLOWINSKI, J. AND BEAUJOAN, J.C. (1992) Possible existence of a new tachykinin receptor subtype in the guinea-pig ileum. *Peptides* **13**, 383-388.

45. RADHAKRISHNAN, V., AND HENRY, J.L. (1991) Novel substance P antagonist, CP 96,345 blocks responses of cat spinal dorsal horn neurons to noxious cutaneous stimulation and to substance P. *Neurosci Lett.* **132**, 39-43.

46. REGOLI, D., DRAPEAU, G., DION, S. AND D'ORLEANS-JUSTE, P. (1986) in *Substance P and neurokinins,* Montreal '86, eds. J.L. Henry et al. Springer-Verlag, New York.

47. SNIDER, R.M., CONSTANTINE, J.W., LOWE, III J.A., LONGO, K.P., LEBEL, W.S., WOODY, H.A., DROZDA, S.E., DESAI, M.C., VINICK, F.J., SPENCER, R.W. AND HESS, H.J. (1991) A potent nonpeptide antagonist of the substance P (NK-1) receptor. *Science* **251**, 435-437.

48. STEWART, J.M., HALL, M.E., HARKINS, J., FREDERICKSON, R.C.A., TERENIUS, L., HOKFELT, T. AND KRIVOY, W.A. (1982) A fragment of substance P with speicific central activity : SP(1-7). *Peptides* **3**, 851-857.

49. THOMPSON, S.W.N., DRAY, A. AND URBAN, L. (1993) The contribution of tachykinin receptor activation to C-fibre-evoked responses in the neonatal rat spinal cord in vitro. *J. Physiol.* **459**, 464P.

50. VAN GIERSBERGEN, P.L.M, SHATZER, S.A., HENDERSON, A.K., LAI J., NAKANISHI, S., YAMAMURA, H.I. AND BUCK, S.H. (1991) Characterization of a tachykinin peptide NK-2 receptor transfected into murine fibroblast B82 cell. *Proc. Natl. Acad .Sci. USA* **88**, 1661-1665.

51. YAMAMOTO, T. AND YAKSH, T.L. (1991) Stereospecific effects of a nonpeptidic NK-1 selective antagonist CP 96,345 : antinociception in the absence of motor dysfunction. *Life Sci.* **49**, 1955-1963.

52. XU, X.J., DALSGAARD, C.J. AND WIESENFELD-HALLIN, Z. (1992) Intrathecal CP 96,345 blocks reflex facilitation induced in rats by substance P and C-fiber conditioning stimulation. *Eur.J. Pharmacol.* **216**, 337-344.

53. XU X.J., MAGGI, C.A AND WIESENFELD-HALLIN, Z. (1991) On the role of NK-2 tachykinin receptors in the mediation of spinal reflex excitability in the rat. *Neuroscience* **44**, 483-490.

SYNAPTIC ACTIVATION BY THE RELEASE OF PEPTIDES

J.L. Henry and V. Radhakrishnan
Departments of Physiology and Psychiatry, McGill University
3655 Drummond St., Montreal, Quebec, H3G 1Y6
CANADA

INTRODUCTION

This survey will review some of the recent evidence which indicates that activation of primary afferent fibres provokes synaptically-elicited responses in the spinal cord which are due to activation of peptide receptors and therefore, by inference, that peptide release has occurred. Such responses are, perhaps, most clearly demonstrated from extracellular and intracellular electrophysiological studies *in vivo*. In fact, these *in vivo* studies also indicate a specificity of the actions of at least some of these peptides to certain modalities of sensory impression, most notably nociception. Furthermore, spinal reflex studies not only confirm a role of peptides in the transfer of nociceptive information, but they also indicate that release is sufficient to cause physiologically relevant changes. This survey will also touch upon two further aspects pertaining to the functional role of synaptically released peptides. One is the mechanisms by which peptide receptor activation is expressed and the other is the interaction of peptide systems with other transmitter systems.

The basic tenets of this field rely on clear definition of the functional properties of dorsal horn neurons and on the explicit nature of the response to peptide administration. Therefore, the anatomical and functional properties which characterize these neurones and responses to exogenous administration of peptides will first be described in detail. Then, evidence will be surveyed in which synaptically-elicited responses may be depressed by antagonists to peptide receptors. Finally, evidence on interactions of substance P receptor activation with nitric oxide activation will be presented.

NATO ASI Series, Vol. H 79
Cellular Mechanisms of Sensory Processing
Edited by Laszlo Urban
© Springer-Verlag Berlin Heidelberg 1994

ANATOMICAL CLASSIFICATION OF NEURONS IN THE SPINAL DORSAL HORN

The grey matter of the spinal cord has been divided into ten laminae on the basis of the cytoarchitectural properties of the neurons.[81] These divisions of the grey matter likely reflect differences in the functional properties of the respective neurons and physiological studies have given some validity to this likelihood. The sensory spinal cord is generally thought to be comprised of the first six laminae, those in the dorsal horn. Lamina I, also called the marginal layer or zone, contains flattened cells of 20-60 μm diameter oriented in a horizontal plane, as well as an assortment of smaller neurons.[27,53] While these neurons are generally thought to be mainly locally projecting neurons[7,52] many project to the brain stem[54,55] and thalamus[42,51,54] and may also participate in "propriospinal" connections to other segments of the spinal cord. The predominant input to these neurones is from Aδ fibers. Receptive fields are larger than those associated with primary afferents, due to the convergence of primary afferents onto second order neurons. Lamina II, which is also called the substantia gelatinosa, is comprised of two types of cell, the central cell and the limiting cell, as first identified by Cajal in 1909. The central cell, also termed the islet cell by Gobel[28] is widespread throughout the lamina and is a radially-oriented small cell (diameter of 7-14 μm), with extensive dendritic arbors arising laterally from the cell body; this cell is believed to serve primarily a projection function.[29] The limiting cell, also termed the stalked cell by Gobel, is slightly larger (diameter of 10-15 μm) and lies mainly in the outer part of the substantia gelatinosa. The axon and dendrites of this cell are oriented vertically and the axon extends into lamina I. Identified cells with dendrites limited to the outer part of lamina II receive excitatory inputs from C fibers innervating mechanical nociceptors or heat sensitive receptors, while those with dendrites confined to the inner layer are excited by C fibers activated by innocuous mechanical stimuli.[52] Cells with dendrites in the inner layer of lamina II which also extend into lamina III are innervated by A fibers responding to innocuous stimulation.[52] An excitatory input appears to come from noxious stimulation but an inhibitory input from innocuous mechanical stimulation to cells at the border of laminae I and II has also been reported;[6] this relationship has given rise to the suggestion that the level of excitability of these neurons may depend on the relative amounts of innocuous and noxious inputs. The deeper laminae, III to VI, are generally lumped together as the nucleus proprius. These deeper laminae are distinguished by the presence of large numbers of myelinated axons and relatively large neuronal cell bodies of 20-80 μm. Dendrites extend medially, laterally and dorsally into the substantia gelatinosa.[6] Neurons of lamina III comprise a heterogeneous population of non-nociceptive cells,[56] some projecting to suprasegmental levels.[6] Cells in laminae III and IV are activated predominantly by innocuous mechanical stimuli, including a major input from hair mechanoreceptors. Large diameter, Aß afferent fibers, which convey innocuous sensory inputs, terminate mainly in laminae III-IV,[6,56] as do Aδ D-hair afferents.[6] On the other hand, Aδ and C fiber nociceptive afferents, in addition to projecting to superficial laminae as indicated above, also project to lamina V,[52,96] including peptide-containing afferents.[84] Lamina V neurones also receive inputs from the larger diameter, Aß fiber, non-nociceptive afferents. Lamina V contains neurons which project to supraspinal structures.

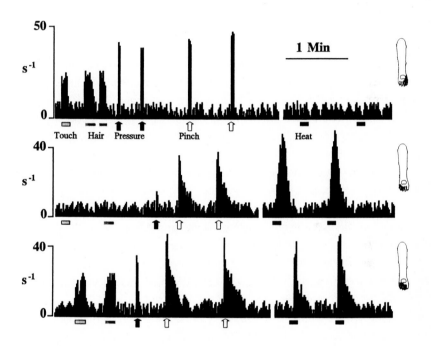

Figure 1. Functional classification of dorsal horn neurons. Ratemeter records showing the firing frequency of three different neurons to various cutaneous stimuli. The **top panel** shows the responses of a *non-nociceptive neuron* to stimulation of the receptive field in the hind paw (shown on right). This unit responded to non-noxious stimuli such as touch, hair and pressure. The response to pinch stimuli did not include an afterdischarge. The **middle panel** shows the response of a *nociceptive specific neuron*. Note the characteristic prolonged afterdischarge following pinch and noxious heat stimuli. The **bottom panel** shows the response of a *wide dynamic range neuron* which responded to both noxious and non-noxious stimuli.

FUNCTIONAL CLASSIFICATION OF NEURONS IN THE SPINAL DORSAL HORN

Figure 1 illustrates typical responses of three dorsal horn neurons in the cat to controlled natural stimulation of the cutaneous receptive field. An important feature which typifies a nociceptive response to a noxious stimulus is the prolonged discharge which outlasts the period of application of the stimulus; non-nociceptive responses end abruptly as illustrated in Figure 1. While several types of classification of dorsal horn neurons exist, the one receiving the greatest use is a classification based on the responses to natural cutaneous stimulation. Thus, the types may be referred to as "non-nociceptive neurons", which respond only to innocuous stimulation of the skin, "nociceptive specific neurons", which respond only to noxious stimulation, and "wide dynamic range neurons", which respond to both innocuous and noxious stimulation.

To define the functional properties of each dorsal horn neuron, a rigorous battery of tests is normally run. Each neuron is normally classified functionally on the basis of responses to natural cutaneous stimulation and on the basis of the response to electrical stimulation of the receptive field or of dissected nerves. In our experiments, natural stimuli include the following: (**1.**) An air stream regulated by an automatically controlled Vincent Assoc. Inc R11170 iris diaphragm to achieve reproducible puffs of air to activate groups of hairs in defined regions of the skin. (**2.**) Mechanical stimulation of single hairs using a feedback-controlled mechanical stimulator (Chubbuck stimulator)[8]; displacements of the stimulator can range from 1 to 1000 μm. This has been used to activate single guard hairs or single down hairs, without touching the skin, in which case the probe stimulated both guard and down hairs, the respective responses can be separated physiologically (De Koninck and Henry, manuscript submitted). (**3.**) Low threshold stimuli applied via the Chubbuck stimulator either to glabrous skin or to skin from which the fur has been removed; as the tip size, the force and the displacement can be controlled or monitored and as the probe can be stepped and held at various positions along its excursion, parametric studies can be carried out in which excitability of the neuron can be compared to the properties of the applied stimulus. (**4.**) High threshold stimuli produced by the Chubbuck stimulator probe applied with higher force against a raised section of skin backed by a metal platform. Again, the tip size and the force can be monitored to provide intensity/response curves for neurons sensitive to this type of stimulation. Successive stimuli can be separated by variable intervals to minimize adaptation or sensitization. **5.** Thermal stimulation (including innocuous warming and cooling as well as noxious heating) using a feedback-controlled heating device (Thermal Devices, Inc.). In this case testing is done using 20 s holding temperatures at 6°C steps from an adapting temperature of 34°C up to 52°C and 20 s holding temperatures at 4°C steps down to 6°C. This paradigm is minimally affected by sensitization, fatigue, hysteresis or long-term adaptation.[10] The mean discharge frequency at each temperature can be sampled. (**6.**) Vibration using the Chubbuck stimulator (frequencies of up to 240 Hz, displacements of 200-500 µm). This has been used extensively in studies from our laboratory.[20,87-91] (**7.**) Electrical stimulation of the receptive field or exposed nerves, to yield precise information on the latencies of the various components of the responses.

Complete classification of a neuron may be done in extracellular recording experiments. Thus, neurons can be classified on the basis of the latency of their response to electrical stimulation of sensory nerves, on the precise physiological response to natural activation of cutaneous receptors and on the basis of their antidromic response to electrical stimulation of sites of projection or termination. During classification while recording extracellularly, identification of inhibitory inputs can be achieved only if the neuron exhibits a reproducible excitatory response to peripheral stimulation, if it has some on-going discharge or if it is induced to discharge by local administration of excitatory agents (eg. by extracellular iontophoresis of glutamate).

During intracellular recording, however, it becomes particularly appropriate to quantitate the responses to noxious cutaneous stimuli, as the neurons characteristically exhibit a slow, prolonged depolarization in response to such stimuli. [19,21] The following criteria must be met before recording is considered to be acceptable: a) penetration with a shift in the DC potential of at least 40 mV, b) a recovery from injury spiking within a few seconds, c) a stable resting membrane potential of 50-65 mV and d) spikes with overshoot. To construct response functions, the areas under the curves of these depolarizations can be compared to the various intensities of the noxious stimuli described above. Additional properties which can be analyzed to complete classification include detailed analysis of postsynaptic potentials such as reversal potential, change in input resistance, etc. [20,87]

Despite the difficulty of recording intracellularly *in vivo*, it is possible to characterize synaptic responses in terms of their electrophysiological properties (*e.g.* change in input resistance, reversal potential, sensitivity to intracellular ion substitution and dependence on intracellular mechanisms), which can provide information about the nature of the chemical transmitter by which the responses are provoked. Figure 2 illustrates two types of synaptically elicited response from natural stimulation of the cutaneous receptive field. Each of these responses can be characterized in terms of their time course, reversal potential and sensitivity to intracellular ion substitution or channel blockers. The combined blockade of the response with an antagonist and the electrophysiological characterization of the membrane mechanisms involved in mediating a response provides evidence of the direct action of a given chemical on the postsynaptic neuron. The combination of these results with the ultrastructural localization of such a chemical in presynaptic profiles in relation to the intracellularly labelled neuron then provides substantial evidence of the involvement of a specific chemical in a specific synaptic function.

On the basis of these criteria, dorsal horn neurons are classified into functional groups. Wide dynamic range neurons characteristically show a brisk, transient response to low threshold mechanical stimuli and an afterdischarge in response to noxious stimuli, this latter response being due to a slow depolarization of the neuron, perhaps imposed by relatively slow acting chemical mediators of synaptic transmission. This is the most commonly encountered type of cell in the dorsal horn, especially in laminae I, II and V. Single pulse electrical stimulation of the cutaneous receptive field elicits early and late evoked spikes in the wide dynamic range neuron, which correspond to inputs from large and small diameter afferents,

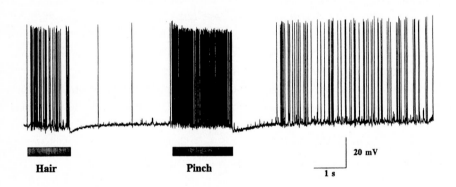

Figure 2. An intracellular record showing the responses of a wide dynamic range neuron to stimulation of hairs and to pinch. Note the brief inhibition of the response immediately after the pinch stimulus. The phase of afterdischarge follows this period of inhibition. Note also the lack of any such after discharge following the hair stimulation. Resting membrane potential: -64 mV.

respectively.[34,35] Cutaneous receptive fields usually consist of a central region which responds to low and high threshold stimulation, surrounded by a larger region from which a response can be elicited only by noxious stimuli. In some cases a third, "inhibitory surround" region is observed, from which stimuli depress the excitability of the neuron.

Nociceptive specific neurons show a late component in the response to single pulse electrical stimulation of the skin. These neurons respond only to noxious stimulation. Receptive fields tend to be relatively small compared to other dorsal horn neurons[21] and responses may be elicited by noxious mechanical and/or thermal stimuli. Responses to noxious stimuli show the typical afterdischarge described above.

Non-nociceptive neurons usually have relatively large receptive fields[21] and respond optimally to innocuous stimulation of the skin, although they of course also show non-specific responses to noxious stimulation due to non-specific activation of their respective cutaneous receptors. For instance, a pinch stimulus can activate the mechanoreceptors responding to touch and/or pressure stimuli but the response of these non-nociceptive neurons, unlike the wide dynamic range neurons, do not show the afterdischarge when the stimulus reaches the noxious range. These neurons are found most predominantly in laminae III and IV,[21] although some may also be found in the inner part of lamina II.

As indicated above, the morphological divisions of the grey matter are correlated with functional differences in the properties of neurons. Lamina I contains cells which respond to noxious and non-noxious thermal and mechanical stimuli.[9,11,43,82,83] Cells of lamina II appear to be grouped functionally according to their localization, as those in deep lamina II do not respond to noxious stimuli while those in outer lamina II respond specifically to these stimuli.[52] Neurons of laminae III-IV are non-nociceptive cells.[56] Laminae III-IV receive some Aδ fibres, from D hair follicles, and lamina V receive some high threshold mechanoceptors.[6,52] Deeper laminae, particularly lamina V, receive nociceptive primary sensory information, as detected by the occurrence of clusters of substance P immunoreactive fibres in lamina V.[84]

SUBSTANCE P AS THE PROTOTYPIC PEPTIDE

There is now considerable evidence of the involvement of substance P in the processing of sensory information in the region of the first sensory synapse.

[17,33,36,67,72] Immunocytochemically, it has been shown to occur in intrinsic fibers and in either unmyelinated or thinly myelinated sensory fibers that terminate mainly in laminae I and II[18,41] and also in lamina V.[84] Substance P is released in the spinal cord *in vivo* specifically upon activation of nociceptive sensory fibers[5,23,26,97] and nociceptive reflexes which are blocked by NK-1 receptor antagonists have been elicited in physiological studies.[14,19,75,107,108] Substance P is reported to have an excitatory effect in the dorsal horn, an effect associated specifically with nociceptive neurons. [32] This specificity prompted the suggestion that substance P is involved as an excitatory agent in the transmission of nociceptive information early in sensory pathways,[32] a suggestion which has generally been borne out by subsequent experimental evidence,[74,79,93] including a role in mediating nociceptive inputs in the trigeminal system.[39] Substance P-induced excitation of nociceptive neurons has recently been shown to be depressed by a novel, non-peptide substance P antagonist.[75]

In terms of actions at the cellular level, substance P has been proposed to decrease a K^+ conductance,[44,49,63,64,68] possibly of the M type.[68] More recently, however, substance P has been suggested to cause an increase in a Ca^{2+}-sensitive inward current[65]. Repetitive electrical stimulation of dorsal roots in the rat spinal slice *in vitro* causes a slow, prolonged depolarization which shows cross-desensitization to substance P[99] and which can be depressed by substance P antagonists.[80] Finally, in an isolated rat whole-spinal cord preparation, substance P antagonists have been shown to block slow depolarizing ventral root potentials to high intensity electrical stimulation of sensory nerves.[1,70,71]

Spinal reflex experiments have also indicated a possible role of substance P in nociception. Intrathecal administration of substance P in the rat produces a transient decrease in reaction time to tail withdrawal from a noxious radiant heat stimulus.[12,15,106,107,110] This decrease is followed by a rebound overshoot; this overshoot, but not the earlier phase of the response, is blocked by naloxone,[106] suggesting the activation of an opioid mechanism at the spinal level, due either to the substance P or to the substance P-induced activation of spinal nociceptive pathways. Noxious cutaneous stimulation produces a response similar to administration of substance P, including the naloxone-reversible component, and the facilitation is reduced by a substance P antagonist.[109]

SYNAPTIC ACTIVATION - EXTRACELLULAR ELECTROPHYSIOLOGICAL STUDIES

Figure 3 illustrates a typical response to iontophoretic application of substance P in extracellular recording experiments. For comparative purposes, responses to glutamate and to natural stimulation of the cutaneous receptive field are also shown. The most noticeable difference between the response to substance P and to the other stimuli is the slow nature of the response; it is slow to begin, normally taking 20-40 s in onset, and prolonged, normally outlasting the period of application by 30-90 s. Responses to glutamate typically begin within 2-3 s of the onset of application and stop abruptly when the ejecting current is ended. In early experiments, the slow

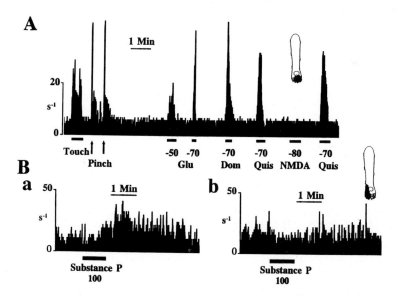

Figure 3. **A.** Response of a wide dynamic range neuron to cutaneous stimuli and to iontophoretic applications of excitatory amino acid agonists such as glutamate (Glu), domoate (Dom), quisqualate (Quis) and NMDA. The values shown above the drugs indicate the strength (nA) and polarity of the iontophoretic currents used. Note the briskness of the responses seen after each application of these agents. **B/a.** Response of a wide dynamic range neuron to iontophoretic application of substance P. Note the delayed onset and the slow, prolonged discharge of the response. **B/b.** Response of the same neuron to substance P after the administration of CP-96,345 (0.5 mg/kg, i.v.).

time course of this response prompted the suggestion that substance P may not be acting as a chemical mediator of fast synaptic responses[38] but may be acting as a slower regulator of the excitability of dorsal horn neurons.[32] In terms of functional significance, the original suggestion that substance P excitation is associated only with nociceptive (ie. nociceptive specific and wide dynamic range) neurons[32] has generally been supported by subsequent electrophysiological evidence.[92]

This response to iontophoretic application of substance P is inhibited by NK-1 receptor antagonists such as CP-96,345.[75] Figure 3 shows that in the presence of CP-96,345, iontophoretic application of substance P fails to produce the typical excitatory response. Thus, upon systemic administration, the NK-1 receptor antagonist has access to the spinal dorsal horn where it reduces the response of nociceptive neurons to substance P.

The involvement of NK-1 receptors in mediating nociceptive responses of dorsal horn neurons to noxious natural stimuli is illustrated in Figure 4. For neurons which are excited by iontophoretic application of substance P, nociceptive responses to noxious thermal stimulation of the cutaneous receptive field are inhibited by the antagonist.[75]

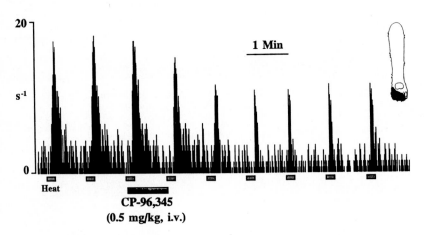

Figure 4. Effect of CP-96,345 on the response of a wide dynamic range neuron to noxious thermal stimulation of the cutaneous receptive field. Note the reduction in the afterdischarge following the administration of CP-96,345.

The response of a nociceptive neuron to noxious thermal stimulation is generally comprised of two components. Initially there is a rapid increase in the rate of firing, leading to a peak in the response which usually lasts 2-3 s. This is followed by a slow and prolonged afterdischarge which outlasts the period of the stimulus; during this afterdischarge the activity slowly returns to the baseline values. It is important to note that although following administration of CP-96,345, there is an inhibition of both components of the response to noxious thermal stimulation, the predominant effect is on the late phase of the response, the afterdischarge.[75]

The predominant effect on the afterdischarge suggests that substance P, or at least the endogenous ligand for the NK-1 receptor, acts predominantly to evoke the late phase of the synaptically-elicited response. The initial, more brisk phase of the evoked response may be elicited by activation of excitatory amino acid receptors, perhaps predominantly the non-NMDA type of glutamate receptor. The decrease produced by CP-96,345 in the magnitude of the early phase of the nociceptive response may be attributable to the facilitatory effect of substance P on responses to excitatory inputs which we and others have reported.[12,22,37,78,85,106,107,109,110]

It is important to point out that at a dose of CP-96,345 which blocks the response to iontophoretic application of substance P, there remains some residual afterdischarge to the noxious cutaneous stimulus. Therefore, it is suggested that this residual response may be mediated via the action of some other excitatory agent. Excitatory amino acids and other peptides come to mind as potential mediators of this residual afterdischarge.

In conjunction with this depression of the nociceptive response of dorsal horn neurons which are excited by iontophoretic application of substance P, it is important to note that not all nociceptive neurons respond to substance P.[32,75] In these cases, the nociceptive response to the noxious thermal stimulus was not altered. This reinforces the suggestion above that other chemical mediators may be responsible for nociceptive inputs to dorsal horn neurons, but these data also indicate that some nociceptive responses may be independent of NK-1 receptor activation.

In addition, CP-96,345 inhibited the responses of nociceptive units to noxious mechanical stimulation.[75] Here again, the inhibition brought about by CP-96,345 was predominantly of the late afterdischarge rather than of the initial fast phase. CP-96,345 failed to affect the responses of dorsal horn neurons to non-noxious mechanical stimuli (Fig. 5). This would therefore suggest that substance P mediates only nociceptive responses and this is favoured by the report that substance P excites mainly the nociceptive specific and wide dynamic range neurons.[32]

SYNAPTIC ACTIVATION - INTRACELLULAR ELECTROPHYSIOLOGICAL STUDIES

Noxious stimulation of the cutaneous receptive field evokes a prolonged afterdischarge associated with a slow, prolonged depolarization that lasted 20 s to

10 min. This specific nociceptive response, can be mimicked by electrical stimulation of sensory fibers at intensities which recruit C fibers.[19] A train of high intensity electrical stimuli of the sensory nerve produced a slow, prolonged

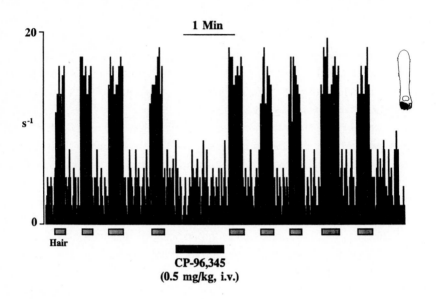

Figure 5. Effect of CP-96,345 on the response of a non-nociceptive neuron to stimulation of hairs in the receptive field. The response was not significantly altered following the administration of CP-96,345.

depolarization of the dorsal horn cells (Figure 6), that was comparable to the response obtained following a sustained noxious mechanical stimulation. This suggests that sustained activation of nociceptive afferent fibers is necessary to provoke the after-excitation and that it is not due to any peripheral injury. The time course of this response is comparable to the typically slow excitation observed with iontophoretic application of substance P on sensory neurons.[32,64,69] This slow, prolonged depolarization is also typically associated with an apparent increase in membrane conductance as has been observed with the effects of exogenous application of substance P under current clamp conditions.[64,66,69] This increase in input resistance contrasts with the marked decrease in resistance observed during the train, which is presumably due to a barrage of fast EPSPs. A decrease in the amplitude of the slow depolarization was observed at hyperpolarized potentials and an increase was observed at depolarized potentials, again resembling the response to exogenous application of substance P *in vitro* .[64,69] On the other hand, instead of a train, when a single electrical stimulus was given the EPSPs, elicited at a latency

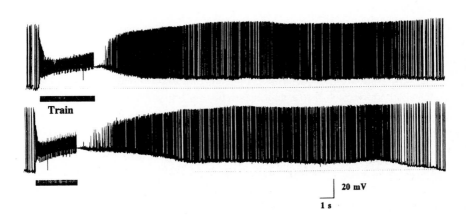

Figure 6. Intracellular record showing the response of a wide dynamic range neuron to a train of maximum intensity electrical stimulation (20 Hz, 3 ms pulse width for 8 s) of superficial peroneal nerve. Note the depolarization during the stimulus and the gradual return to baseline over time which depended on the duration of stimulus period. Also note the increase in firing rate following the stimulus. The responses were repeatable. Resting membrane potential: -60 mV.

consistent with conduction in C fibers, showed a reversal potential comparable to more classical EPSPs, such as those of the non-NMDA excitatory amino acid type. [19,95,111]

The slow, prolonged depolarization evoked by sustained noxious cutaneous stimulation or by a train of electrical stimuli to a sensory nerve could be blocked by the substance P antagonist CP-96,345, suggesting that these components of the response were mediated by substance P.[19] The fast initial excitation seen during the stimuli was unaffected. Fast EPSPs in response to single stimuli and recorded at latencies consistent with conduction in C fibers were also unaffected. These results indicated that substance P is released in response to a sustained noxious stimulation but not following a single or brief stimulus.

CELLULAR MECHANISM OF SUBSTANCE P ACTION ON DORSAL HORN NEURONS - IMPLICATION OF A NITRIC OXIDE STEP

While substance P action on nociceptive neurons appears to include effects on K^+ and Ca^{2+} currents, as discussed above, other cellular events may also be provoked. Peripherally, substance P-induced relaxation of rabbit aortic rings[50] and vasodilation in dogs[73] are antagonized by an endothelial nitric oxide synthase inhibitor,[59] suggesting the mediation of substance P effects through the release of endothelial nitric oxide. The first evidence that nitric oxide may play a role in central nervous system was provided by Garthwaite et al.[25] who reported that activation of NMDA receptors gives rise to the release of nitric oxide in cerebellar neurons. Nitric oxide is derived from L-arginine by the action of the enzyme nitric oxide synthase present in brain synaptosomes[4,47,48] leading to a Ca^{2+}-dependent increase in intracellular cyclic guanosine monophosphate (cGMP).[25] Histochemical studies have indicated the presence of a nitric oxide synthase predominantly in the superficial layers of spinal dorsal horn, but not in the ventral horn, suggesting a possible role in sensory mechanisms.[24,100] A role of nitric oxide specifically in nociception is evident from the finding that nitric oxide synthase inhibitors exhibit antinociceptive properties in various animal models of nociception.[45,57,58,61]

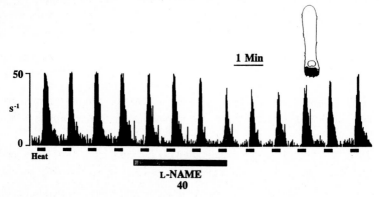

Figure 7. Effect of iontophoretically applied L-NAME on the response of a wide dynamic range neuron to noxious thermal stimulation.

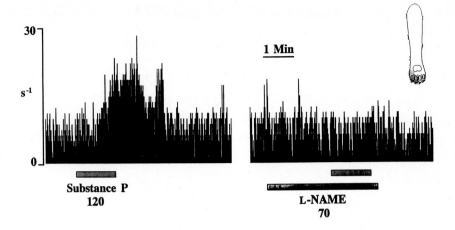

Figure 8. Effect of iontophoretically applied L-NAME on the response of a wide dynamic range neuron to iontophoretically applied substance P. Note the inhibition of the response to substance P in the presence of L-NAME.

We have recently demonstrated that the nitric oxide synthase inhibitor, N^G-nitro-L-arginine methyl ester (L-NAME) attenuates the responses of dorsal horn neurons to noxious thermal (Fig. 7) and mechanical stimulation.[76] This inhibition may not be attributed to any peripheral action of L-NAME, since both systemic and iontophoretic administration of L-NAME were effective. Both the initial, fast and the later, slow, prolonged afterdischarge components of the response were inhibited. The inhibition appears to be independent of changes in blood pressure because, following systemic administration of L-NAME, there was only a rise in blood pressure (owing to an inhibition of nitric oxide synthase enzyme in the endothelial cells) and not a fall. Also, the baseline firing rate was unaffected indicating that L-NAME does not interfere with normal synaptic transmission or with the basal excitability of the neurons. The effects of L-NAME appear to be enantiomer-specific, as D-NAME, the inactive isomer is without effect.

The responses of dorsal horn neurons to noxious cutaneous stimulation are, therefore, inhibited both by substance P antagonists and by the nitric oxide synthase inhibitor. As activation of NMDA receptors induces nitric oxide synthesis[25] and as hyperalgesic states induced by NMDA are antagonized by nitric oxide synthase

246

inhibitors,[45,57] it is conceivable that blockade of noxious thermal and mechanical responses by L-NAME in our paradigm may be due to an antagonism of NMDA receptor-mediated effects. Indeed, the responses of dorsal horn neurons to iontophoretic application of NMDA, but not quisqualate are attenuated by L-NAME.[76] Our data also indicate that NMDA antagonists such as ketamine and 2-amino-5-phosphonovaleric acid (APV) fail to alter the responses of dorsal horn neurons to noxious cutaneous stimulation in a similar paradigm.[77] Stated otherwise, these data therefore indicate a different mechanism, apart from NMDA receptor activation, for the initiation of the nitric oxide pathway.

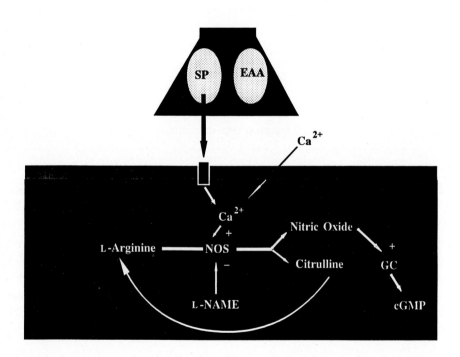

Figure 9. Schematic representation of substance P-induced activation of the nitric oxide pathway. SP: Substance P; EAA: Excitatory amino acid; NOS: Nitric oxide synthase; GC: soluble guanylate cyclase.

Considering the facts that the responses of dorsal horn neurons to noxious cutaneous stimulation are affected both by substance P antagonists and by L-NAME, and that peripheral vasodilator actions of substance P are antagonized by nitric oxide synthase inhibitors,[50,73] we tested the effect of L-NAME on the responses of dorsal horn neurons to iontophoretically applied substance P (Figure 8). The results indicated a blockade of substance P effects by L-NAME[76] suggesting that responses of dorsal horn neurons to substance P are mediated via a nitric oxide mechanism. Activation of nitric oxide synthase is Ca^{2+}-dependent and substance P is known to increase the intracellular Ca^{2+} in dorsal horn neurons.[65,103] To visualize the processes involved, the possible steps in this substance P-activated nitric oxide mechanism are summarized in Figure 9.

Electrophysiological and behavioural studies have indicated that the second phase of formalin response is preferentially inhibited by nitric oxide synthase inhibitors.[30,60,62] Our data have shown that this phase is also inhibited by a substance P antagonist[108] consistent with the notion that nitric oxide is an intracellular mediator of NK-1 receptor activation.

CONCLUSIONS

Though the present review has considered substance P as a prototypic peptide in nociceptive transmission in the spinal cord, the role of other peptides cannot be ignored. Immunohistochemical studies have shown the co-existence of substance P with calcitonin gene-related peptide (CGRP) in primary afferent terminals in the dorsal horn and a role of CGRP in nociception has also been experimentally supported.[2,3,13,16,31,40,86,94,98,104] Recent evidence also implicates cholecystokinin in primary afferent transmission,[46,101] galanin[13,94,101,102] and vasooactive intestinal polypeptide,[13,105] though localized in primary afferent terminals in the dorsal horn, may not mediate direct excitation of sensory neurons.[94] Certainly, there is abundant evidence that neuropeptides released from primary afferents play a pivotal role in the mediation of sensory signals, especially nociceptive inputs.

REFERENCES

1. AKAGI H., KONISHI S., OTSUKA M. AND YANAGISAWA M. (1985) The role of substance P as a neurotransmitter in the reflexes of slow time courses in the neonatal rat spinal cord. *Br. J. Pharmacol.* **84**, 663-673.

2. ALVAREZ F.J., KAVOOKJIAN A.M. AND LIGHT A.R. (1993) Ultrastructural morphology, synaptic relationships, and CGRP immunoreactivity of physiologically identified C-fiber terminals in the monkey spinal cord. *J. Comp. Neurol.* **329**, 472-490.

3. BIELLA G., PANARA C., PECILE A. AND SOTGIU M.L. (1991) Facilitatory role of calcitonin gene-related peptide (CGRP) on excitation induced by substance P (SP) and noxious stimuli in rat spinal dorsal horn neurons. An iontophoretic study in vivo. *Brain Res.* **559**, 352-356.

4. BREDT D.S., HWANG P.M. AND SNYDER S.H. (1990) Localization of nitric oxide synthase indicating a neural role for nitric oxide. *Nature* **347**, 768-770.

5. BRODIN E., LINDEROTH B., CAZELIUS B. AND UNGERSTEDT V. (1987) In vivo release of substance P in cat dorsal horn studied with microdialysis. *Neurosci. Lett.* **76**, 357-362.

6. BROWN A.G. (1981) *Organization in the spinal cord.* Springer Verlag, New York.

7. CERVERO F., IGGO A. AND MOLONY V. (1979) Ascending projections of nociceptor-driven lamina I neurons in the cat. *Exp. Brain Res.* **35**, 135-149.

8. CHUBBUCK J.G. (1966) Small motion biological stimulator. *APL Tech. Dig.* **6**, 18-23.

9. CRAIG A.D. AND DOSTROVSKY J.O. (1991) Thermoreceptive lamina I trigeminothalamic neurons project to the nucleus submedius in the cat. *Exp. Brain Res.* **85**, 470-474.

10. CRAIG A.D. AND HUNSLEY S.J. (1991) Morphine enhances the activity of thermoreceptive cold-specific lamina I spinothalamic neurons in the cat. *Brain Res.* **558**, 93-97.

11. CRAIG A.D. AND KNIFFKI K.D. (1985) Spinothalamic lumbosacral lamina I cells responsive to skin and muscle stimulation in the cat. *J. Physiol. (Lond.)* **365**, 197-221.

12. CRIDLAND R.A. AND HENRY J.L. (1986) Comparison of the effects of substance P, neurokinin A, physalaemin and eledoisin in facilitating a nociceptive reflex in the rat. *Brain Res.* **381**, 93-99.

13. CRIDLAND R.A. AND HENRY J.L. (1988) Effects of intrathecal administration of neuropeptides on a spinal nociceptive reflex in the rat: VIP, galanin, CGRP, TRH, somatostatin and angiotensin II. *Neuropeptides* **11**, 23-32.

14. CRIDLAND R.A. AND HENRY J.L. (1988) Facilitation of the tail-flick reflex by noxious cutaneous stimulation in the rat: antagonism by a substance P analogue. *Brain Res.* **462**, 15-21.

15. CRIDLAND R.A. AND HENRY J.L. (1988) Intrathecal administration of substance P in the rat: spinal transection or morphine blocks the behavioural responses but not the facilitation of the tail flick reflex. *Neurosci. Lett.* **84**, 203-208.

16. CRIDLAND R.A. AND HENRY J.L. (1989) Intrathecal administration of CGRP in the rat attenuates a facilitation of the tail flick reflex induced by either substance P or noxious cutaneous stimulation. *Neurosci. Lett.* **102**, 241-246.

17. CUELLO A.C. (1987) Peptides as neuromodulators in primary sensory neurons. *Neuropharmacology* **7**, 971-979.

18. CUELLO A.C. AND KANAZAWA I. (1978) The distribution of substance P immunoreactive fibers in the rat central nervous system. *J. Comp. Neurol.* **178**, 129-156.

19. DE KONINCK Y. AND HENRY J.L. (1991) Substance P-mediated slow EPSP elicited in dorsal horn neurons *in vivo* by noxious stimulation. *Proc. Natl. Acad. Sci. USA* **88**, 11344-11348.

20. DE KONINCK Y. AND HENRY J.L. (1992) Peripheral vibration causes an adenosine-mediated postsynaptic inhibitory potential in dorsal horn neurons of the cat spinal cord. *Neuroscience* **50**, 435-443.

21. DE KONINCK Y., RIBEIRO-DA-SILVA A., HENRY J.L. AND CUELLO A.C. (1992) Spinal neurons exhibiting a specific nociceptive response receive abundant substance P-containing synaptic contacts. *Proc. Natl. Acad. Sci. USA* **89**, 5073-5077.

22. DOUGHERTY P.M. AND WILLIS W.D. (1991) Enhancement of spinothalamic neuron responses to chemical and mechanical stimuli following combined micro-iontophoretic application of N-methyl-D-aspartic acid and substance P. *Pain* **47**, 85-93.

23. DUGGAN A.W., HENDRY I.A., MORTON C.R., HUTCHISON W.D. AND ZHAO Z.Q. (1988) Cutaneous stimuli releasing immunoreactive substance P in the dorsal horn of the cat. *Brain Res.* **451**, 261.

24. DUN N.J., DUN S.L., FORSTERMANN U. AND TSENG L.F. (1992) Nitric oxide synthase immunoreactivity in rat spinal cord. *Neurosci. Lett.* **147**, 217-220.

25. GARTHWAITE J., CHARLES S.L. AND CHESS-WILLIAMS R. (1988) Endothelium-derived relaxing factor release on activation of NMDA receptors suggests role as intracellular messenger in the brain. *Nature* **336**, 385-388.

26. GO V.L.W. AND YAKSH T.L. (1987) Release of substance P from the cat spinal cord. *J. Physiol. (Lond.)* **391**, 141-167.

27. GOBEL S. (1978) Golgi studies of the neurons in layer 1 of the dorsal horn of the medulla (trigeminal nucleus caudalis). *J. Comp. Neurol.* **180**, 375-394.

28. GOBEL S. (1978) Golgi studies of the neurons in layer II of the dorsal horn of the medulla (trigeminal nucleus caudalis). *J. Comp. Neurol.* **180**, 395-414.

29. GOBEL S., FALLS W.A., BENNETT G.J., ABDELMOUMENE M., HAYASHI H. AND HUMPHREY E. (1980) An EM analysis of the synaptic connections of horseradish peroxidase-filled stalked cells and islet cells in the substantia gelatinosa of adult cat spinal cord. *J. Comp. Neurol.* **194**, 781-807.

30. HALEY J.E., DICKENSON A.H. AND SCHACHTER M. (1992) Electrophysiological evidence for a role of nitric oxide in prolonged chemical nociception in the rat. *Neuropharmacology* **31**, 251-258.

31. HAYES E.S. AND CARLTON S.M. (1992) Primary afferent interactions: Analysis of calcitonin gene-related peptide-immunoreactive terminals in contact

with unlabeled and GABA-immunoreactive profiles in the monkey dorsal horn. *Neuroscience* **47**, 873-896.

32. HENRY J.L. (1976) Effects of substance P on functionally identified units in cat spinal cord. *Brain Res.* **114**, 439-451.

33. HENRY J.L. (1982) Relation of substance P to pain transmission: neurophysiological evidence. *Ciba. Found. Symp.* **9**, 206-224.

34. HENRY J.L. (1982) Pharmacological studies on the prolonged depressant effects of baclofen on lumbar dorsal horn units in the cat. *Neuropharmacology* **21**, 1085-1093.

35. HENRY J.L. (1982) Effects of intravenously administered enantiomers of baclofen on functionally identified units in lumbar dorsal horn of the spinal cat. *Neuropharmacology* **21**, 1073-1083.

36. HENRY J.L. (1993) Participation of substance P in spinal physiological responses to peripheral aversive stimulation. *Regul. Pept.* **(in press)**.

37. HENRY J.L. AND BEN ARI Y. (1976) Actions of the p-chlorophenyl derivative of GABA, Lioresal, on nociceptive and non-nociceptive units in the spinal cord of the cat. *Brain Res.* **117**, 540-544.

38. HENRY J.L., KRNJEVIC K. AND MORRIS M.E. (1975) Substance P and spinal neurons. *Can. J. Physiol. Pharmacol.* **53**, 423-432.

39. HENRY J.L., SESSLE B.J., LUCIER G.E. AND HU J.W. (1980) Effects of substance P on nociceptive and non-nociceptive trigeminal brain stem neurons. *Pain* **8**, 33-45.

40. HENRY M.A., NOUSEK-GOEBL N.A. AND WESTRUM L.E. (1993) Light and electron microscopic localization of calcitonin gene-related peptide immunoreactivity in lamina II of the feline trigeminal pars caudalis/medullary dorsal horn: A qualitative study. *Synapse* **13**, 99-107.

41. HÖKFELT T., KELLERTH J.-O., NILSSON G. AND PERNOW B. (1975) Substance P: localization in the central nervous system and in some primary sensory neurons. *Science* **190**, 889-891.

42. HYLDEN J.L.K., HAYASHI H., DUBNER R. AND BENNETT G.J. (1986) Physiology and morphology of the lamina I spinomesencephalic projection. *J. Comp. Neurol.* **274**, 505-515.

43. HYLDEN J.L.K., NAHIN R.L., TRAUB R.J. AND DUBNER R. (1989) Expansion of receptive fields of spinal lamina I projection neurons in rats with unilateral adjuvant-induced inflammation: the contribution of dorsal horn mechanisms. *Pain* **37**, 229-243.

44. KATAYAMA Y. AND NORTH R.A. (1978) Does substance P mediate slow synaptic excitation within the myenteric plexus. *Nature* **274**, 387-388.

45. KITTO K.F., HALEY J.E. AND WILCOX G.L. (1992) Involvement of nitric oxide in spinally mediated hyperalgesia in the mouse. *Neurosci. Lett.* **148**, 1-5.

46. KLEIN C.M., COGGESHALL R.E., CARLTON S.M. AND SORKIN L.S. (1992) The effects of $A\delta$ and C-fiber stimulation on patterns of neuropeptide immunostaining in the rat superficial dorsal horn. *Brain Res.* **580**, 121-128.

47. KNOWLES R.G., PALACIOS M., PALMER R.M.J. AND MONCADA S. (1989) Formation of nitric oxide from L-arginine in the central nervous system: a transduction mechanism for stimulation of the soluble guanylate cyclase. *Proc. Natl. Acad. Sci. USA* **86**, 5159-5162.

48. KNOWLES R.G., PALACIOS M., PALMER R.M.J. AND MONCADA S. (1990)

Kinetic characteristics of nitric oxide synthase from rat brain. *Biochem. J.* **269**, 207-210.

49. KRNJEVIC K. (1977) Effects of substance P on central neurons in cats. In *Substance P* (Eds. von Euler U.S. and Pernow B.), pp. 217-230. Raven Press, New York.

50. LEWIS M.J. AND HENDERSON A.H. (1987) A phorbol ester inhibits the release of endothelium-derived relaxing factor. *Eur. J. Pharmacol.* **137**, 167-171.

51. LIGHT A.R. (1992) *The initial processing of pain and its descending control: spinal and trigeminal systems.* Karger, Basel.

52. LIGHT A.R. AND PERL E.R. (1979) Spinal termination of functionally identified primary afferent neurons with slowly conducting myelinated fibers. *J. Comp. Neurol.* **186**, 133-150.

53. LIMA D. AND COIMBRA A. (1986) A Golgi study of the neuronal population of the marginal zone (lamina I) of the rat spinal cord. *J. Comp. Neurol.* **244**, 53-71.

54. LIMA D. AND COIMBRA A. (1988) The spinothalamic system of the rat: Structural types of retrogradely labelled neurons in the marginal zone (Lamina I). *Neuroscience* **27**, 215-230.

55. LIMA D. AND COIMBRA A. (1990) Structural types of marginal (lamina I) neurons projecting to the dorsal reticular nucleus of the medulla oblongata. *Neuroscience* **34**, 591-606.

56. MAXWELL D.J., FYFFE R.E.W. AND RETHELYI M. (1983) Morphological properties of physiologically characterized lamina III neurons in the cat spinal cord. *Neuroscience* **10**, 1-22.

57. MELLER S.T., DYKSTRA C. AND GEBHART G.F. (1992) Production of endogenous nitric oxide and activation of soluble guanylate cyclase are required for N-methyl-D-aspartate- produced facilitation of the nociceptive tail-flick reflex. *Eur. J. Pharmacol.* **214**, 93-96.

58. MELLER S.T., PECHMAN P.S., GEBHART G.F. AND MAVES T.J. (1992) Nitric oxide mediates the thermal hyperalgesia produced in a model of neuropathic pain in the rat. *Neuroscience* **50**, 7-10.

59. MONCADA S., PALMER R.M.J. AND HIGGS E.A. (1991) Nitric oxide: Physiology, pathophysiology, and pharmacology. *Pharmacol. Rev.* **43**, 109-142.

60. MOORE P.K., BABBEDGE R.C., WALLACE P., GAFFEN Z.A. AND HART S.L. (1993) 7-nitro indazole, an inhibitor of nitric oxide synthase, exhibits anti-nociceptive activity in the mouse without increasing blood pressure. *Br. J. Pharmacol.* **108**, 296-297.

61. MOORE P.K., OLUYOMI A.O., BABBEDGE R.C., WALLACE P. AND HART S.L. (1991) L-N^{G}-nitro arginine methyl ester exhibits antinociceptive activity in the mouse. *Br. J. Pharmacol.* **102**, 198-202.

62. MORGAN C.V.J., BABBEDGE R.C., GAFFEN Z., WALLACE P., HART S.L. AND MOORE P.K. (1992) Synergistic anti-nociceptive effect of L-N^{G}-nitro arginine methyl ester (L-NAME) and flurbiprofen in the mouse. *Br. J. Pharmacol.* **106**, 493-497.

63. MURASE K., NEDELJKOV V. AND RANDIC M. (1982) The actions of neuropeptides on dorsal horn neurons in the rat spinal cord slice preparation: an intracellular study. *Brain Res.* **234**, 170-176.

64. MURASE K. AND RANDIC M. (1984) Actions of substance P on rat spinal dorsal

horn neurons. *J. Physiol. (Lond.)* **346**, 203-217.

65. MURASE K., RYU P.D. AND RANDIC M. (1986) Substance P augments a persistent slow inward calcium-sensitive current in voltage-clamped spinal dorsal horn neurons of the rat. *Brain Res.* **365**, 369-376.

66. NEWTON B.W., UNGER J. AND HAMILL R.W. (1990) Calcitonin gene-related peptide and somatostatin immunoreactivities in the rat lumbar spinal cord: Sexually dimorphic aspects. *Neuroscience* **37**, 471-489.

67. NICOLL R.A., SCHENKER C. AND LEEMAN S.E. (1980) Substance P as a transmitter candidate. *Ann. Rev. Neurosci.* **3**, 227-268.

68. NOWAK L.M. AND MACDONALD R.L. (1981) Substance P decreases a potassium conductance of spinal cord neurons in cell culture. *Brain Res.* **214**, 416-423.

69. NOWAK L.M. AND MACDONALD R.L. (1982) Substance P: ionic basis for depolarizing responses of mouse spinal cord neurons in cell culture. *J. Neurosci.* **2**, 1119-1128.

70. NUSSBAUMER J.-C., YANAGISAWA M. AND OTSUKA M. (1989) Pharmacological properties of a C-fibre response evoked by saphenous nerve stimulation in an isolated spinal cord-nerve preparation of the newborn rat. *Br. J. Pharmacol.* **98**, 373-382.

71. OTSUKA M. AND YANAGISAWA M. (1988) Effect of a tachykinin antagonist on a nociceptive reflex in the isolated spinal cord-tail preparation of the newborn rat. *J. Physiol. (Lond.)* **395**, 255-270.

72. OTSUKA M. AND YANAGISAWA M. (1990) Pain and neurotransmitters. *Cell. Mol. Neurobiol.* **10**, 293-302.

73. PERSSON M.G., HEDQVIST P. AND GUSTAFSSON L.E. (1991) Nerve-induced tachykinin-mediated vasodilatation in skeletal muscle is dependent on nitric oxide formation. *Eur. J. Pharmacol.* **205**, 295-301.

74. PIERCEY M.F. AND EINSPAHR F.J. (1980) Use of substance P partial fragments to characterize substance P receptors of cat dorsal horn neurons. *Brain Res.* **187**, 481-486.

75. RADHAKRISHNAN V. AND HENRY J.L. (1991) Novel substance P antagonist, CP-96,345, blocks responses of spinal dorsal horn neurons to noxious cutaneous stimulation and to substance P. *Neurosci. Lett.* **132**, 39-43.

76. RADHAKRISHNAN V. AND HENRY J.L. (1993) L-NAME blocks responses to NMDA, substance P and noxious cutaneous stimuli in cat dorsal horn. *NeuroReport* **4**, 323-326.

77. RADHAKRISHNAN V. AND HENRY J.L. (1993) Excitatory amino acid receptor mediation of sensory inputs to functionally identified dorsal horn neurons in cat spinal cord. *Neuroscience* **(in press)**.

78. RANDIC M., HECIMOVIC H. AND RYU P.D. (1990) Substance P modulates glutamate-induced currents in acutely isolated rat spinal dorsal horn neurons. *Neurosci. Lett.* **117**, 74-80.

79. RANDIC M. AND MILETIC V. (1977) Effect of substance P in cat dorsal horn neurons activated by noxious stimuli. *Brain Res.* **128**, 164-169.

80. RANDIC M., RYU P.D. AND URBAN L. (1986) Effects of polyclonal and monoclonal antibodies to substance P on slow excitatory transmission in rat spinal dorsal horn. *Brain Res.* **383**, 15-27.

81. REXED B. (1952) The cytoarchitectonic organization of the spinal cord in the cat. *J. Comp. Neurol.* **96**, 415-495.

82. RÉTHELYI M., LIGHT A.R. AND PERL E.R. (1989) Synaptic ultrastructure of functionally and morphologically characterized neurons of the superficial spinal dorsal horn of cat. *J. Neurosci.* **9**, 1846-1863.

83. RIBEIRO-DA-SILVA A., DE KONINCK Y., CUELLO A.C. AND HENRY J.L. (1992) Enkephalin-immunoreactive nociceptive neurons in the cat spinal cord. *NeuroReport* **3**, 25-28.

84. RUDA M.A., BENNETT G.J. AND DUBNER R. (1986) Neurochemistry and neural circuitry in the dorsal horn. In *Peptides and Neurological disease. Prog. Brain Res., Vol. 66* (Eds. Emson P.C., Rossor M. and Tohyama M.), pp. 219-268. Elsevier Science Publishers, Amsterdam.

85. RUSIN K.I., RYU P.D. AND RANDIC M. (1992) Modulation of excitatory amino acid responses in rat dorsal horn neurons by tachykinins. *J. Neurophysiol.* **68**, 265-286.

86. RYU P.D., GERBER G., MURASE K. AND RANDIC M. (1988) Calcitonin gene-related peptide enhances calcium current of rat dorsal root ganglion neurons and spinal excitatory synaptic transmission. *Neurosci. Lett.* **89**, 305-312.

87. SALTER M.W., DE KONINCK Y. AND HENRY J.L. (1992) ATP-sensitive K+ channels mediate an IPSP in dorsal horn neurons elicited by sensory stimulation. *Synapse* **11**, 214-220.

88. SALTER M.W. AND HENRY J.L. (1987) Evidence that adenosine mediates the depression of spinal dorsal horn neurons induced by peripheral vibration in the cat. *Neuroscience* **22**, 631-650.

89. SALTER M.W. AND HENRY J.L. (1988) Tachykinins enhance the depression of spinal nociceptive neurons caused by cutaneously applied vibration in the cat. *Neuroscience* **27**, 243-249.

90. SALTER M.W. AND HENRY J.L. (1990) Physiological characteristics of responses of wide dynamic range spinal neurons to cutaneously applied vibration in the cat. *Brain Res.* **507**, 69-84.

91. SALTER M.W. AND HENRY J.L. (1990) Differential responses of nociceptive vs. non-nociceptive spinal dorsal horn neurons to cutaneously applied vibration in the cat. *Pain* **40**, 311-322.

92. SALTER M.W. AND HENRY J.L. (1991) Responses of functionally identified neurons in the dorsal horn of the cat spinal cord to substance P, neurokinin A and physalaemin. *Neuroscience* **43**, 601-610.

93. SASTRY B.R. (1979) Substance P effects on spinal nociceptive neurons. *Life Sci.* **24**, 2169-2178.

94. SATOH M., KURAISHI Y. AND KAWAMURA M. (1992) Effects of intrathecal antibodies to substance P, calcitonin gene-related peptide and galanin on repeated cold stress- induced hyperalgesia: Comparison with carrageenan-induced hyperalgesia. *Pain* **49**, 273-278.

95. SCHNEIDER S.P. AND PERL E.R. (1988) Comparison of primary afferent and glutamate excitation of neurons in the mammalian spinal dorsal horn. *J. Neurosci.* **8**, 2062-2073.

96. SUGIURA Y., LEE C.L. AND PERL E.R. (1986) Central projections of identified, unmyelinated (C) afferent fibers innervating mammalian skin. *Science* **234**, 358-361.

97. THERIAULT E., OTSUKA M. AND JESSELL T. (1979) Capsaicin-evoked release of substance P from primary sensory neurons. *Brain Res.* **170**, 209-213.

98. TRAUB R.J., ALLEN B., HUMPHREY E. AND RUDA M.A. (1990) Analysis of calcitonin gene-related peptide-like immunoreactivity in the cat dorsal spinal cord and dorsal root ganglia provide evidence for a multisegmental projection of nociceptive C-fiber primary afferents. *J. Comp. Neurol.* **302**, 562-574.

99. URBAN L. AND RANDIC M. (1984) Slow excitatory transmission in rat dorsal horn: possible mediation by peptides. *Brain Res.* **290**, 336-341.

100. VALTSCHANOFF J.G., WEINBERG R.J. AND RUSTIONI A. (1992) NADPH diaphorase in the spinal cord of rats. *J. Comp. Neurol.* **321**, 209-222.

101. VERGE V.M.K., XU X.-J., LANGEL ., HÖKFELT T., WIESENFELD-HALLIN Z. AND BARTFAI T. (1993) Evidence for endogenous inhibition of autotomy by galanin in the rat after sciatic nerve section: Demonstrated by chronic intrathecal infusion of a high affinity galanin receptor antagonist. *Neurosci. Lett.* **149**, 193-197.

102. WIESENFELD-HALLIN Z., XU X.-J., LANGEL ., BEDECS K., HÖKFELT T. AND BARTFAI T. (1992) Galanin-mediated control of pain: Enhanced role after nerve injury. *Proc. Natl. Acad. Sci. USA* **89**, 3334-3337.

103. WOMACK M.D., MACDERMOTT A.B. AND JESSELL T.M. (1988) Sensory transmitters regulate intracellular calcium in dorsal horn neurons. *Nature* **334**, 351-353.

104. WOOLF C. AND WIESENFELD-HALLIN Z. (1986) Substance P and calcitonin gene-related peptide synergistically modulate the gain of the nociceptive flexor withdrawal reflex in the rat. *Neurosci. Lett.* **66**, 226-230.

105. XU X.-J. AND WIESENFELD-HALLIN Z. (1991) An analogue of growth hormone releasing factor (GRF), (Ac-Try[1], D-Phe[2])-GRF-(1-29), specifically antagonizes the facilitation of the flexor reflex induced by intrathecal vasoactive intestinal peptide in rat spinal cord. *Neuropeptides* **18**, 129-135.

106. YASHPAL K. AND HENRY J.L. (1983) Endorphins mediate overshoot of substance P-induced facilitation of a spinal nociceptive reflex. *Can. J. Physiol. Pharmacol.* **61**, 303-307.

107. YASHPAL K. AND HENRY J.L. (1984) Substance P analogue blocks SP-induced facilitation of a spinal nociceptive reflex. *Brain Res. Bull.* **13**, 597-600.

108. Yashpal K., Radhakrishnan V., Coderre T.J. and Henry J.L. (1993) CP-96,345, but not its stereoisomer, CP-96,344, blocks the nociceptive responses to intrathecally administered substance P and to noxious thermal and chemical stimuli in the rat. *Neuroscience* **52**, 1039-1047.

109. YASHPAL K., RADHAKRISHNAN V. AND HENRY J.L. (1991) NMDA receptor antagonist blocks the facilitation of the tail flick reflex in the rat induced by intrathecal administration of substance P and by noxious cutaneous stimulation. *Neurosci. Lett.* **128**, 269-272.

110. YASHPAL K., WRIGHT D.M. AND HENRY J.L. (1982) Substance P reduces tail-flick latency: implications for chronic pain syndromes. *Pain* **14**, 155-167.

111. YOSHIMURA M. AND JESSELL T. (1990) Amino acid-mediated EPSPs at primary afferent synapses with substantia gelatinosa neurons in the rat spinal cord. *J. Physiol. (Lond.)* **430**, 315-335.

TRH AND SUBSTANCE P INCREASE RAT MOTONEURONE EXCITABILITY THROUGH A BLOCK OF A NOVEL K+ CONDUCTANCE

A. Nistri, N.D. Fisher and G. Baranauskas
Biophysics Sector, International School for Advanced Studies (SISSA)
Via Beirut 4, 34013 Trieste
Italy

INTRODUCTION

Immunocytochemical studies of the fine localization of endogenously-occurring TRH and substance P in the mammalian spinal cord have shown that these two peptides are present in the terminals of fibres descending from the raphe nucleus and which establish synaptic contacts with the proximal dendrites of motoneurons.[1,7]. Other nerve cells containing these peptides are found in the spinal dorsal horn.

Both TRH and substance P possess strong depolarising effects on motoneurons.[9,12] These responses usually have a slow onset/offset and display desensitization upon closely-spaced applications. Although phenomenologically similar, these responses are supposed to be mediated by specific receptor sites for TRH and substance P.[3,13] Intracellular recording from spinal neurons has suggested that the mechanism underlying the action of these peptides involved the block of a K+ current[11,16]. Experiments carried out in our laboratory to characterise further the ionic basis of the action of these peptides will be described in the present report.

NATO ASI Series, Vol. H 79
Cellular Mechanisms of Sensory Processing
Edited by Laszlo Urban
© Springer-Verlag Berlin Heidelberg 1994

EXPERIMENTAL PROCEDURES

Experiments were performed using 6-12 day old rats (both sexes). Under urethane anaesthesia the spinal cord was removed and dissected out with its roots attached. It was subsequently transferred to a recording chamber and continuously superfused with a salt solution containing (mM) NaCl 113, KCl 4.5, $MgCl_2.7H_2O$ 1, $CaCl_2$ 2, $NaHCO_3$ 25 and glucose 11, and gassed with 95% O_2/5% CO_2 (pH 7.4). Miniature suction electrodes were used to deliver stimuli to or to record responses from ventral or dorsal roots of the lumbar region. Functionally-identified lumbar motoneurons were impaled with 3M KCl, CsCl or 4M K-acetate filled micro-electrodes. Discontinuous current clamp or single electrode voltage clamp was performed at a sampling rate of $\approx$ 2kHz with an Axoclamp 2A amplifier. The headstage output was routinely monitored to ensure optimisation of capacitance compensation and sampling frequency. Drugs were applied by fast superfusion (7 ml/min). All voltage clamp experiments were run in the presence of 1 µM tetrodotoxin (TTX) in order to block voltage-activated sodium currents.

RESULTS

The database of the present investigation comprised 105 motoneurons with a resting potential of -71±1 mV.

Current clamp data

TRH elicited membrane depolarizations and repetitive firing of action potentials (Figure 1, Top). Responses persisted for several min after washout and were reproducible when applications were spaced by $\approx$ 45 min. In the presence of TRH the amplitude of electrotonic potentials induced by constant current pulses was usually increased indicating a rise in cell input resistance. However, this phenomenon was masked whenever repetitive firing and synaptic activity occurred and in some cells (see the example of Figure 1) could only be observed during early washout. Figure 1 (bottom) shows the relation between TRH concentrations and

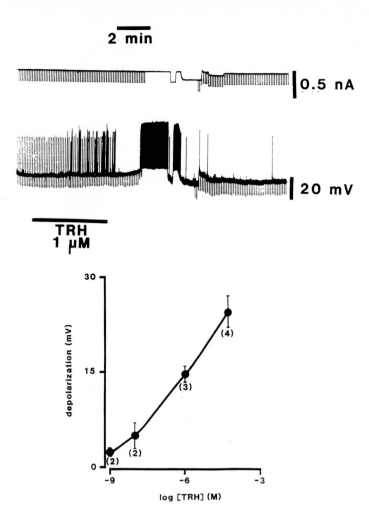

Figure 1. Effects of TRH on rat motoneurons. **Top:** Current clamp tracings (current above; voltage below) showing slow onset/offset of response to TRH. Note that manual repolarization immediately blocked firing and that during washout there was an input resistance increase. Note that true action potential amplitude was truncated due to the limited frequency response of the pen recorder. Resting membrane potential was -71 mV. **Bottom:** Plot of log concentrations of TRH *vs.* amplitude of membrane depolarization (mV). Number of cells is given in brackets.

ensuing membrane depolarizations (measured at a steady state interspike level whenever sustained firing developed). The threshold dose was ≈ 1 nM and no apparent response saturation was detected up to 50 μM. The comparatively shallow slope of this graph suggests that in control medium the response amplitude was probably determined by the combination of direct as well as indirect actions of this peptide. These effects were due to TRH itself and not to its bio-transformation into active metabolites since application of high concentrations of the principal

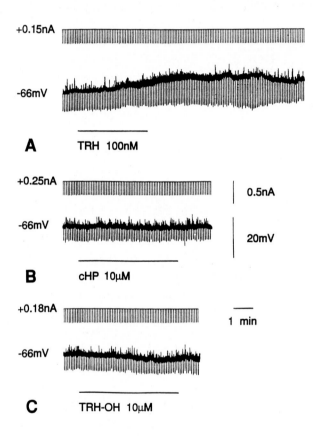

Figure 2. Current clamp recordings of the responses of a motoneuron to: **A** 100 nM TRH, **B** 10 μM cHP, and **C** 10 μM TRH-OH. cHP and TRH-OH apparently elicited no response (see bottom traces of B and C respectively) despite being applied for a longer time (see horizontal bars) and in concentrations 100-fold greater than that of TRH.

compounds of this class, namely histidylprolinediketopiperazine (cHP) or the deamidated form of TRH (TRH-OH) was ineffective (Figure 2). It is noteworthy that in Figure 2 TRH evoked a large rise in input resistance which could be clearly observed as the associated membrane depolarization did not reach threshold for firing. Substance P also produced a sustained depolarization of motoneurons (Figure 3) but was weaker than TRH since the dose threshold was $\approx$ 100 nM, and at 1 µM concentration the effect of substance P was only 60 % of that of 1 µM TRH. Substance P receptor sites are heterogeneous since they comprise at least three pharmacologically distinct classes[8] termed NK1, NK2 and NK3. Preliminary studies were thus performed to test the responsiveness of motoneurons to synthetic analogues selective for each of these receptor types. The NK1 agonist substance P methylester (200 nM) produced large and sustained depolarizations in each cell tested. The NK3 agonist [Me-Phe[7]]-NKB (200nM) was also a potent excitant of all motoneurons examined while [Ala[8]]-NKA (200nM), a NK2 agonist, depolarised $\approx$70% of the neurons. These observations suggest that in the neonatal rat spinal cord all three classes of receptor were functionally expressed. Responses of motoneurons to exogenously-applied neuropeptides might include direct and indirect actions, the latter originating from interneurons. In order to help to distinguish between these two possibilities, experiments were carried out in TTX (1 µM) solution which blocked propagated afferent activity. Figure 4 shows that in the presence of TTX TRH still typically elicited a delayed depolarization. Because of the suppression of neuronal firing it was possible to observe an input resistance increase. The latter was not caused merely by the effect of membrane depolarization on intrinsic voltage-dependent conductances since depolarising the membrane potential (by steady D.C. current injection) to its resting value preserved the observed rise in input resistance. Similar data were obtained with substance P, allowing the conclusion that both TRH and substance P exert a large part of their action directly on motoneurons. The effectiveness of substance P agonists in TTX solution was a more complex issue. The action of NKA was virtually absent after exposure to TTX, indicating that NK2 receptors were presumably located only on interneurons. The effect of NKB was preserved in about 20 % of the cells tested, suggesting a predominant (although not exclusive) contribution of interneurons to the responses to this agent. The action of substance P methylester was maintained in all cells tested, suggesting that motoneuron NK1 receptors were probably responsible for most of the postsynaptic effects of substance P. This notion will require validation using selective receptor antagonists.

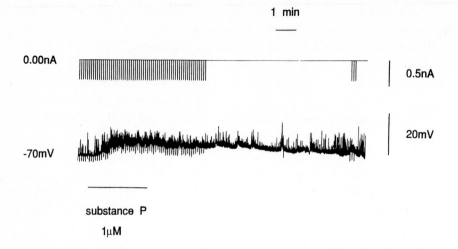

Figure 3. Current clamp recording of a motoneuron responding to substance P. Input resistance was monitored by injecting current pulses of -0.4 nA through the microelectrode at 0.2 Hz (top trace). Initial resting potential was -70 mV. Application of substance P (see horizontal bar) elicited a response that was characterised by a delayed depolarization associated with increased neuronal activity, seen as a thickened baseline.

In summary, TRH and substance P directly depolarised motoneurons and since this phenomenon was accompanied by a measurable rise in input resistance, it seemed likely that some inhibitory conductance mechanism was blocked by these peptides. This possibility was then explored with voltage clamp studies.

Voltage clamp data

Figure 5 shows the effect of TRH on a motoneuron held at a membrane potential of -65 mV. In control solution depolarising or hyperpolarising voltage steps elicited current responses with minimal time or voltage dependent relaxations. In the presence of TRH (1 µM) there was a development of a sustained inward current (see downward shift of baseline) with an associated fall in input conductance at its holding potential as shown by the smaller amplitude of the initial current jump induced by a voltage command. Curiously though, the initial amplitude of the current relaxed to a

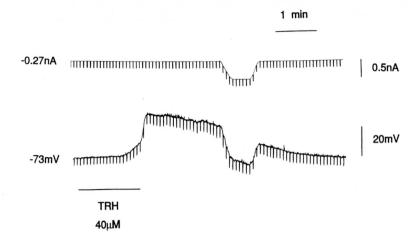

Figure 4. A current clamp record of a motoneuron responding to 40 µM TRH in the presence of 3 µM tetrodotoxin. The cell was hyperpolarised to a membrane potential of -73 mV by a steady current of -0.27 nA and input resistance was monitored by passing current pulses of -0.2 nA through the microelectrode at 0.2 Hz (top trace). Application of TRH (see horizontal bar) elicited a slow depolarization associated with an increase in input resistance, as indicated by the larger voltage responses to the current pulses. Just after the cell had depolarised in response to TRH it was momentarily hyperpolarised to near its original membrane potential by manipulation of the holding current. During this manoeuvre the input resistance was shown to be higher than in control conditions in a manner independent of the membrane potential.

new steady-state level, attained usually within 150 ms. The graph of Figure 5 depicts current/voltage relations in control or TRH solution. The two lines intersected at approximately -100 mV which was therefore taken as the apparent level of reversal potential. Subtracting steady-state control data from those in TRH solution yielded a plot (triangles) of the net inward current generated by the peptide (I_{TRH}). Pooled results from twelve neurons gave a maximal amplitude of I_{TRH} between -50 and -40 mV. Reversal of I_{TRH} could be observed only in 44 % of cells (27/61) and had an average value of -107±3 mV. For neurons displaying I_{TRH} reversal it was possible to construct a plot of chord (ionic) conductance vs. membrane potential (where the chord conductance is obtained by dividing I_{TRH} by the difference between holding potential and reversal potential). The plot had a bell-like shape with a maximum around -60 mV, suggesting a voltage-dependent block by TRH of an intrinsic membrane conductance. The latter was identified as being due to K^+ in view of the Nernstian shift of I_{TRH} reversal when extracellular K^+ was raised[10]. No comparable changes were found when 80 % of extracellular Na^+ was replaced by

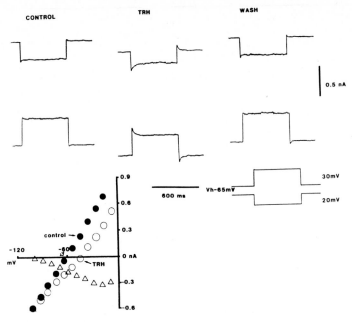

CONTROL   TRH   WASH

Figure 5. Effects of TRH on a voltage clamped motoneuron. **Top:** Currents elicited by depolarising or hyperpolarising steps (calibrated in terms of amplitude) from a holding potential (Vh) of -65 mV. Responses are DC mounted to indicate the level of holding current. TRH (1 μM) reduced initial steps suggesting a decreased input conductance and elicited time-dependent relaxations. Leak currents were not subtracted. Washout responses were obtained after _ 30 min. **Bottom:** Current/voltage plot obtained for steady-state currents in control (filled circles) or TRH (open circles) solution. Open triangles show I_{TRH} (obtained by subtracting control data from those in the presence of TRH). Note apparent reversal near -110 mV and plateau at ≈-40 mV.

tetraethylammonium (TEA) or the recording electrode contained acetate instead of Cl⁻. We therefore suggested that TRH inhibited a background K⁺ current which was termed $I_{K(T)}$[10]. The pharmacological sensitivity of $I_{K(T)}$ was rather unexpected. Figure 6 shows that a combination of TEA, 4-aminopyridine plus intracellular Cs⁺ did not block the action of TRH; carbachol solution was also ineffective (Figure 7). A similar lack of antagonism by extracellular Cs⁺ (2 mM) or apamin (200 nM) was found. The only K⁺ channel blocker observed to depress TRH-mediated responses was Ba²⁺ (1.5 mM; equimolar replacement of Ca²⁺). Figure 8A shows that Ba²⁺ depressed I_{TRH} (filled squares) although not completely, leaving a resistant component (filled triangles). The Ba²⁺ sensitive component (crosses) was obtained by subtraction of these two plots. On average the reduction in I_{TRH} by Ba²⁺ amounted to nearly 50 % and the Ba²⁺ sensitive current consistently displayed

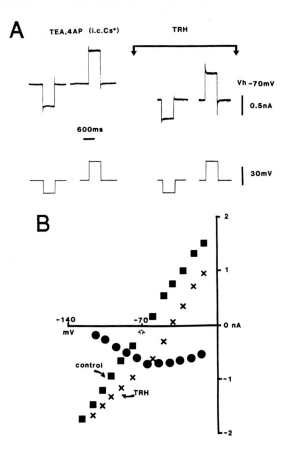

Figure 6. Effects of TRH on a voltage clamped motoneuron in the presence of K+ channel blockers. **A.** Currents (top) produced by voltage steps (bottom) before or during application of 1 µM TRH. The bath solution contained 20 mM TEA, 2 mM 4-aminopyridine (4AP) while the cell was loaded intracellularly with a Cs+ (i.c. Cs+) microelectrode. Note that the TRH effect was fully developed at the holding potential (Vh; -70 mV). **B.** Current/voltage graph plotted as for Fig. 5, bottom.

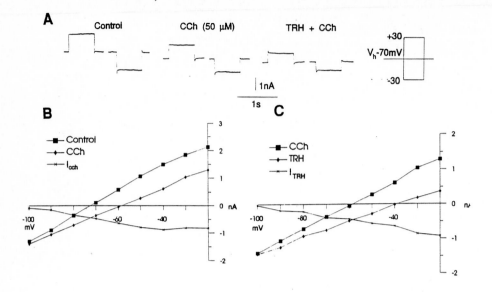

Figure 7. Carbachol (CCh) did not prevent the action of TRH. **A.** Currents elicited by voltage steps (calibrated in terms of amplitude) from a holding potential (Vh) of -70 mV. Carbachol induced a steady inward current with a conductance decrease but no significant time-dependent relaxations. TRH (1 µM) applied in the continuous presence of carbachol, was still able to induce an additional inward current with a conductance decrease. **B** and **C** present current/voltage graphs for carbachol and carbachol + TRH, respectively..

reversal at -110 mV. Cd^{2+} (0.2-0.5 mM; equimolar replacement of Ca^{2+}) also depressed, albeit incompletely, I_{TRH} (on average by 48 %). Figure 8B shows that the residual current in Cd^{2+} solution (filled triangles) also displayed reversal potential and voltage-sensitivity similar to the Ba^{2+}-sensitive component. Therefore it seems likely that TRH induced an inward current via a dual mechanism, namely block of a Ba^{2+}-sensitive K^+ current ($I_{K(T)}$) and activation of a Cd^{2+}-sensitive (presumably Ca^{2+}-dependent) cationic current.

Substance P produced effects quite similar to those of TRH, consisting in the development of a slow inward current with a fall in input conductance. Figure 9 shows average current/voltage plots before and during application of substance P to seven motoneurons. Reversal of the substance P-induced current was very near to -100 mV.

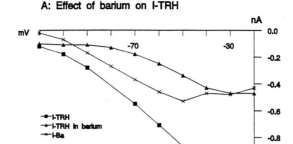

A: Effect of barium on I-TRH

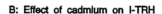

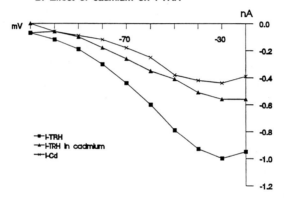

B: Effect of cadmium on I-TRH

Figure 8. The effect of extracellular Ba^{2+} or Cd^{2+} on I_{TRH}. **A:** The presence of Ba^{2+} reduced the magnitude of I_{TRH}. The plots of I_{TRH} obtained in standard solution (squares) and in the presence of 1.5 mM Ba^{2+} (triangles; direct replacement of Ca^{2+}) were significantly different at tested membrane potential values positive to -90 mV ($P<0.05$; paired t-test). A plot of the component of I_{TRH} blocked by Ba^{2+} ($I_{TRH(Ba)}$) is also shown (crosses). This was obtained by subtracting the control I_{TRH} plot from that produced in Ba^{2+}. $I_{TRH(Ba)}$ had an estimated reversal potential near -110 mV. **B:** The presence of Cd^{2+} also reduced the magnitude of I_{TRH}. The plots of I_{TRH} in control conditions (squares) and in the presence of 0.5 mM Cd^{2+} (triangles; direct replacement of Ca^{2+}) were significantly different at tested membrane potential values positive to -70 mV. A plot of the fraction of I_{TRH} blocked by Cd^{2+} ($I_{TRH(Cd)}$) is also shown (crosses; calculated as for $I_{TRH(Ba)}$ above). Note that the fraction of I_{TRH} not blocked by Cd^{2+} had an apparent reversal potential near -110 mv. Data are means from four cells.

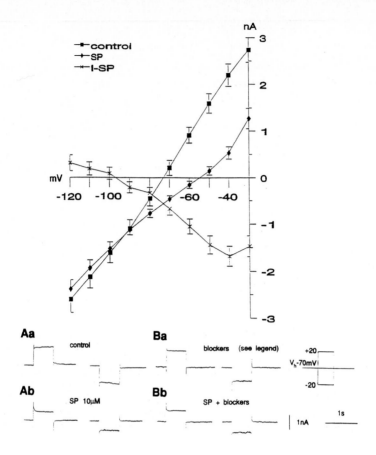

Figure 9. Effects of substance P (SP) on a voltage clamped motoneuron. **Top:** Average current/voltage plots of steady state currents for seven cells in control conditions and in the presence of 10 µM SP. Crosses indicate the plot of I_{SP} obtained by subtracting the control plot (squares) from the SP plot (diamonds). I_{SP} was maximal at -40 mV and reversed polarity near -95 mV. The difference between each set of points for membrane potentials positive to -90 mV was statistically significant (P<0.05; paired t-test). **Bottom:** The action of substance P was not blocked by extracellular Cs^+, TEA and 4-AP. Sample current responses to 600ms voltage commands (calibrated in terms of amplitude) from the holding potential (V_h) of -70mV are shown on a fast time-base in the presence of: control solution (omitting PO_4^{3-} to prevent salt precipitation with Cd^{2+}; **Aa**); 10 µM substance P (SP; **Ab**); 2 mM Cs^+, 20 mM TEA and 2 mM 4-AP containing solution (blockers; **Ba**); and blockers and SP (**Bb**). Note that the addition of substance P to the medium in the presence of the blockers induced an input resistance increase.

Constructing a plot of chord conductance *vs.* membrane potential in the presence of this peptide gave a bell-shape relation with a peak at -50 mV. The tracings of Figure 9 indicate that TEA, Cs^+ and 4-aminopyridine did not suppress the action of substance P, while Ba^{2+} (1.5 mM) blocked the response at membrane potentials positive to -70 mV[4]. Experiments are in progress to ascertain the role of Ca^{2+} in the action of substance P.

DISCUSSION

The isolated spinal cord preparation of the neonatal rat is a useful model system for intracellular studies of the action of peptides, although the relative immaturity of the tissue might produce effects somewhat different from those found in adult neurons. While the excitation elicited by TRH or substance P is qualitatively similar to that observed *in vivo* in the adult mammalian spinal cord,[5,17] the pharmacological profile of responses to substance P agonists cannot be directly compared with that of adult cells in view of the lack of intracellular studies of these agents on mature motoneurons. Hence, on neonatal motoneurons preliminary data suggest the prevailing presence of NK1 receptors with a minority of NK3 receptors (the NK2 receptor system being apparently confined to interneurons). As far as TRH receptors are concerned, it seems that they are fully expressed on these cells in view of their high sensitivity to this compound.

The excitatory action of TRH and substance P was investigated under voltage clamp conditions and found to be very similar. Two essentially distinct mechanisms appear to contribute to the observed responses: a) voltage dependent block of a background K^+ current ($I_{K(T)}$[10]) which could also be inhibited by Ba^{2+} and had a reversal potential near -100 mV; b) activation of a Ca^{2+}-sensitive cationic (presumably non-specific) current which was blocked by Cd^{2+} and had a comparatively positive reversal potential (although not directly measured). The relative preponderance of one of the two mechanisms in different cells would account for the variability in the reversal level of the peptide-evoked responses, although in a significant number of cases the detection of I_{TRH} reversal implied only a small contribution by the cationic current to the overall response. Experimental conditions similar to these have recently been modelled by Shen and North[14] to explain the dual action of acetylcholine on brainstem neurons. The pharmacological characteristics of $I_{K(T)}$, including its resistance to TEA, 4-aminopyridine, Cs^+, carbachol and apamin preclude its identification with other well-established K^+ currents of central neurons.[15] The curious time-dependent current relaxations observed in TRH or substance P solution may be interpreted as due to the voltage-dependent nature of the block of this conductance as suggested by the highly non-linear chord conductance plots. According to this interpretation, step depolarizations would enhance the block (thus ensuring an inward relaxation) while step hyperpolarizations would decrease the block (thus causing an outward relaxation). Recent experiments on guinea-pig facial motoneurons have confirmed that TRH mainly acted by suppressing a sustained K^+ current[2] but it is difficult to ascribe this phenomenon to block of $I_{K(T)}$ in view of the apparent lack of current relaxations and its incomplete pharmacological characterization.

Substance P seems to share most of the effects of TRH, although it is expected to bind to a distinct family of membrane receptors. Similarity of action would then imply common effector mechanisms as also indicated by a recent study in which occlusion of effects was found upon co-application of the two peptides.[4] A challenge for further investigations will be the identification of the site(s) where convergence of the signal transduction process[6] for TRH and substance P occurs. Finally, clarification of the physiological significance of the peptidergic signals for excitatory neurotrasmission on motoneurons is warranted: this goal will be greatly aided by future availability of selective peptide receptor antagonists.

ACKNOWLEDGEMENTS: We are grateful to Dr. C. Maggi (Menarini Pharmaceuticals, Florence) for gifts of the substance P analogues. This work was supported by grants from INFM, CNR and "Science" Plan of the EEC. N.D.F. holds a postdoctoral fellowship from the INFM-EEC Human Capital and Mobility Programme.

REFERENCES

1. ARVIDSSON, U., CULLHEIM, S., ULFHAKE, B., BENNETT, G.W., FONE, K.C.F., CUELLO, A.C., VERHOFSTAD, A.A.J., VISSER, T.J. AND HÖKFELT, T. (1990) 5-Hydroxytryptamine, substance P, and thyrotropin-releasing hormone in the adult cat spinal cord segment L_7:immunohistochemical and chemical studies. *Synapse* **6,** 237-270.

2. BAYLISS D.A., VIANA, F. AND BERGER, A.J. (1992) Mechanisms underlying excitatory effects of thyrotropin-releasing hormone on rat hypoglossal motoneurons in vitro. *J. Neurophysiol.* **68,** 1733-1745.
3. CHARLTON, C.G. AND HELKE, C.J. (1985) Characterization and segmental distribution of [^{125}I]Bolton-Hunter-labeled substance P binding sites in rat spinal cord. *J. Neurosci.* **5,** 1653-1661.
4. FISHER, N.D. AND NISTRI, A. (1993) Substance P and TRH share a common effector pathway in rat spinal motoneurons: an in vitro electrophysiological study. *Neurosci. Lett.* (in press).
5. HENRY, J.L., KRNJEVIC, K. AND MORRIS, M.E. (1975) Substance P and spinal neurons. *Can. J. Physiol. Pharmacol.* **53,** 423-432.
6. HILLE, B. (1992) G protein-coupled mechanisms and nervous signaling. *Neuron* **9,** 187-195.
7. JOHANSSEN, O., HÖKFELT, T., JEFFCOATE, S.L., WHITE, N. AND STERNBERGER, L.A. (1980) Ultrastructural localization of TRH-like immunoreactivity. *Exp. Brain Res.* **38,** 1-10.
8. MAGGI, C.A., PATACCHINI, R., ROVERO, P. AND GIACHETTI, A. (1993) Tachykinin receptors and tachykinin receptor antagonists. *J. Auton. Pharmacol.* **13,** (in press).
9. NICOLL, R.A. (1978) The action of thyrotropin-releasing hormone, substance P and related peptides on frog spinal motoneurons. *J. Pharmacol. Exp. Ther.* **207,** 817-824.
10. NISTRI, A., FISHER, N.D. AND GURNELL, M. (1990) Block by the neuropeptide TRH of an apparently novel K^+ conductance of rat motoneurons. *Neurosci. Lett.* **120,** 25-30.
11. NOWAK, L.M. AND MACDONALD, R.L. (1982) Substance P: Ionic basis for depolarising responses of mouse spinal cord neurons in cell culture. *J. Neurosci.* **2,** 1119-1128.
12. OTSUKA, M. AND KONISHI, S. (1974) Electrophysiology of mammalian spinal cord *in vitro. Nature* **252,** 733-734.
13. SHARIF, N.A. AND BURT, D.R. (1985) Limbic, hypothalamic, cortical and spinal regions are enriched in receptors for thyrotropin-releasing hormone: evidence from [^{3}H] ultrafilm autoradiography and correlation with central effects of the tripeptide in rat brain. *Neurosci. Lett.* **60,** 337-342.
14. SHEN, K.-Z. AND NORTH, R.A. (1992) Muscarine increases cation conductance and decreases potassium conductance in rat locus coeruleus neurons. *J. Physiol.* **455,** 471-485.
15. STORM, J.F. (1990) Potassium currents in hippocampal pyramidal cells. *Prog. Brain Res.* **83,** 161-187.
16. TAKAHASHI, T. (1985) Thyrotropin-releasing hormone mimics descending slow synaptic potentials in rat spinal motoneurons. *Proc. R. Soc. Lond. B.* **225,** 391-398.
17. WHITE, S.R. (1985) A comparison of the effects of serotonin, substance P and thyrotropin-releasing hormone on excitability of rat spinal motoneurons in vivo. *Brain Res.* **335,** 63-70.

DYNAMIC CHANGES IN THE SENSORY SYSTEM

INFLUENCES OF THE CHEMICAL ENVIRONMENT ON PERIPHERAL AFFERENT NEURONS

Andy Dray
Sandoz Institute for Medical Research
5 Gower Place, London WC1E 6BN
United Kingdom

INTRODUCTION

Fine afferent fibers respond to a number of potentially harmful physiological stimuli including pressure, heat and a variety of noxious chemicals. Particularly striking is the repertoir of endogenous chemicals to which the afferent nerve terminal may be exposed and to which it is sensitive: as if it were specialized to "taste" its environment. The present discussion will focus, in the main, on pathophysiological chemical factors; as these have received most attention, particularly regarding the activation and sensitization of peripheral nociceptors following tissue injury and inflammation. In addition there are other cellular regulatory factors, often derived from target tissues, which are important for development and for maintaining the normal phenotype of afferent neurons. These substances may be present to a greater or lesser extent following tissue damage, inflammation or nerve injury and have a major influence in determining the long term properties of sensory neurons and other nearby cells. Important to all these chemical stimuli are the ways in which they interact at the nerve membrane to transduce and transmit their signals.

This article will not detail the actions of each individual chemical, rather an attempt will be made to describe features which groups of substance have in common and which relate to their site and mechanism of action. This will be illustrated with suitable examples from the literature.

NATO ASI Series, Vol. H 79
Cellular Mechanisms of Sensory Processing
Edited by Laszlo Urban
© Springer-Verlag Berlin Heidelberg 1994

PHYSIOLOGICAL AND PATHOPHYSIOLOGICAL FACTORS

Some of these substances have been summarized in Figure 1. These have been grouped according to their source or circumstances of production. Thus a number of substances are produced or released following tissue injury, including bradykinin, serotonin, prostanoid products (prostaglandins, leukotrienes, hydroxyacids) of arachidonic acid metabolism and protons. During the stimulation of fine afferent nerve terminals the release of a number of neuropeptides (e.g., neurokinins, somatostatin), may be evoked.[16,20] These peptides can affect nerve-terminal (sensory, sympathetic) excitability directly or indirectly via the release of neuroactive substances from mast cells, other immune cells or from the vasculature. Products of immune cell (eg macrophages) activity include a number of cytokines particularly IL1, IL6 IL8 and TNFα each of which has been shown to produce behavioral hyperalgesia.[8,9] However it is unclear whether these substances affect sensory nerve excitability directly. More likely they stimulate the production or release of other agents such as prostanoids or growth factors which then sensitize nociceptors to exogenous stimuli. Interestingly immune cells also synthesize a number of opioid peptides including endorphin and enkephalin.[33] These substances may act on opioid receptors which are expressed on the peripheral terminals of afferent fibers during nerve damage or inflammation.[33] Activation of these opioid receptors may inhibit activity or excite[7] sensory neurons. A number of cellular and chemical factors may be released from blood vessels (eg kinins, NO, immune cells, platelets). This may arise following vascular injury or following the stimulation of vascular endothelial cells by neurogenic factors resulting in plasma extravasation and neurogenic inflammation. During inflammation, reflex or local chemical stimulation of sympathetic nerve fibers may also release sympathetic transmitters as well as other chemicals such as prostanoids.[22] Finally neurotrophic factors, exemplified by NGF, may be synthesised by target tissues normally innervated by afferent and sympathetic nerve terminals. However synthesis may be dramatically increased during inflammation in which case these factors may also be derived from many types of reactive cells. This multiplicity of chemical agents not only affect sensory neurons but also change the activity of surrounding tissues and other neurons eg sympathetic post ganglionic fibers. As a consequence there is vast potential for signal amplification and modulation due to the the initiation of cascades of chemically induced events, synergistic interactions between different substances and interactions between neural and non-neural systems.

CHEMICAL AND CELLULAR FACTORS AFFECTING SENSORY NEURON ACTIVITY

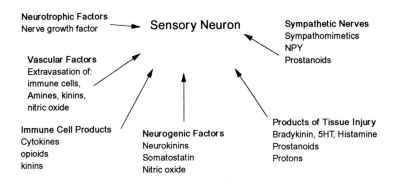

Figure 1. Summary of some of the chemical factors which alter the excitability of chemosensitive sensory neurons.

TRANSDUCTION

Sensory transduction and transmission of chemical signals in the somatosensory system involves similar steps to those described for other sensory processes such as olfaction and gustation.[31] These mechanisms, shown in figure 2, require a detector, usually a membrane receptor protein, which can be characterized pharmacologically or with molecular biological techniques. During signal transduction amplification processes exist by which certain chemical signals sensitize afferent nerve terminals to the effects of other stimuli thus enhancing signal generation. Ultimately signal generation is brought about by the chemically induced increase in membrane ion permeability at the peripheral nerve terminal. This leads to the activation of voltage gated cation channels, depolarization, and the generation of action potentials which leads to the propagation of nerve impulses into the spinal cord. Here further amplification and modulation of somatosensory signals occurs.

TRANSDUCTION OF CHEMICAL SIGNALS BY SOMATOSENSORY NEURONES

CHEMICAL MEDIATORS

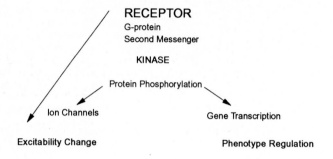

Figure 2. Transduction of chemical signals by sensory neurons. Exogenous chemicals or endogenous mediators act via receptors to affect cellular excitability. Others affect biochemical processes and alter gene transcription.

RECEPTORS

As mentioned earlier chemical receptors on afferent nerve terminals can be characterized pharmacologically using selective agonists and antagonists. In some cases receptors have been identified, sequenced and cloned using molecular biological methods. As in other excitable membranes, receptors are most commonly coupled via G-proteins and second messenger systems (cAMP, cGMP, IP3) to affect the regulation of intracellular ions and alter membrane ion channel activity respectively, thereby altering membrane ionic permeability. Activation of protein kinase can also affect ion channels by the phosphorylation of ion channel proteins. These aforementioned effects produce changes in cellular excitability. In addition protein kinase induced phosphorylation of cellular transcription factors can serve to regulate the phenotype of sensory neurons. As a result the activity of RNA polymerases may increase or decrease the production of mRNA for coding the synthesis of various peptides and proteins . With such changes the potential exists for producing longer lasting changes in cell excitability and biochemistry as well as inducing structural modification of cell cytoarchitecture. Finally some receptors have been shown to be coupled directly with membrane ion channels and in this case receptors may indeed be an integral part of the ion channel protein complex.

In common with other excitable cells, several types of ion channels are expressed in sensory neurons.[24] Two major types of sodium channel exist. One is sensitive to blockade by TTX, as in other neurons: the other channels are TTX-insensitive. In the latter cells the activation and inactivation of membrane sodium conductance is slower. Several types of potassium channel are also found. These comprise the delayed rectifier, as in most neurons, which is responsible for rapid membrane repolarization after the generation of the action potential. Another type of fast, transient, potassium channel open rapidly during depolarization and are important for maintaining nerve excitability. Certain types of sensory neuron, especially those of the vicera, possess a calcium activated potassium conductance mechanism which is responsible for the prolonged after-spike hyperpolarization important for keeping this type of cell quiescent for long periods. Inflammatory mediators can block this conductance mechanism and thereby allow these cells to fire repetitively following an initial action potential.[38] This has been suggested as a likely cellular mechanism for inflammatory hyperalgesia.[26]

As in other neurons there are three major types of voltage dependent calcium channels. These comprise: T-channels which have a low activation threshold and generate a transient current. These make a significant contribution to the excitability of sensory neurons. N-channels have a higher activation threshold and are important in signal propagation for they are involved in the release of neurochemicals from sensory neurons both in the periphery and also in the spinal cord during synaptic transmission. N-channels can be blocked with some degree of selectivity by ω-conotoxin. Finally, L-channels have the highest activation threshold and remain open for longer. These can also be characterized pharmacologically because of their susceptibility to dihydropyridines and also can be blocked by a number of chemical transmitters (opioids, GABA).

RECEPTORS COUPLED DIRECTLY WITH ION CHANNELS

Several substances including serotonin ($5HT_3$ receptors), capsaicin and protons affect nerve excitability by interacting directly with the receptor - ion channel complex.

Protons and capsaicin

Protons are able to activate a variety of sensory neurons including those with myelinated fibers as well as those with poorly myelinated or unmyelinated fibers. Activation of the latter groups of fibers accounts for the known effects of protons to induce a sharp stinging pain following local injections and to contribute to the sensation of aching and discomfort following tissue acidosis after muscle excercise. The pH of the extracellular environment is also known to fall in several pathophysiological conditions such as hypoxia/anoxia as well as in inflammation. Indeed the pH of synovial fluid from inflamed joints is significantly more acid than that from normal joints and has been measured as low as pH 6.6-6.8. It may also be that the pericellular pH around sensory terminals is even more acidic than the bulk fluid and that constant formation of protons, because of local metabolic activity, provides an important stimulus for regulating the sensitivity and excitability of sensory nerve terminals.

Two types of proton-induced depolarization have been studied in sensory neurons. One type of depolarization is associated with a rapid, transient increase in membrane cation permeability and is evoked by pH changes in the normal physiological range. The second type of depolarization is associated with a more prolonged increase in membrane permeability and is evoked by a greater lowering of the extracellular pH, similar to that which gives rise to the sustained nerve activation. This type of depolarization shows a much slower rate of inactivation, can be sustained for several minutes[4] and is likely to make a significant contribution to any prolonged nociceptive response. This type of membrane depolarization is also likely to be the basis for the prolonged sensory neuron activation seen with low pH solutions[32] and for the enhanced responsiveness of mechanosensitive afferent fibers.

Several characteristics of the prolonged increase in membrane permeability produced by protons are shared by capsaicin, but not by other sensory neuron activators such as GABA or ATP.[4] Capsaicin, an exogenous chemical, is a major pungent principle in *Capsicum* peppers. It is distinguished by its uniquely specific action on polymodal nociceptors and heat sensitive sensory neurons. Thus like protons, capsaicin activates nociceptors to elicit a sensation of burning pain. Activated of neuropeptide containing afferent fibers also results in autonomic effects either through reflex actions on the viscera, through the release of sensory neuropeptides, or via the release of other substances from the microvasculature following the induction of plasma protein extravasation.[16,20] There is compelling evidence showing that capsaicin interacts with a specific membrane receptor. Thus the effects of capsaicin are cell specific and there is a clear structure-activity relationship that can be demonstrated using chemical analogues of capsaicin. Most convincing is the demonstration that the effects of capsaicin can be antagonised competitively by a newly discovered antagonist, capsazepine.[13]

The presence of an ion channel in nociceptive neurons which is uniquely sensitive to capasicin raises questions about its normal physiological role. So far no endogenous capsaicin-like molecule has been indentified, but the sustained proton-evoked current shows a striking similarity to that evoked by capsaicin.[3] Furthermore the expression of the responses to both agents is controlled by nerve growth factor (NGF). The interaction between capsaicin and its receptor opens an ion channel that is permeable to both monovalent and divalent cations.[3] The resultant ion flow produces an inward membrane current that depolarizes and activates the neuron. Although protons can activate the capsaicin operated ion channels the binding site for protons and capsaicin appear to differ as capsazepine, a competitive capsaicin antagonist, has no effect on the sensory nerve activation by protons. However proton induced neuropeptide release from viceral sensory neurons has been shown to be inhibited by capsazepine.[19] Finally a number of second messengers can be generated by capsaicin in sensory neurons although this is thought to be secondary to the increase in calcium permeability and rise in intracellular free calcium.

RECEPTORS COUPLED WITH G-PROTEINS AND SECOND MESSENGERS

Several examples of this type of receptor exist on afferent nerve terminals; these include receptors for opioids,[7] $5HT_1$ and $5HT_2$ receptors,[28] prostaglandin receptors[29] and bradykinin (BK) receptors. One of the most comprehensively studied receptors on sensory neurons is that to bradykinin and the features of this will be described in more detail.

Bradykinin

Bradykinin, is a nonapeptide formed by proteolytic (kallikrein enzymes) cleavage of circulating and tissue derived precursor proteins, the kininogens. It is thought to be made only during adverse conditions including local tissue anoxia, tissue injury and inflammation. In addition bradykinin production can be induced in several different types of cells by the actions of other mediators e.g. cytokines such as IL1. Bradykinin stimulates nociceptive nerve terminals and causes pain. In this respect it is the most potent endogenous algogenic substance known. In addition to activating sensory fibers directly (skin, joint, muscle), bradykinin sensitizes them to other stimuli, including mechanical stimulation.[26] Indeed there is a strong synergism between the excitatory action of bradykinin and the effects of other algogenic substances, such as prostaglandins and 5-hydroxytryptamine. Bradykinin induces a number of secondary effects including release of prostaglandins, degranulation of mast cells to release histamine and other inflammatory mediators, and chemotactic effects to attract immune cells to sites of tissue injury. Postganglionic sympathetic neurons are also excited by bradykinin and activation of these fibers is considered to be of importance in mediating some of the inflammatory actions of bradykinin both in skin and joint inflammation.[6] Bradykinin is somewhat ubiquitous in its actions since it also produces contraction or relaxation of visceral and vascular smooth muscle and secretion from epithelial cells.[14]

The effects of bradykinin are mediated via two main classes of receptor (B1 and B2) which can be defined pharmacologically.[15] The B1 receptor is selectively activated by des-Arg[9]-bradykinin, which can be formed from bradykinin by the action of a tissue peptidase while another analogue which does not occur naturally, des-Arg[9]-Leu[8]-bradykinin, acts as a selective B1 receptor antagonist. The B1 receptor is constitutively expressed in certain vascular tissues, but in other tissues it appears only to be expressed (or unmasked) under conditions of inflammation. The physiological significance of this behavior is not yet clear. Much more is known of the B2 receptor which accounts for the majority of the pharmacological effects of bradykinin. Selective antagonists of B2 receptors which are peptide analogues, have been used to show that bradykinin makes a significant contribution to inflammatory pain and hyperalgesia and that the direct effects of bradykinin on sensory neurons are mediated by B2 receptors.[14] However under conditions where inflammatory hyperalgesia persists for a few days or longer, there may be a major contribution of B1 receptors to the hyperalgesia.[14,25]

Both molecular cloning and biochemical studies indicate that the B2 receptor is coupled to other effector molecules via a G-protein[14]. Furthermore in sensory neurons, the main biochemical pathway through which bradykinin acts involves the G protein-mediated activation of phospholipase C, which generates two intracellular second messengers, 1,4,5- inositol-trisphosphate (IP3) and diacylglycerol (DAG) by cleavage of membrane phospholipids[14,26]. IP3 stimulates the release of intracellular calcium, and produces a rise in the free calcium concentration within the cell. The main effect of diacylglycerol is to activate protein kinase C (PKC), leading to the phosphorylation of various intracellular proteins including membrane ion channels. Indeed Burgess et al.[5] showed that bradykinin-induced depolarization of sensory neurons, and the associated calcium entry, could be reduced or abolished by inhibition or down-regulation of PKC, and could be mimicked by phorbol esters, which activate protein kinase C. Further PKC plays a key role in the excitation of sensory fibers since staurosporine, a protein kinase C inhibitor, attenuated afferent fiber stimulation by bradykinin in the skin[14] but did not inhibit the bradykinin-evoked depolarization of afferent fiber terminals in the spinal cord.[26] This suggests that PKC is unlikely to be the only mechanism involved in the excitatory effect of bradykinin. One observation that is difficult to explain is that bradykinin inhibits voltage-gated calcium currents in sensory neurons, this effect being ascribed to activation of PKC[14a]. This is hard to reconcile with the well-documented ability of bradykinin to evoke neuropeptide release from sensory neurons[14] which would require an increased calcium permeability. Recent studies show however that bradykinin B2 receptor activation stimulates cobalt uptake into sensory neurons indicating that a receptor coupled increase in extracellular calcium can occur.[23a]

The release of intracellular calcium by IP3 seems to make little contribution to the activation of sensory neurons by bradykinin. However intracellular free calcium may contribute towards the regulation of calcium-activated potassium channels, which normally show a low susceptibility to opening. Indeed other calcium-dependent effects of bradykinin in sensory neurons, such as neuropeptide release and generation of cGMP[5], require the presence of extracellular calcium which enters the cell through voltage-activated channels. Sensory neurons also generate arachidonic acid in response to bradykinin, through an indirect mechanism via activation of phospholipase C and metabolism of DAG[26]. In many other types of cell however bradykinin directly activates phospholipase A2 to generate prostanoid production. Indeed bradykinin induced excitation of sensory neurons is partly mediated through the actions of prostaglandins release from other tissues. In keeping with this, cyclooxygenase inhibitors reduce the excitation of nociceptors by bradykinin[29].

NERVE GROWTH FACTOR and SENSORY NEURONS

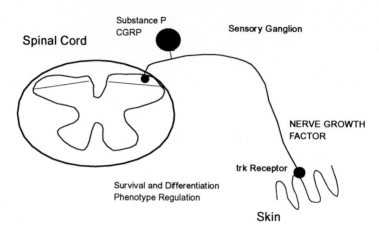

Figure 3. Nerve growth factor (NGF) and sensory neuron activity. NGF derived from target tissues acts on a tyrosine kinase (trk) receptor on sensory neurons. After transportation to the cell body in the sensory ganglion, NGF effects gene transcription and alters peptide (substance P and CGRP) synthesis.

The excitatory effect of bradykinin on sensory neurons[5,21] is associated with an inward (depolarising) current and an increase in membrane conductance, mainly to sodium ions. The increase in excitability of viceral sensory neurons is however associated with the inhibition of a long-lasting spike after-hyperpolarisation induced by a calcium dependent potassium conductance mechanisms which is regulated by a cAMP dependent process. Normally the slow-AHP following a single action potential produces a state of inexcitability, which limits the number of action potentials that can be evoked[38]. Inhibition of the slow-AHP by bradykinin (and prostaglandin) induced c-AMP formation allows the cell to fire repetitively when it is depolarised and this mechanism could account for nociceptor sensitization.

The activity of B2 receptors is regulated by a cGMP dependent mechanism which induces receptor desensitization. Thus BK stimulated IP3 production and BK induced activation of sensory neurons is reduced in the presence of cGMP.[21] Moreover this cGMP dependent mechanism may be initiated by the action of nitric oxide (NO) since inhibitors of nitric oxide synthase (NOS) attenuate bradykinin induced desensitization.[21]

GROWTH FACTORS (NEUROTROPHINS)

A number of neurotrophic factors exist including nerve growth factor (NGF), brain derived nerve growth factor (BDNF), neurotrophin-3, neurotrophin-5 and cilliary neurotrophic factor (CNTF). NGF has perhaps been the most extensively characterized (Figure 3) and is produced in limited amounts by a range of cell types and peripheral target tissues (e.g. fibroblasts, keratinocytes, Schwann cells[10]. NGF and other neurotrophic factors act on a specific membrane receptor in sensory neurons, trk-A, that belongs to the tyrosine kinase family of receptors. Following activation the NGF-receptor complex is transported to the cell body where gene transcription is altered by activation of specific transcription factor such as Oct-2.[40] In the early stages of development NGF is essential for the survival of sensory and sympathetic neurons but is no longer required for survival of adult neurons. In addition NGF promotes the development of neurons. Thus treatment of neonates with anti-NGF prevents the differentiation of Aδ fibers into high thereshold mechanoreceptors[27]. In adults however NGF is able to influence the properties of sensory neurons by regulating gene expression and the encoding of a number of important cellular proteins. Thus NGF induces an increase of mRNA for substance P and CGRP[18] and a corresponding increase in their synthesis, transport and neuronal concentration[12]] Furthermore NGF may regulate the expression of membrane receptors (eg capsaicin)[39] and ion channels (proton activated ion channel, the TTX resistant Na$^+$ channel).[2] Consequently exposure to NGF is essential for the expression of cellular excitability changes while its removal results in a large reduction or complete loss of evoked excitability. NGF may also induce structural modification in sensory neurons. Thus following partial denervation of the skin NGF may promote axonal sprouting and thereby increasing in the peripheral receptive field.[11] Such a phenomenon could also occur at the central terminals of nociceptive neurons exposed to abnormally high levels of NGF. If so, it would explain the increased strength of synaptic connections between sensory and dorsal horn neurons after experimental elevation of NGF in vivo;[17] although other mechanisms such as release of increased amounts of neuropeptides (e.g. substance P) could also play an important role. Structural regenerative changes following peripheral nerve injury may also involve the stimulation of growth proteins such as GAP-43[35] and it seems possible that NGF may be involved in the expression of this. However this seems unlikely since NGF receptors on sensory neurons are reduced following sciatic nerve injuries[36] and sensory neuropeptide markers such as SP and CGRP, which are usually increased following NGF treatment, are reduced by peripheral nerve transection.[37] Interestingly under these conditions sensory neurons upregulate the synthesis of other peptides and proteins (NPY, VIP, nitric oxide synthase) while noradrenergic axons sprout into the DRG.[22] Clearly trophic signaling other than that by NGF is involved.

Besides maintaining the expression of sensory neuronal phenotype, NGF is also important in pathophysiological conditions such as inflammatory pain. Thus increased levels of NGF have been measured in inflammatory injuries, in blister fluid, in pleurisy, in keratinocytes after skin injury with UV irradiation and in the synovial fluid from patients with rheumatoid arthritis.[1] therefore the production of abnormal amounts of NGF may be responsible for the increased chemosensitivity and exaggerated responsiveness in nociceptive pathways during inflammatory hyperalgesia. Indeed such findings are consistent with experimental studies showing that injection of NGF leads to increased sensitivity to noxious stimuli while animals exposed to anti-NGF antibodies have a reduced response to painful and inflammatory stimuli.[17]

During tissue damage and inflammation there is likely to be substantial interplay between sensory and sympathetic nerves, invading immune cells as well as resident tissue cells. NGF contributes futher to this interplay by promoting the differentiation of eosinophils, basophils and mast cells and by stimulating IgM secretion from B-lymphocytes and releasing histamine and lipid mediators (LTC_4) from human basophils. Conversely NGF synthesis may be stimulated by cytokines such as IL-1β and TNFa produced during inflammation. Substance P released from the sensory nerves further stimulates the production of cytokines.[26] Thus, NGF can initate a cascade of events which stimulate a number of positive feedback loops between neuropeptides, cytokines and immune cells in chronic inflammation.

In addition to the long term effects of NGF described above which are mediated by changing gene expression, some short term effects have also been described. An amino terminal octapeptide cleaved from NGF by an endogenous endopeptidase has been thought responsibe for a rapidly occurring mechanical hyperalgesia following NGF. The basis for this hyperalgesia is unclear, although the finding that the response is abolished by sympathectomy implies an interaction between sensory and sympathetic nerves.[34] More recently NGF has been shown to produce hyperalgesia to a heat stimulus which occurs within minutes. This is thought to involve mast cells degranulation and the release of bradykinin or 5HT.[30] However it is unclear whether these latter effects relate to the pathophysiological effects of endogenous NGF, since the amounts administered experimentally were far in excess of the concentrations found in inflamed tissues.

CONCLUSIONS

The preceding discussion has emphasised the importance of the chemical environment for sensory neurons from the standpoint of normal physiology where the milieu is responsible for regulating the moment to moment state of excitability. Overlaid are the more long-term changes that are provided by alterations in gene expression; usually determined by trophic and growth factors secreted from target tissues or other supporting cell. Under adverse conditions such as inflammation and tissue injury, adaptive processes take place which increase cell sensitivity and amplify potentially adverse signals. This process can be viewed as both reactive (to exogenous stimuli) but also interactive since there is a dynamic chemical exchange between chemicals secreted by "afferent" nerve fibers which affect the function of surrounding tissues and the chemical signals that surrounding (or circulating) tissues generate. So far the rather simplistic image of the sensory nerve terminal being bathed by a "soup " of chemical mediators has prevailed. This should be displaced by a view that the presentation of chemicals to the nerve terminal is likely to be organised. Indeed interactions between tissues and sensory nerve terminals are likely to be highly regulated. For instance chemo-attractive and specific cellular adhesion molecules make it likely that certain cell types eg mast cells, macrophages exchange signals at specific loci on the sensory nerve terminal (hot spots). Many such interactions would be occurring simultaneously. In addition we are soon likely to make further discoveries concerning the heterogeneity (both functional and biochemical) of chemosensitive afferent fibers; presently we are hampered by methodological limitations with which to resolve the function and chemistry of individual fine fibers. It is clear that the multitude of chemical entities which affect sensory neurons undergo molecular interactions via receptors coupled with other cell regulatory intermediates as discussed above. In this respect we are beginning to describe the boundaries between the mechanisms responsible for the moment to moment adaptations in cell function and those processes which allow the sensory elements long-term choices (favourable and unfavourable) about future viability and excitability. Appreciation of the extensive range of responsiveness that sensory neurons are capable should make us cautious about relating details of *in vitro* and *in vivo* studies, where experimental conditions impose de facto phenotype alterations.

REFERENCES

1. ALOE, L., TUVERNI, M.A., CARCASSI, U. AND LEVI-MONTALCINI, R. (1992) Nerve growth factor in the synovial fluid of patients with chronic arthritis. *Brain Res.*, **570**, 6-67.

2. AGUYO, L.G., WEIGHT F.F., AND WHITE, G, (1991) TTX-insensitive action potentials and excitability of adult sensory neurons cultured in serum- and exogenous nerve growth factor-free medium. *Neurosci. Lett.* **121**, 88-92.

3. BEVAN, S., FORBES, C.A. AND WINTER, J. (1993) Protons and capsaicin activate the same ion channels in rat isolated dorsal root ganglion neurones. *J. Physiol.* **459,** 401P.

4. BEVAN, S. AND YEATS, J. (1991) Protons activate a cation conductance in a sub-population of rat dorsal root ganglion neurones. *J. Physiol.* **433**, 145-161.

5. BURGESS, G.M., MULLANEY, J., MCNEIL, M., DUNN, P. AND RANG, H. P. (1989) Second messengers involved in the action of bradykinin on cultured sensory neurones. *J. Neurosci.* **9**, 3314-3325.

6. CODERRE, T.J., BASBAUM, A.I., AND LEVINE, J.D. (1989) Neural control of vascular permeability; interaction between primary afferents, mast cells, and sympathetic efferents. *J. Neurophysiol.* **62,** 48-58.

7. CRAIN, S.M. AND SHEN, K-F. (1990) Opioids can evoke direct receptor-mediated excitatory effects on sensory neurons. *Trends Pharmacol.* **11**, 77-81.

8. CUNHA, F.Q., POOLE, S., LORENZETTI, B.B., AND FERREIRA, S.H. (1992) The pivotal role of tumor necrosis factor a in the development of inflammatory hyperalgesia. *Brit. J. Pharmacol.* **107**, 660-664.

9. CUNHA, F.Q., LORENZETTI, B.B., POOLE, S., AND FERREIRA, S.H. (1991) Interleukin-8 as a mediator of sympathetic pain. *Brit. J. Pharmacol.* **104,** 765-767.

10. DAVIES, A. (1991) Cell death and the trophic requirements of developing sensory neurons. In: Sensory Neurons: Diversity, Development and Plasticity. ed. S.A. Scott. Oxford University Press: New York.

11. DIAMOND, J., HOLMES, M. AND COUGHLIN, M, (1992) Endogenous NGF and nerve impulses regulate the collateral sprouting of sensory axons in the skin of the adult rat. *J. Neurosci.* **12,** 1454-1466.

12. DONNERER, J., SCHULIGOI, R. AND STEIN, C. (1992) Increased content and transport of substance P and calcitonin gene-related peptide in sensory nerves innervating inflamed tissue: evidence for a regulatory function of nerve growth factor *in vivo. Neuroscience* **49**, 693-698.

13. DRAY, A. (1992) Neuropharmacological mechanisms of capsaicin and related substances. *Biochem. Pharmacol.* **44**, 611-615.

14. DRAY, A. AND PERKINS, M. (1993) Bradykinin and inflammatory pain. *Trends Neurosci* **16**, 99-104.

14a. EWALD, D.A., MATTHIES, J.G., PERNEY, T.M. WALKER, M.W. AND MILLER, RJ. (1988) The effect of down regulation of protein kinase C on the inhibition of dorsal root ganglion neuron Ca^{2+} current by neuropeptide Y. *J. Neurosci.* **8**. 2447-2451.

15. FARMER, S. G. AND BURCH, R.M. (1992) Biochemical and molecular pharmacology of kinin receptors. *Ann. Rev. Pharmacol.* **32**, 511-536.

16. HOLZER, P. (1988) Local effector functions of capsaicin-sensitive sensory nerve endings: involvement of tachykinins, calcitonin gene-related peptide, and other neuropeptides. *Neuroscience* **24**, 739-768.

17. LEWIN, G.R. AND MENDELL, L.M. (1992) NGF induced heat and mechanical hyperalgesia in adult rats. *Soc. Neurosci.* **18**, 130

18. LINDSAY, R.M. AND HARMAR, A.J. (1989) Nerve growth factor regulates expression of neuropeptide genes in adult sensory neurons. *Nature* **337,** 362-364.

19. LOU, Y-P. AND LUNDBERG, J.M. (1992) Inhibition of low pH evoked activation of airway sensory nerves by capsazepine, a novel capsaicin-receptor antagonists. *Biochem. Biophys. res. Comm.* **189**, 537-544.

20. MAGGI, C.A. AND MELI, A. (1988) The sensory-efferent function of capsaicin-sensitive neurons. *General Pharmacology* **19**, 1-43.

21. MCGEHEE, D.S., GOY ,M.F. AND OXFORD, G.S. (1992) Involvement of the nitric oxide-cyclic GMP pathway in the desensitization of bradykinin responses of cultured rat sensory neurons. *Neuron* **9**, 315-324.

22. MCLACHLAN, E.M., JANIG, W., DEVOR, M. AND MICHAELIS, M. (1993) peripheral nerve injury triggers noradrenergic sprouting within dorsal root ganglia. *Nature* **363**, 543-546.

23. MCMAHON, S. B. (1991) Mechanisms of sympathetic pain. *Brit. Med. Bull.* **47**, 584-600.

23a. NAGY, I., PABLA, R., MATESZ, C., DRAY, A., WOOLF, C.J. AND URBAN, L. (1993) Cobalt uptake enables identification of capsaicin- and bradykinin-sensitive subpopulation of dorsal root ganglion cells in vitro. *Neuroscience* (in press)

24. NOWYCKY, M. (1992) Voltage gated ion channels in dorsal root ganglion neurons. In: Sensory Neurons: Diversity, Development and Plasticity. ed. Scott, S.A. Oxford University Press: New York.

25. PERKINS, M.N., CAMPBELL, E. AND DRAY, A. (1993) Anti-nociceptive activity of the B_1 and B_2 receptor antagonists desArg[9]Leu[8]Bk and HOE 140, in two models of persistent hyperalgesia in the rat. Pain, 53, 191-197.

26. RANG, H.P., BEVAN, S. AND DRAY, A. (1991) Chemical activation of nociceptive peripheral neurones. *Br. Med. Bull.* **47**, 534-548.

27. RITTER, A.M., LEWIN, G.R., KREMER, N.E. AND MENDELL, L.M. (1991) Requirement for nerve growth factor in the development of myelinated nociceptors in vivo. *Nature* **350**, 500-502.

28. RUEFF, A. AND DRAY, A. (1992) 5-Hydroxytryptamine-induced sensitization and activation of peripheral fibres in the neonatal rat are mediated via different 5-hydroxytryptamine-receptors. *Neuroscience* **50**, 899-905.

29. RUEFF, A. AND DRAY, A. (1993) Sensitization of peripheral afferent fibres in the in vitro neonatal rat spinal cord-tail by bradykinin and prostaglandins. *Neuroscience*, **54**, 527-535.

30. RUEFF, A., LEWIN, G.R. AND MENDELL, L.M. (1993) Peripheral and central mechanisms of NGF-induced hyperalgesia in adult rat. *Soc Neurosci.* **19**, (in press)

31. SHEPHERD, G.M. (1991) Sensory transduction: entering the mainstream of membrane signaling. *Cell* **67,** 845-851.

32. STEEN, K.H., REEH, P.W., ANTON, F., AND HANDWERKER, H.O. (1992) Protons selectively induce lasting excitation and sensitization to mechanical stimuli of nociceptors in rat skin, in vivo. *J. Neurosci.* **12**, 86-95.

33. STEIN, C. (1991) Peripheral analgesic actions of opioids. *Pain and Symptom Management* **6,** 119-124.

34. TAIWO Y.O., LEVINE, J.D., BURCH, R.M., WOO, J.E. AND MOBLEY W.C. (1991) Hyperalgesia induced in the rat by the amino-terminal octapeptide of nerve growth factor. *Proc. Nat. Acad. Sci. USA* **88**, 5144-5148.

35. VAN DER ZEE, C.E.E.M., NIELANDER, H.B., VOS, J.P., DA SILVA, S.L., VERHAAGEN, J., OESTREICHER, A.B., SCHRAMA, L.H., SCHOTMAN, P., AND GISPEN, W.H. (1989) Expression of growth-associated protein B-50 (GAP-43) in dorsal root ganglia and in sciatic nerve during regenerative sprouting. *J. Neurosci.,* **9**, 3505-3512.

36. VERGE, V.M.K., MERLIO, J.-P., GRONDIN, J., ERNFORS, P., PERSSON, H., RIOPPELLE, R.J., HOKFELT, T., AND RICHARDSON, P.M. (1992) Colocalization of NGF binding sites, trk mRNA, and low-affinityNGF receptor mRNA in primary sensoy neurons: responses to injury and infusion of NGF. *J. Neurosci.,* **12**, 4011-4022.

37. VERGE, V.M.K., XU, Z., XU, X-J AND WIESENFELD-HALLIN, Z. (1992) Marked increase in nitric oxide synthase mRNA is dorsal root ganglia after peripheral axotomy: in situ hybridization and functional studies. *Proc. Nat Acad sci USA* **89**, 11617-11621.

38 WEINREICH, D. AND WONDERLIN, W.F. (1987) Inhibition of calcium-dependent spike after-hyperpolarization increases excitability of rabbit visceral sensory neurones. *J. Physiol.* **394,** 415-427.

39. WINTER, J., FORBES, C.A., STERNBERG, J. AND LINDSAY, R.M. (1988) Nerve growth factor (NGF) regulates adult rat cultured dosrsal root ganglion neuron responses to the excitotoxin capsaicin. *Neuron,* **1**, 973-981.

40. WOOD J.N., LILLYCROP, K.A., DENT, K.L. NINKINA, N.N., BEECH, M.M., WILLOUGHBY, J.J., WINTER, J. AND LATCHAM, D.S. (1992) Regulation of expression of the neuronal POU protein Oct-2 by nerve growth factor. *J. Biol. Chem.,* **267**, 17787-17791.

SILENT PRIMARY AFFERENTS

Robert F. Schmidt and H.-G. Schaible
Physiologisches Institut, Universität Würzburg
Röntgenring 9, D-8700 Würzburg
F.R.G.

INTRODUCTION

Under experimental conditions silent neurons are frequently encountered

When recording from single neurons of the peripheral and central nervous system of vertebrates many are being encountered which are silent at rest und unresponsive to the particular stimuli used be the experimenter. Therefore, these units are usually discarded. For instance, in a study of 534 single preganglionic units of the cervical sympathetic trunk of the cat with conduction velocities ranging from less than 0.5 m/s to 20 m/s about 70% were not spontaneously active and did not exhibit evoked discharges upon somatic nerve stimulation, whereas 25% had both properties, and the other five percent had one or the other property.[12] Both in the myelinated and the unmyelinated fiber range (72% and 28% of the samples respectively) similar proportions of silent units were found.

On a more anecdotal basis there exist many accidental observations of silent cells. For instance when searching with a microelectrode suitable for intracellular recording for single unit activity in the gray substance of the spinal cord, not too rarely units are encountered which display nothing but a large and stable resting potential regardless of the experimental manipulations to which the spinal cord is being exposed. Such units may well be glia cells but the experienced experimenter often has little doubt that the ease of the impalement and the size and stability of the membrane potential is typical for recording from a large neuron rather than from a tiny glia cell. But again, with no available technique to let these units "speak up", they are quickly left alone.

NATO ASI Series, Vol. H 79
Cellular Mechanisms of Sensory Processing
Edited by Laszlo Urban
© Springer-Verlag Berlin Heidelberg 1994

Investigations of single primary afferent units in sensory nerves or in dorsal roots usually reveal a certain proportion of afferent fibers which despite their electrical identification cannot be excited by adequate natural stimulation. Except for the ambiguity with unmyelinated afferents in peripheral nerves (which with an average chance of some 50% may be preganglionic autonomic efferents) the lack of responsiveness of such units is usually attributed to missing the peripheral receptive field of the unit or to inadequate or subthreshold natural stimulation. Usually such units are not even mentioned in the reports coming out of such studies, except perhaps in the data on the total number of units isolated. As a rule they are not even included in the compiled conduction velocity histograms of the sample (cf.,[15] for a striking exception see below[4]).

Articular silent afferent units in the normal joint

In our first extensive study of the responses of fine medial articular nerve (MAN) afferents to passive movements of the knee joint in the cat[16,17] we found, somewhat surprisingly, that in addition to group III (conduction velocity 2.5-20 m/s) and group IV units (conduction velocity <2,5 m/s) which according to their response behavior to movements were ideal candidates for nociceptors, there was a considerable percentage of units which had either much lower, i.e. (non-noxious) threshold, or which were not excited by any movements although their local receptive fields could be clearly identified.

In our total sample of 36 group III and 46 group IV units, the ones with very low threshold comprised 30.5% and 13% respectively, whereas the unresponsive ones were 22% and 43,5% of our sample, respectively (i.e. 28 units altogether). With one exception these units had conduction velocities below 5 m/s. Since they were all activated by high-intensity local pressure stimuli[15] we considered them to be nociceptors for the reception of local noxious stimuli, but we remarked that "it remains an open question what other sensory function they may subserve". And we added: "It may be speculated that in the course of inflammation, many become sensitive to joint movements".

A couple of years later we were investigating the fine afferent units innervating the dorsal aspect of the cat's knee joint via the posterior articular nerve (PAN). In these experiments the number of afferents (particularly in the group IV range, without responding to local stimulation and to any movements of the knee joint) was so extremely low that for several weeks we were seriously questioning our experimental approach, and consequently dissected these units not only from the sciatic nerve but also from the dorsal roots in order to avoid recording from preganglionic sympathetic units.[4] Nevertheless the number of responding units remained small: recordings from sciatic nerve filaments revealed responses to local mechanical stimulation of the joint in only 3 of 41 group IV units and in 12 of 18 group III units. In recordings from dorsal root filaments 4 of 11 group IV units and 7 of 13 group III units were activated by local stimulation of the joint tissue. Four group IV units (recorded from dorsal root filaments) responded only to rotation against the resistance of the tissue, whereas the majority of the fibers did not respond even to forceful movements. Group III units with local mechanosensitivity in the normal joint reacted strongly or weakly to movements in the working range of the joint or only to movements against resistance of the tissue. Thus, group III units in the PAN were similar in their response pattern to those in the MAN whereas their vast majority of the PAN group IV units were mechanoinsensitive thus providing a dramatic difference to those in the MAN (see above).

At the time these recordings were done, we were well aware of the possibility that our failure to active group IV PAN units in normal joints reflects other factors than the lack of sensitivity of these afferents. It might have been, for example, that the group IV receptor structures were inaccessible or were injured in our experiments, or that with the peripheral recordings we simply had a relatively small number of afferent units in our sample. However, for reasons discussed at that time we felt that each of these factors could be ruled out.[4]

In inflamed joint the percentage of mechanosensitive units is much larger than in normal joints: evidence for sensitization

Nearly all fine afferent units in the MAN from inflamed joints had low thresholds to movements (group III 89%, group IV 72%), and most units responded well to flexion and extension.[18] The responses were mostly tonic in character and adapted slowly or not at all when the joint was held in a new position. And, very much in contrast to the situation in normal joints (see above), afferent units with local mechanoreceptive fields which could not be excited by any physiological or noxious joint movement, were only very occasionally seen in the sample from inflamed joints: only one out of 38 group III and 2 out of 29 group IV units fell into this group.

The inflammation-induced changes in the overall response behavior of fine afferent units were even more striking in those sampled from the PAN: in recordings from sciatic nerve filaments, responses to local mechanical stimulation were seen in 14 of 36 group IV units (against 3 out of 41 from normal joints, see above), and the majority of fibers with detectable mechanical receptive fields responded strongly to gentle or to noxious movements.[4] We concluded that in the normal joint group IV units make very little contribution to the sensory input but as the joint becomes inflamed a large fraction of them becomes responsive to mechanical stimulation. This indicates that most of group IV units serve as nociceptors but only under tissue-damaging conditions.

In the inflamed joints, several other signs of sensitization of MAN and PAN fibers could be recognized: e.g. in the MAN resting activity was observed in 75% of the group III and 83% of the group IV units. Discharges were irregular and of high frequency.[3,18] Both the percentages of units with resting activity and the discharge frequency were more than twice as high as in the control sample. Furthermore, the receptive fields were larger than those in the control units and the average number of receptive fields per unit found in inflamed joints considerably exceeded that in normal joints. Interestingly, no systematic drop in von Frey thresholds was seen when comparing the control sample with the inflamed one, a result which was in contrast to that obtained in rat joints with chronic Freund's adjuvant arthritis where a general drop of von Frey threshold had been observed.[5,10]

Direct observation of the sensitization of silent articular afferents during experimental arthritis

The results discussed so far led us to conclude that an inflammatory lesion of the joint causes sensitization of high-threshold (nociceptive) afferents, sensitization of low-threshold (non-nociceptive) afferents and induction of mechanosensitivity in units without movement-induced sensitivity or without any mechanosensitivity. However, the comparison of samples of afferent units from normal and inflamed joints leaves some uncertainty about inflammation-induced changes in the discharge behavior of individual articular units. Therefore we studied the effects of inflammation on these afferents while recording from them prior to inflammation and thereafter during the developement of arthritis. This approach also allowed to determine the time course of sensitization that could not be analyzed previously.[19,20]

In these studies we divided the unresponsive units in 3 categories: 1) units which did not respond to movements but had receptive fields and responded to KCl (1 group III, 3 group IV units); 2) units that responded neither to movements nor to local mechanical stimulation (no detectable receptive field) but showed a typical response to KCl (2 group III and 14 group IV units); and 3) units without mechansosensitivity and no clear response to KCl (8 group IV units). Resting activity was absent in all classes.

Units of all 3 categories became sensitized during the course of inflammation, some of them to the point that they developed resting activity and vigorous responses to movements in the working range of the joint.

In category 1 group III units showed some impulses to extension of the joint but there was no resting activity during the development of the inflammation. One of the 3 group IV units responded to flexion and extension and exhibited resting discharge at about 150 min after the injection of kaolin. The response properties of the other 2 units did not change.

In category 2 one of the 2 group III and 5 of the 14 group IV units developed responsiveness to gentle mechanical stimuli during inflammation. Receptive fields became detectable in the patellar or medial region of the knee, and excitation by flexion and/or extension was induced. In addition these units developed spontaneous discharges. Four other group IV units were also sensitized but not as pronounced as the units described above. They became responsive only to movements against the resistance of the tissue and did not develop resting discharges. However, in 3 of these units receptive fields became detectable in the patellar or medial region of the inflamed knee. In a further group IV unit the inflammation induced spontaneous discharges but not mechanosensitivity. The other 4 group IV units as well as the remaining one group III unit did not develop any afferent activity during the inflammation.

Of the 8 group IV units, unresponsive to mechanical stimuli and to KCl (category 3), one unit developed a detectable receptive field and some resting discharges but no response to movements. During the control period this unit had an atypical response (1-4 impulses) to KCl. All other units remained unresponsive throughout the recording period.

Thus, over a period of some five years (1983-1988[4,15-20]) the existence of mechanoinsensitive, i.e. silent primary afferents in the articular nerves of the cat's knee joint slowly but steadily emerged in the course of our experiments. It became obvious that there is most likely a continuity of mechanical thresholds for articular fine afferents both under physiological and under pathophysiological conditions. Under physiological conditions the spectrum of mechanical thresholds is rather evenly distributed, whereas under pathophysiological conditions, such as an experimental arthritis, all units become sensitized and the spectrum of thresholds is skewed, i.e. most units can now be actived by stimulation which under normal condition is completely innoxious.

Silent primary afferent units in various tissues

Meanwhile an ever increasing number of research reports provides more and more evidence that silent afferent units seem to be widespread in mammalian peripheral nerves. A first brief review on this topic published in 1990 by McMahon and Koltzenburg[13] summarizes reports on the existence of silent primary afferents.[7,8] In recent years silent afferent units were described in the colon of the cat,[1,2,11] and in the skin of the rat[6] and the monkey.[14]

More recently additional support for the existence of silent afferent units has come forward with *in vivo* and *in vitro* studies of the skin of the rat[9], and in afferent units of the cat's and rat's veins and perineurium (Jänig, personal communication). In human subjects Torebjörk and Handwerker (personal communication) using microneurographic recordings from skin nerves have detected a considerable percentage of fine afferent units which could not be activated by mechanical stimuli until the skin was irritated by mustard oil or by comparable procedures.

Thus, in summary, silent primary afferent units may be an universal feature of the somato-afferent system of mammals, and, presumably, of other vertebrates. Many details of their functional characteristics and their possible afferent and efferent functions have still to be elucidated. For instance, many of the mechanoinsensitive units can be activated by chemical stimulation, particularly by close i.a. injection of algesic substances such as bradykinin, but whether such stimuli have any physiological significance is open for discussion. Furthermore, no evidence is available yet whether silent afferents have more prominent efferent functions than other fine afferent units. There is, however, little doubt that they form a special population of fine afferent units which only comes into play under pathophysiological conditions thus providing a special alarm system to inform the organism on particularly threatening noxious situations.

SUMMARY

Silent (mechanoinsensitive) primary afferent units have first been described in nerves innervating the knee joint of the cat. They are a substantial subpopulation of the fine afferent fibers of groups III (A δ) and IV (C) of the medial and posterior articular nerves. There properties are being described and its is shown that they became sensitized in the course of pathophysiological processes in the tissue (such as an experimental arthritis) to respond to (formerly) nonnoxious stimuli (e.g. movements in the normal working range of the joint). Evidence will be quoted that makes it likely that silent afferent units form a widespread if not an universal component of the somatoafferent system in mammals.

REFERENCES

1. BAHNS, E., ERNSBERGER, U., JÄNIG, W. AND NELKE, A. (1986) Discharge properties of mechanosensitive afferents supplying the retroperitoneal space, *Pflugers Arch.* **407,** 519-525.
2. BAHNS, E., HALSBAND, U. AND JÄNIG, W., (1987) Responses of sacral visceral afferents from the lower urinary tract, colon and anus to mechanical stimulation, *Pflugers Arch.* **410,** 296-303.
3. COGGESHALL, R.E., HONG, K.A., LANGFORD, L.A., SCHAIBLE, H.-G. AND SCHMIDT, R.F., Discharge characteristics of fine medial articular afferents at rest and during passive movements of inflamed knee joints, *Brain Res.* **272** (1983) 185-188.
4. GRIGG, P., SCHAIBLE, H.-G., SCHMIDT, R.F. (1986) Mechanical sensitivity of group III and IV afferents from PAN in normal and inflamed cat knee, *J. Neurophysiol.* **55,** 635-643.
5. GUILBAUD, G., IGGO, A. AND TEGNER, R. (1985) Sensory receptors in ankle joint capsules of normal and arthritic rats, *Exp Brain Res.* **58,** 29-40.
6. HANDWERKER, H.O., KILO, S. AND REEH, P.W. (1991) Unresponsive afferent nerve fibres in the sural nerve of the rat, *J. Physiol.* **435,** 229-242.
7. HÄBLER, H.-J., JÄNIG, W. AND KOLTZENBURG, M. (1988) A novel type of unmyelinated chemosensitive nociceptor in the acutely inflamed bladder, *Agents and Actions* **25,** 219-221.
8. HÄBLER, H.-J., JÄNIG, W. AND KOLTZENBURG, M. (1990) Activation of unmyelinated afferent fibres by mechanical stimuli and inflammation of the urinary bladder in the cat, *J. Physiol.* **425,** 545-562.
9. HÄBLER, H.J., JÄNIG, W. AND KOLTZENBURG, M. (1990) Activation of unmyelinated afferent fibres by mechanical stimuli and inflammation of the urinary bladder in the cat, *J. Physiol.* **425,** 545-562.
10. IGGO, A., GUILBAUD, G. AND TEGNER, R. (1984) Sensory mechanisms in

arthritic rat joints. In L. Kruger and J.C. Liebeskind (Eds.) *Advances in pain research and therapy. Vol.16*, New York: Raven Pres, pp. 83-93.

11. JÄNIG, W. AND KOLTZENBURG, M. (1991) Receptive properties of sacral primary afferent neurons supplying the colon, *J. Neurophysiol.*, **65**, 1067-1077.

12. JÄNIG, W. AND SCHMIDT, R.F. (1970) Single unit responses in the cervical sympathetic trunk upon somatic nerve stimulation, *Pflugers Arch.* **314**, 199-216.

13. MCMAHON, S. AND KOLTZENBURG, M. (1991) Novel classes of nociceptors: beyond Sherrington, *Trends Neurosci.* **13**, 199-201.

14. MEYER, R.A., DAVIS, K.D., COHEN, R.H., TREEDE, R.-D. AND CAMPBELL, J.N. (1991) Mechanically insensitive afferents (MIAs) in cutaneous nerves of monkey, *Brain Res.* **561**, 252-261.

15. SCHAIBLE, H.-G. AND SCHMIDT, R.F. (1983) Activation of groups III and IV sensory units in medial articular nerve by mechanical stimulation of knee joint, *J. Neurophysiol.* **49**, 35-44.

16. SCHAIBLE, H.-G. AND SCHMIDT, R.F. (1983) Responses of fine medial articular nerve afferents to passive movements of knee joint, *J. Neurophysiol.* **49** 1118-1126.

17. SCHAIBLE, H.-G. AND SCHMIDT, R.F. (1984) Mechanosensibility of joint receptors with fine afferent fibres, *Exp. Brain Res.* **9**, 284-297.

18. SCHAIBLE, H.-G. AND SCHMIDT, R.F. Effects of an experimental arthritis on the sensory properties of fine articular afferent units, *J. Neurophysiol.* **54**, (1985) 1109-1122.

19. SCHAIBLE, H.-G. AND SCHMIDT, R.F. (1988) Direct observation of the sensitization of articular afferents during an experimental arthritis. In R. Dubner, G.F. Gebhardt and M.R. Bond (Eds.) *Pain research and clinical management series, proceedings of the Vth world congress on pain*, Elsevier Science Publisher, Amsterdam, pp. 44-50.

20. SCHAIBLE, H.-G. AND SCHMIDT, R.F. (1988) Time course of mechanosensitivity changes in articular afferents during a developing experimental arthritis., *J. Neurophysiol.* **60**, 2180-2195.

SENSORY NEURONS AND PLASTICITY: THE ROLE OF IMMEDIATE EARLY GENES.

Carmen De Felipe, Robert Jenkins and Stephen P. Hunt
MRC Laboratory of Molecular Biology, Division of Neurobiology
Hills Road, Cambridge CB2 2QH
United Kingdom

INTRODUCTION

The protooncogenes c-fos and c-jun, code for transcriptionally active nuclear proteins that may play a central role in the long term response of neurons and glial cells to stimulation and damage. Fos and Jun are also 'immediate early genes' (IEGs) which were originally described as a class of genes that were rapidly induced in cells stimulated with growth factors.[11]

c-jun and *c-fos* are members of a family of closely related proteins which possess a leucine zipper through which they form homo- or heterodimers that will bind to DNA and act as transcriptional regulators.[31] However, the control of *c-jun* gene expression and protein activity is complex and may involve transcriptional, combinatorial, temporal and posttranslational mechanisms, which vary between different cell types (see[25,30] for reviews).

c-jun has been shown to heterodimerize with *c-fos*, to form the AP1 transcription factor, other fos related proteins and with members of the CREB/ATF (cyclic AMP response element binding protein/activating transcription factor) family of binding proteins, or to form Jun-Jun homodimers.[30] In this form, molecules such as *c-jun* and *c-fos*, are able to bind to DNA domains in a sequence-specific manner and modulate gene transcription.[16] Different combinations of proteins can possess different DNA binding specificities, affinities and transcriptional activities. Jun-Fos heterodimers possess both an increased DNA binding activity and trans-activating activity when compared with Jun-Jun homodimers. Following stimulation of neurons, neuronal cell lines or glial cells, with phorbol esters, polypeptide

NATO ASI Series, Vol. H 79
Cellular Mechanisms of Sensory Processing
Edited by Laszlo Urban
© Springer-Verlag Berlin Heidelberg 1994

hormones, growth factors, cytokines or neurotransmitters the expression of c-jun and *c-fos* mRNA may follow 'immediate early' gene kinetics.[41,45,53] This is characterised by a rapid, but transient, expression of *c-jun* mRNA following stimulation and is not dependant upon new protein synthesis. However in certain situations the induction of *c-jun* expression can be both delayed and prolonged. For example during the differentiation of F9 carcinoma cells with retinoic acid or in the neuronal response to axonal damage described below.[26,33,46,57] Experimental investigations of the maintained expression of *c-jun* in non-neuronal cells have suggested that the positive autoregulation of *c-jun* expression though an AP1 site on the promoter of *c-jun* itself may play a key role in translating a transient stimulus into a long term response.[1,57] Whether such a mechanism operates in neurons is far from clear.

In this chapter we describe the rapid and transient postsynaptic expression of Fos and Jun in the nervous system as IEGs and the slower, longer lasting expression of *c-jun* that accompanies neuronal damage and the process of regeneration.

RAPID CHANGES IN GENE EXPRESSION IN THE SPINAL CORD

We previously described the rapid induction of Fos and a wide range of other genes in a subset of spinal cord neurons as a result of sensory stimulation. We found that noxious stimulation was crucial for a change in gene expression within neurons of the dorsal horn.[23,53] A brief noxious stimulus results, within 1-2 hours, in the induction of Fos protein and in the mRNA and protein for a large number of other genes, including *c-jun*, within superficial and deep neurons of the ipsilateral dorsal horn. Activation of non-nociceptive low threshold afferents results in the induction of Fos in a subpopulation of neurons in the intermediate layers of the dorsal horn which are not generally labelled following noxious stimulation. Induction of *c-fos* and *c-jun* was never seen within sensory neurons in the dorsal root ganglion (DRG) even following electrical stimulation. Similarly we have rarely seen Fos immunoreactivity within neurons in areas of termination of large diameter, low threshold, primary sensory fibers, including the dorsal column nuclei and the ventral horn.

Expression of IEGs within the dorsal horn following sensory stimulation is generally a transient event with levels of mRNA for *c-fos, c-jun* and NGFI-A (Zif 268, krox-24) returning to basal levels within 4-6 hours. We have also described a pattern of Fos staining that changes over time following either noxious stimulation or crush of the sciatic nerve. By 24 hours this pattern has changed radically and positive neurons are now seen bilaterally but predominantly within deeper layers of the dorsal horn, emphasising the dynamic, changing pattern of IEG expression set up within the spinal cord following a brief but relevant stimulus.[52]

It has frequently been suggested that the appearance of *c-fos* and *c-jun* together leads to a change in expression of the neuropeptide genes dynorphin and enkephalin both of which possess AP1 or AP1-like binding sequences in their promoters. The expression of both of these neuropeptide genes is massively increased following a peripheral inflamatory lesion or in an adjuvant model of arthritis, and with a time course compatible with a preceeding Fos/Jun activation. Alternatively it has been suggested that the physiological sequelae within the spinal cord of a brief C-fiber volley, including 'wind-up', changing size and shape of receptive field and reduced reflex thresholds, could be the result of molecular changes such as those described here.[17,24]

At this point it should be reemphasised that we failed to find any evidence for rapid, immediate-early changes in gene transcription in the DRG itself under any of the stimulation paradigms described above including direct electrical stimulation of the nerve. However, when the nerve was either crushed or sectioned we were able to detect a massive increase in *c-jun*, but not *c-fos*, expression occuring at 24h, but not at 2h.

LONGER TERM CHANGES IN C-JUN EXPRESSION

A number of recent studies have implicated the *c-jun* protooncogene in the control of growth and differentiation in a variety of cell types including neurons and glial cells.[6,9,13,14,26,33,54,56] Following axon damage or block of axonal transport in peripheral sensory or motor neurons in the rat, there is a delayed expression of *c-jun* protein and mRNA, which is maintained until the nerve has fully regenerated.[26,33] Damage to the sciatic nerve induces expression of *c-jun* protein and mRNA within DRG cells and motor neurons that give rise to that nerve.[26,33] Similar expression of *c-jun* was also seen in nigrostriatal and rubrospinal neurons following lesion of their axons.[28,29] General axonal transport block, induced by the application of colchicine to the sciatic nerve, resulted in the expression of *c-jun* in both large and small diameter fibres, suggesting that the absence of a transported factor may play a role in the expression of *c-jun* in sensory neurons. *c-jun* expression was maintained if the axons were prevented from regenerating. However, the role of *c-jun* in the maintenance of the regenerative response is unclear and we therefore designed a number of experiments to test the hypothesis that *c-jun* expression is related to regeneration or growth of axons rather than simply axonal damage.

In a recent study[27] we investigated four lesion paradigms associated with different degrees of primary sensory axon growth (Figure 1). These were (i) peripheral nerve lesion, which allows for successful regeneration of the damaged axons back to their targets; (ii) dorsal root section (rhizotomy), which is associated with a slow regrowth of at least some of the damaged axons, but a failure of these to penetrate the spinal cord; (iii) peripheral nerve section, which allows nearby intact sensory neurons to undergo collateral sprouting into denervated peripheral tissue. Previous work suggests that large axons (conducting in the Aβ range) do not undertake any significant sprouting, whereas some fine axons do. In this study we ligated the sciatic nerve (which projects through dorsal root ganglia L4, L5, L6), and looked for a reaction in the nearby intact saphenous nerve afferents (most of which are derived from the adjacent L3 dorsal root ganglion); (iv) dorsal root section which offers the opportunity for nearby intact dorsal root axons to collaterally sprout into the denervated CNS neuropil. The available evidence suggests that such collateral sprouting occurs to a very limited extent.

Sciatic nerve lesion at 24h but not 2h, resulted in a massive expression of c-jun in the nuclei of all damaged sensory neurons (Figure 2) as has previously been described in detail.[26,33] Similar results were seen in ganglion L3 following saphenous nerve section. From 24 hours the expression of *c-jun* was approximately constant until the time of reinnervation of target, at which point it declined to control levels. *c-jun* protein was also expressed in Schwann cell nuclei of the sciatic nerve segment, distal but not proximal to the nerve lesion (De Felipe and Hunt, unpublished).

In contrast to nerve section, dorsal root section induced a small and variable expression of *c-jun* in damaged ganglia. Nevertheless the number of cells showing *c-jun* immunoreactivity was significantly greater than that seen in L4/L5 ganglia contralateral to the lesioned ganglia or following a sham lesion. No significant change in *c-jun* expression was seen in DRG L3 following L4/L5 dorsal root section but lesion of the sciatic nerve resulted in the appearance of *c-jun* immunoreactivity in L3 DRG cells from 24 hours to 32 days post-lesion. The response of the DRG cell to axotomy of the central process was thus far less dramatic and occured to only a minor extent (Figure 2).

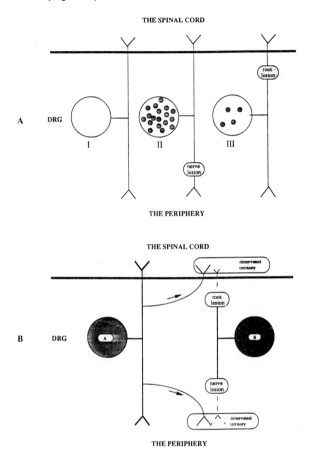

Figure 1. The diagrams summarise the experimental lesion paradigms and the types of collateral sprouting and accompanying increased c-jun expression that occurs after lesion of the central or peripheral processes of DRG cells.

a)   I, represents the intact DRG; II, represents a DRG after section of the peripheral processes (sciatic or saphenous lesion); III, represents a DRG after the section of the dorsal root. c-jun immunopositive cells are represented by shaded circles.

b)   illustrates the direction of peripheral and central collateral sprouting (arrows) from adjacent DRGs (A) to denervated territory due to lesion of one of the processes of an adjacent cell (B). Section of the sciatic nerve results in substantial expression in DRGs L4,L5 (which give rise to the nerve) and more limited expression in L3 which probably reflects growth of L3 axons into denervated sciatic territory. The c-jun response to dorsal root section is much weaker and there is very little collateral sprouting (see text).
(From Jenkins et al., 1993c)

The literature surrounding neuronal change following damage to the dorsal root is controversial. In contrast to the result of peripheral nerve lesion, chromatolysis is not seen[12] and there are no changes in growth associated protein (GAP 43) levels.[55] However, levels of neurofilament (NF) gene mRNA are reduced for a number of weeks and tubulin levels increased (also[21]), although the changes were of shorter duration and smaller magnitude than those seen following division of the peripheral process. However, the levels of NF gene expression was only measured in large diameter DRG cells, which represent a minor subpopulation of these ganglion cells. In our material, *c-jun* expression was not restricted to a particular size of neuron.

The limited *c-jun* response to central root section is of particular interest as it has previously been demonstrated that the rate of regeneration of crushed dorsal root axons can be substantially facilitated by a prior conditioning crush of the peripheral process, or by inflammation near the neuronal cell body.[38,44] We suggest that the generalized activation of c-jun, by peripheral nerve damage, augments the rather weak increase in expression of the gene by the initial crush of the central process, leading to the greatly enhanced regenerative response.

A similar logic could explain the enhanced growth of intact dorsal root axons into previously denervated areas of the dorsal horn.[55] These so-called "spared root" preparations indicate that intact root fibres have a barely detectable capacity to sprout into adjacent denervated territory, but that this capacity can be dramatically improved following crush or cut of the peripheral process. We would argue that the increased expression of *c-jun* protein caused by peripheral nerve damage may be important in increasing the efficacy of the central growth process.

It is also of considerable interest to know whether the *c-jun* response is correlated with axon damage alone, or with neuronal growth. Our demonstration that *c-jun* expression is elevated in the L3 DRG after sciatic nerve section suggests the latter. There is no evidence of axons of the L3 DRG projecting through the sciatic nerve, so changes in this ganglion are likely to reflect expression in undamaged neurons. There is considerable, if somewhat conflicting, evidence that some collateral sprouting of intact afferents can occur into denervated tissue. After sciatic nerve section and ligation, fine, but not coarse, axons in the saphenous nerve are reported to progressively invade some of the sciatic territory.[15] The elevation of c-jun in a limited number of cells, particularly small cells, in the L3 DRG, is therefore well-correlated with such sprouting, although we are not able to provide direct evidence that the c-jun positive neurons are indeed those which grow into the denervated area.

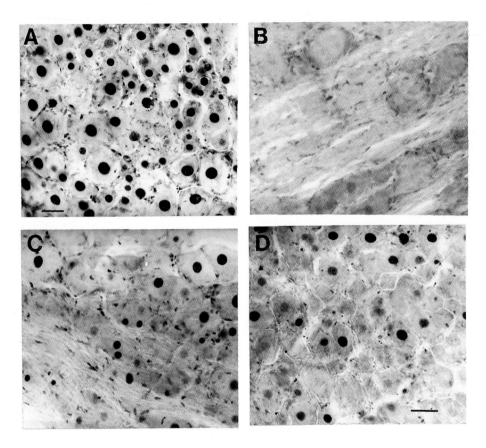

Figure 2. Illustrates the expression of c-jun immunopositive DRG cells following various lesion paradigms.
a)   c-jun immunoreactivity in a section of L4 DRG ipsilateral to a sciatic nerve lesion (4 days post-lesion).
b)   A section of L4 DRG contralateral to a sciatic nerve lesion immunostained for c-jun (4 days post-lesion).
c)   c-jun immunoreactivity in a section of L4 DRG 7 days after dorsal root section.
d)   c-jun immunoreactivity in a section of L3 DRG 4 days after sciatic nerve lesion. Scale bar = 25mm.
(From Jenkins et al.[29])

The effects of rhizotomy on adjacent, intact, sensory neurons are also consistent with the notion that *c-jun* expression is related to growth rather than damage alone. In this case, the evidence is that the intact axons show, at the most, a very limited ability to sprout centrally, as discussed above, and we observed only a small and non-significant increase in c-jun positive cells in the L3 DRG after L4/L5 rhizotomy.

The observation that in peripheral nerve, axoplasmic block was as effective as axon section, or ligation, in causing an increased *c-jun* expression in neurons, led us to suggest that the *c-jun* response may have resulted in part from deprivation of axonally transported target factors.[27-29] The most obvious candidates are the neurotrophins, nerve growth factor (NGF) and brain derived neurotrophic factor (BDNF), which are known to be retrogradely transported in sensory neurons.[22] Indeed, exogenously applied NGF has been shown to reverse the changes in peptide and growth factor receptor expression seen following peripheral nerve section in rat.[19,49] To look at these possibilities more closely we established primary cultures of adult dorsal root ganglion cells and their supporting satellite and Schwann cells and investigated the signals and intracellular events that lead to and modify c-jun expression (De Felipe and Hunt, unpublished).

THE REGULATION OF C-JUN EXPRESSION IN VITRO

High levels of *c-jun* protein and mRNA were also found in both neurons and Schwann cells when cultured in either defined medium or in the presence of serum suggesting that the results of axotomy *in vivo* on both neurons and glial cells could be maintained or reconstructed *in vitro* (Figure 3).

Before monitoring the effects of growth factors on c-jun levels in our cultures, we used in situ hybridization to check for the presence of the neurotrophin trk family of receptors on our sensory neurons in culture and found that growth factor receptor mRNA was differentially expressed by sensory neurons (De Felipe and Hunt unpublished).

We maintained cultures in defined medium with NGF or BDNF for a 5 day period. *c-jun* mRNA levels were not changed by addition of growth factors at any time point in either neurons or Schwann cells. Similarly, the total number of *c-jun* positive neurons (and neuronal survival) was unaffected by growth factor treatment and no changes in *c-jun* protein immunofluorescence levels was found in neurons after treatment with any of these compounds. The intensity of GAP43 staining in neurons was similarly unaffected by growth factor treatment.

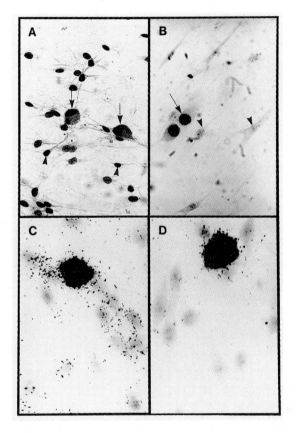

Figure 3. The majority of neurons and glial cells (Schwann cells and satellite cells) express c-jun protein (A,B) and mRNA (C,D) in vitro. In these photomicrographs taken after 7 days in culture, c-jun protein and mRNA was seen in both glial satellite cells (arrowheads) and neurons (arrows). 24h following treatment with diButyrylcAMP the levels of c-jun were substantially reduced in glial cells but not neurons. This was true for both protein (B) and mRNA (D,). Scale bar=30 μm.

To determine the influence of second messenger candidates on the expression of *c-jun* in DRG cells in culture, levels of *c-jun* mRNA and protein were studied after phorbol 12-mystirate 13-acetate (PMA) treatment, which stimulates protein kinase C, or stimulation of protein kinase A (PKA) with forskolin which elevates cAMP though adenylate cyclase activation or by addition of the membrane permeable analogue of cAMP, dibutyryl cyclic adenosine monophosphate (dBcAMP). The effects of artificially raising or lowering internal calcium levels and of depolarization were also studied.

We found that glial cell but not neuronal levels of *c-jun* protein and mRNA were raised by increasing intracellular calcium levels and lowered by treatment with cAMP or forskolin (Figure 3). High K^+ concentrations, veratridine or tetrodotoxin were added to DRG cultures in order to ask whether depolarization or Na^+ channel activity could induce changes in *c-jun* gene expression. No differences in *c-jun* protein or mRNA were found after these treatments.

DISCUSSION

The protooncogenes *c-fos* and *c-jun* can be induced rapidly and transiently in postsynaptic neurons following stimulation, but *c-jun* can be induced in a more persistant fashion following axon damage. The increased expression of *c-jun* by neurons and glial cells following axotomy can be reproduced and maintained *in vitro* yet the levels of *c-jun* protein and mRNA in neurons and glial cells can be differentially regulated by intracellular second messengers suggesting that different molecular control mechanisms are operative.

We previously suggested that the effectiveness of axoplasmic block in initiating the increased expression of *c-jun* in DRG cells may have been due to loss of a target derived factor such as NGF.[26,27,33] In culture, sensory neurons expressed the tyrosine kinase receptor mRNAs trk, trkB and trk C which code for high affinity receptors for the neurotrophins NGF, BDNF (and NT4) and NT3 respectively and mediate their functions in vivo (see review[10]). NGF high affinity binding sites have been identified on approximately half of the lumbar DRG cells including those containing substance P and calcitonin gene related peptide (CGRP) and some of the larger diameter neurons.[50,51] Furthermore, the loss of trk from sensory neurons following axotomy can be partially reversed by NGF infusion[49] as can the loss of substance P immunoreactivity both *in vivo* and *in vitro*.[19,36,37] BDNF, but not NGF, is expressed by some DRG cells in vivo[18] and in cultured adult sensory neurons BDNF enhances neurite outgrowth but is not required for survival[35]. Our results also suggest that neurotrophin receptors are expressed on sensory neurons even when maintained in serum free medium but, importantly, that the addition of NGF or BDNF to these cultures does not effect the expression of *c-jun* mRNA in neurons or glial cells. These results strongly suggest that the expression of *c-jun* is not related to growth factor starvation but to loss of unknown target derived factors which act to repress *c-jun* expression in the intact nerve. This is not a particularly suprising result if it is accepted that the stimulus for regeneration is the loss of transported factors that follows axon damage. However, while NGF and probably BDNF are able to sustain and encourage cell growth and differentiation and to reverse many of the neurochemical events associated with axon damage, it seems unlikely that absence of these factors could account for the changes in *c-jun* expression seen in axotomised neurons. This suggests therefore that there are both neurotrophin dependant and independant mechanisms operative during regeneration (see also Woolf, this volume).

The effects of increased intracellular calcium levels, or stimulation with second messenger candidates such as cAMP, on *c-jun* levels were entirely within the glial cell population. Stimulation with PMA had no effect at the time points used. However, addition of stable cAMP analogue or forskolin to the cultures resulted in a massive and rapid loss of *c-jun* mRNA from glial cells but with no effect on neuronal levels. These results are similar to those described for the regulation of BDNF expression in Schwann cell cultures but the reverse of those described for NGF mRNA regulation.[42]

Denervation of Schwann cells following peripheral nerve section has been shown to result in a substantially changed pattern of gene expression that is thought to encourage the regeneration of the damaged neuron. Thus, there is an upregulation of low affinity NGF receptor, an increased expression of BDNF and NGF as well as *c-jun* described here[42,48] and an increase in the production of matrix factors.[41] It has also been reported that denervated nerve provides a better substrate for growth of explanted adult DRG cells than intact nerve.[4] We have also shown that DRG cultures grown on Schwann cell beds treated with forskolin or dBcAMP to turn off *c-jun* expression, substantially retards the growth of dissociated sensory neurons.[43] Much of this data would fit with the suggestion that axon-glial cell contact activates a cAMP second messenger system within the glial cell[34] which then inhibits the expression of numerous genes such as *c-jun* and BDNF and discourages further axon growth. The close correlation between the pattern of gene expression seen in denervated Schwann cells, the coordinate expression of the transcription factor *c-jun*, and the co-regulation of many of these genes by cAMP, suggests that *c-jun* may serve a pivotal role in the regenerative process.

The mechanism by which *c-jun* expression is downregulated in glial cells but not neurons is obscure in that most previous reports have suggested that cAMP operates though a CREB protein acting at the cAMP response element (CRE) on the *c-jun* promoter causing increased gene expression.[32] PKA mediated phosphorylation of CREB activates gene transcription, while dephosphorylation inhibits *c-jun* expression. However, recent studies have suggested that the presence of other members of the CREB family could act as transcriptional repressors[5], and genes encoding cAMP-responsive element modulator (CREM) proteins, with antagonist properties, have been described.[20] The presence of IP1, a trans activating inhibitor of AP1 binding to DNA, is likewise inactivated by phosphorylation following stimulation with cAMP,[2] and unlikely to explain the present results although a novel inhibitory interaction may well be operative,[3] at least in Schwann cells.

The function of *c-jun* in neuronal regeneration is also unclear. In the sensory ganglion *in vivo*, section of the dorsal root results only in a weak and variable expression of *c-jun* protein, yet the damaged axons will regenerate to the spinal cord.[27] However this regeneration is greatly facilitated by a conditioning crush to the peripheral branch of the neuron which also results in a massive expression of *c-jun* protein in damaged neurons.[27,44] This suggests that *c-jun* expression can facilitate but is not an absolute requirement for growth in all nerve cells. The mechanisms by which *c-jun* can facilitate growth are unknown. We recently pointed out that the suggestion of a causal relationship between other changes in gene expression seen in sensory neurons following axotomy and *c-jun* expression may be an oversimplification Most of these changes in gene expression were restricted to subsets of sensory neurons and occured at different times after axotomy. For example, the upregulation of GAP 43 expression occurs initially in small diameter sensory neurons and involves larger diameter DRGs only at longer survival times.[47] In contrast, the change in *c-jun* expression was rapid and appeared simultaneously in both small and large sensory neurons within 24 hours, regardless of chemical phenotype.[26,33] Thus it seems unlikely that *c-jun* expression leads directly to changes in the expression of other downstream genes simply by direct interaction with the relevant promoter sequences.

Recent studies suggest that genes such as *c-fos* and *c-jun* can act as selectors of cell responsiveness to external stimuli.[16] We suggest that the activation of *c-jun* could prime neurons and glial cells to respond in a novel way to factors in their environment and so accelerate repair.

REFERENCES

1. ANGEL, P., HATTORI, K., SMEAL, T. AND KARIN, M. (1988) The *jun* proto-oncogene is positively autoregulated by its product, Jun/AP-1. *Cell* **55**, 875-885.
2. AUWERX, J. AND SASSONI-CORSI, P. (1991) IP-1: A dominant inhibitor of fos/jun whose activity is modulated by phosphorylation. *Cell* **64**, 983-993.
3. BAICHWAL, V.R. AND TJIAN, R. (1990) Control of c-Jun activity by interaction of a cell-specific inhibitor with regulatory domain δ: Differences between v- and c-Jun. *Cell* **63**, 815-825.
4. BEDI, K.S., WINTER, J., BERRY, M. AND COHEN, J. (1991) Adult rat dorsal root ganglion neurons extend neurites on predegenerated but not on normal peripheral nerves *in vitro. Eur. J. Neurosci.* **4**, 193-200.
5. BENBROOK, D.M. AND JONES, N.C. (1990) Heterodimer formation between CREB and JUN proteins. *Oncogene* **5**, 295-302.
6. BOS, T.J., F.S. MONTECLARO, F., MITSUOBU, F., BALL, A.R., CHANG, C.H.W., NISHIMURA, T. AND VOGT, P.K. (1990) Efficient transformation of chicken embryo fibroblasts by c-Jun requires structural modification in coding and non-coding sequences. *Genes and Development* **4**, 1677-1687.
7. CARROLL, S.L., SILOS-SANTIAGO, I., FRESE, S.E., RUIT, K.G., MILBRANDT, J. AND SNIDER, W.D. (1992) Dorsal root ganglion neurons expressing *trk* are selectively sensitive to NGF deprivation in utero. *Neuron* **9**, 779-788.
8. CASTELLAZI, M., LOISEAU, L., PIU, F. AND SERGEANT, A. (1993) Chimeric c-Jun containing an heterologous homodimerization domain transforms primary chick embryo fibroblasts. *Oncogene* **8**, 1149-1160.
9. CASTELLAZZI, M., SPYROU, G., LA VISTA, N., DANGY, J.-P., PIU, F., YANIV M. AND BRUN, G. (1991) Overexpression of c-*jun, junB, or junD. Proc. Natl. Acad. Sci, USA* **88**, 8890-8894.
10. CHAO, M.V. (1992) Neurotrophin receptors: A window into neural differentiation. *Neuron* **9**, 583-593.
11. COCHRAN, B.H., REFFEL A.C., AND STILES, C.D. (1983) Molecular cloning of gene sequences regulated by platelet-derived growth factor. *Cell* **33**, 939-947.
12. CRAGG, B. (1970).What is the signal for chromatolysis? *Brain Res.* **23**, 1-21.
13. DE FELIPE, C., JENKINS, R., O'SHEA, R., WILLIAMS, T.S.C. AND HUNT, S.P. (1993) The role of immediate early genes in the regeneration of the central nervous system. *Adv. in Neurol.* New York, Raven Press. 263-271.
14. DE GROOT, R.P., KRUYT, F.A.E., VAN DER SAAG, P.T. AND KRUIJER, W. (1990).Ectopic expression of c-*jun* leads to differentiation of P19 embryonal carcinoma cells. *The EMBO Journal* **9**, 1831-1837.
15. DEVOR, M., SCHONFIELD, D., SELTZER, Z., AND WALL, P.D. (1979) Two modes of cutaneous representation following peripheral nerve injury. *J Comp. Neurol..* **185**, 211-220.

16. DIAMOND, M.I., MINER, J.N., YOSHINAGA, S.K. AND YAMAMOTO, K.R. (1990) Transcription factor interactions: Selectors of positive or negative regulation from a single DNA element. *Science* **249**, 1266-1271.

17. DUBNER, R. AND RUDA, M.A. (1992) Activity dependant neuronal plasticity following tissue injury and inflammation. *Trends Neurosci.* **15**, 96-103.

18. ERNFORS, P. AND PERSSON, H. (1991) Developmentally regulated expression of HDNF/NT-3 mRNA in rat spinal cord motoneurons and expression of BDNF mRNA in embryonic dorsal root ganglion. *Eur. J. Neurosci.* **3**:,953-961.

19. FITZGERALD, M., WALL, P.D., GOEDERT, M. AND EMSON, P.C. (1985) Nerve growth factor counteracts the neurophysiological and neurochemical effects of chronic sciatic nerve section. *Brain Res.* **332**, 131-141.

20. FOULKES, N.S., LAOIDE, B.M., SCHLOTTE F. AND SASSONI-CORSI, P. (1991) Transcriptional antagonist cAMP-responsive element modulator (CREM) down-regulates c-fos cAMP-induced expression. *Proc. Natl. Acad Sci, USA* **88**, 5448-5452.

21. GREENBERG, S.E. AND LASEK, R.J. (1988) Neurofilament protein synthesis in DRG neurons decreases more after peripheral axotomy than central axotomy. *J. Neurosci* **8**, 1739-1746.

22. HENDRY, I.A., THOENEN, H. AND IVERSEN, L.L. (1974) The retrograde axonal transport of nerve growth factor. *Brain Res.* **68**, 103-121.

23. HUNT, S.P., PINI A. AND EVAN, G. (1987) Induction of c-fos like protein in spinal cord neurons following sensory stimulation. *Nature* **328**, 632-634.

24. IADAROLA, M.J., BRADY, L.S., DRAISCI, G. AND DUBNER, R. (1988) Enhancement of dynorphin gene expression in spinal cord following experimental inflammation: Stimulus specificity, behavioural parameters and opioid receptor binding. *Pain* **35**, 313-326.

25. JACKSON, S.P. (1992) Regulating transcription factor activity by phosphorylation. *Trends in Cell Biol.* **2**, 104-108.

26. JENKINS, R. AND HUNT, S.P. (1991) Long term increases in the levels of c-jun mRNA and Jun protein like immunoreactivity in motor and sensory neurons following axon damage. *Neurosci Lett* **129**, 107-111.

27. JENKINS, R., MCMAHON, S.B., BOND, A.B. AND HUNT, S.P. (1993) Expression of c-Jun as a response to dorsal root and peripheral nerve section in damaged and adjacent intact primary sensory neurons in the rat. *Eur. J. Neurosci.* **5**, 751-759.

28. JENKINS, R., O'SHEA, R., THOMAS, K.L. AND HUNT, S.P. (1993) c-jun expression of immediate early genes in substantia nigra neurons following striatal 6-OHDA lesions in the rat. *Neuroscience* **53**, 447-457.

29. JENKINS, R., TETZLAFF, W. AND HUNT, S.P. (1993) Differential expression of immediate early genes in rubrospinal neurons following axotomy in the rat. *Eur. J.Neurosci* **5**, 203-209.

30. KARIN, M. AND SMEAL, T. (1992) Control of transcription factors by signal transduction pathways: The beginning of the end. *Trends in Biochem. Sci.* **17**, 418-422.

31. LAMB, P. AND MCKNIGHT, S.L. (1991) Diversity and specificity in transcriptional regulation: The advantages of heterotypic dimerization. *Trends in Biochem. Sci.* **16**, 417-422.

32. LAMPH, W.W., DWARKI, V.J., OFIR, R., MONTMINY, M. AND VERMA, I.M. (1990) Negative and positive regulation by transcription factor cAMP response element-binding protein is modulated by phosphorylation. *Proc. Natl Acad. Sci. USA* **87**, 4320-4324.

33. LEAH, J.D., HERDEGEN, T. AND BRAVO, R. (1991) Selective expression of Jun proteins following axotomy and axonal transport block in peripheral nerves in the rat; evidence for a role in the regeneration process. *Brain Res.* **566**, 198-207.

34. LEMKE, G. (1990) Glial growth factors. *Seminars in the Neurosciences* **2**, 437-443.

35. LINDSAY, R. M. (1988) Nerve growth factors (NGF, BDNF) enhance axonal regeneration but are not required for survival of adult sensory neurons. *J. Neurosci.* **8**, 2394-2405.

36. LINDSAY, R.M. AND HARMAR, A.J. (1989) Nerve growth factor regulates expression of neuropeptide genes in adult sensory neurons. *Nature* **337**, 362-364.

37. LINDSAY, R.M., LOCKETT, C., STERNBERG, J. AND WINTER, J. (1989) Neuropeptide expression in cultures of adult sensory neurons: Modulation of substance P and calcitonin gene-related peptide levels by nerve growth factor. *Neuroscience* **33**, 53-65.

38. LU, X. AND RICHARDSON, P.M. (1991) Inflammation near the nerve cell body enhances axonal regeneation. *J. Neurosci.* **11**, 972-978.

39. MAKI, Y., T.J. BOS, DAVIES, C., STARBUCK, M. AND VOGT, P.K. (1987) Avian sarcoma virus 17 carries the jun oncogene. *Proc. Natl Acad. Sci. USA* **84**, 2848-2852.

40. MARTINI, R. AND SCHACHNER, M. (1988) Immunoelectron microscopic localization of neural cell adhesion molecules (L1, N-CAM and myelin associated glycoprotein) in regenerating adult mouse sciatic nerve. *J. Cell Biol.* **106**, 1735-1746.

41. MCNAUGHTON, L.A. AND HUNT, S.P. (1992) Regulation of gene expression in astrocytes by excitatory amino acids. *Molec. Brain Res.* **16**, 261-266.

42. MEYER, M., MATSUOKA, I., WETMORE, C., OLSON L. AND THOENEN, H. (1992) Enhanced synthesis of brain-derived neurotrophic factor in the lesioned peripheral nerve: Different mechanisms are responsible for the regulation of BDNF and NGF mRNA. *J. Cell Biol.* **119**, 45-54.

43. PALMER, J.A., DE FELIPE, C., AND HUNT, S.P. (1993) The expression of c-jun is correlated with the facilitation of neurite outgrowth. *Brain Res. Assoc. Abstr.* **10**, 8.

44. RICHARDSON, P. AND ISSA, V.M.K. (1984) Peripheral injury enhances central regeneration of primary sensory neurons. *Nature* **309**, 791-793.

45. SHENG, M. AND GREENBERG, M.E. (1990) The regulation and function of c-*fos* and other immediate early genes in the nervous system. *Neuron* **4**, 477-485.

46. SLEIGH, M.J. (1992) Differentiation and proliferation in mouse embryonal carcinoma cells. *BioEssays* **14**, 769-775.

47. SOMMERVAILLE, T., REYNOLDS, M.L. AND WOOLF, C.J. (1991) Time-dependant differences in the increase in GAP-43 expression in dorsal root ganglion cells after peripheral axotomy. *Neuroscience* **45**, 213-230.

48. TANIUCHI, M., CLARK, H.B. SCHWEITZER, J.B. AND JOHNSON, E.M. (1988) Expression of nerve growth factor receptors by Schwann cells of axotomized peripheral nerves: Ultrastructural location, suppression by axonal contact, and binding properties. *J.Neurosci.* **8**, 664-681.

49. VERGE, V.M.K., MERLIO, J.-P., GRONDIN, J., ERNFORS, P., PERSSON, H., RIOPELLE, R.J., HOKFELT, T. AND RICHARDSON, P.M. (1992) Colocalization of NGF binding sites, trk mRNA, and low-affinity NGF receptor mRNA in primary sensory neurons: Responses to injury and infusion of NGF. *J. Neurosci* **12**, 4011-4022.

50. VERGE, V.M.K., RICHARDSON, P.M., BENOIT, R. AND ROPELLE, R.J. (1989) Histochemical characterisation of sensory neurons with high affinity receptors for nerve growth factor. *J. Neurocytol.* **18**, 583-591.

51. VERGE, V.M.K., R.J. RIOPELLE AND RICHARDSON P.M. (1989) Nerve growth factor receptors on normal and injured sensory neurons. *J. Neurosci.* **9**, 914-922.

52. WILLIAMS, T. S. C., G. I. EVAN AND S. P. HUNT (1990) Changing patterns of c-fos induction in spinal neurons following thermal cutaneous stimulation in the rat. *Neuroscience* **36**, 73-81.

53. WISDEN, W., M. L. ERRINGTON, S. WILLIAMS, S. B. DUNNETT, C. WATERS, D. HITCHCOCK, G. EVAN, T. V. BLISS AND S. P. HUNT (1990) Differential expression of immediate early genes in the hippocampus and spinal cord. *Neuron* **4**, 603-614.

54. WONG, W.-Y., L. HAVARSTEIN, I. M. MORGAN AND P. K. VOgt (1992) c-jun causes focus formation and anchorage-independant growth in culture but is non-tumorigenic. *Oncogene* **7**, 2077-2080.

55. WOOLF, C. J., M. L. REYNOLDS, C. MOLANDER, C. O'BRIEN, R. M. LINDSAY AND L. I. BENOWITZ (1990) The growth-associated protein GAP-43 appears in dorsal root ganglion cells and in the dorsal horn of the rat spinal cord following peripheral nerve injury. *Neuroscience* **34**, 465-478.

56. YAMAGUCHI-IWAI, Y., M. SATAKE, Y. MURAKAMI, M. SAKAI, M. MURAMATSU AND Y. ITO (1990) Differentiation of F9 embryonal carcinoma cells induced by c-jun and activated c-Ha-ras oncogenes. *Proc. Natl. Acad. Sci., USA* **87**, 8670-8674.

57. YANG-YEN, H.-F., R. CHIU AND M. KARIN (1990) Elevation of AP1 activity during F9 cell differentiation is due to increased c-*jun* transcription. *The New Biologist* **2**, 351-361.

MOLECULAR BIOLOGY OF DYNORPHIN GENE EXPRESSION IN RELATIONSHIP TO SPINAL CORD PROCESSING OF PAIN

Michael J. Iadarola and Donna J. Messersmith
Neurobiol. and Anesthesiol. Branch, NIDR, NIH
Bethesda MD, 20892
USA

INTRODUCTION

Peripheral inflammation and experimental neuropathic pain are known to induce a series of fundamental modifications of gene expression in neurons of the spinal cord dorsal horn. In most cases examined to date, the expression of the gene in question is increased.[19-21,28,31-34,41,58,78] Several of the activated genes code for the precursor proteins of neuropeptides which include the dynorphin and enkephalin families of opioid peptides and the tachykinins, substance P and substance K.[10,13,18,23] The increased expression results in an altered pattern of neuropeptide content in spinal cord second order neurons and their terminals.[31-34,37,54,67] However, the exact physiological meaning of the increase in gene expression or peptide content remains somewhat of an open question. The increase likely signifies a greater state of physiological activity in the peptide synthesizing neuron and likely results in a more effective signal transduction through release of greater amounts of peptide. Some of the increases seen in spinal cord, therefore, may modulate or underlie neuronal excitability changes that are established over time in the dorsal horn during inflammation.[30,79]

The processes governing these changes in gene expression can be explored on several levels (a) the physiological/phenomenological (e.g. time course of the increase, dependency on primary afferent innervation, types of injuries or

NATO ASI Series, Vol. H 79
Cellular Mechanisms of Sensory Processing
Edited by Laszlo Urban
© Springer-Verlag Berlin Heidelberg 1994

inflammatory stimuli that may induce the increase, connections of the neurons, etc.); (b) the second messengers and associated receptors and enzymes that may be involved (e.g. signal transduction pathways)(5), and (c) molecular biological and biochemical mechanisms of transcriptional, post-transcriptional or translational control processes.[49,52,63,77] The various physiological/phenomenological aspects have been examined in previous studies from our group[19-21,31-34,37,59,60,67] and by others.[28,46,47,57,58,78] For the dynorphin gene a robust increase in expression commences at about 4 hours after the onset of a peripheral inflammation.[20] The subsequent time course of the mRNA elevation closely parallels the peak and resolution of the peripheral inflammation.[33] The dynorphin mRNA increase occurs in neurons within the superficial laminae (I and II) and in laminae V and VI of the dorsal horn[67] which are the principal spinal cord sites for processing primary afferent nociceptive information. Some of the dynorphin neurons project rostrally but the majority appear to be local circuit neurons.[54] The latter fact is consistent with the measurement of an increase in dynorphin peptide content by radioimmunoassay of extracts of dorsal spinal cord.[31-34,37,47] The lateralized, segmentally-specific increase in dynorphin peptide content mainly reflects accumulation within synaptic vesicles in local nerve terminals.[33,37,54,67]

In this report we focus on the molecular biology of transcription processes controlling dynorphin gene expression.[18,20,35,38,39,41,45,57] In normal spinal cord this gene is expressed at a very low level or is in a partially repressed state.[31] Once a noxious stimulus reaches the spinal cord, if it is of sufficient degree and duration, the dynorphin gene undergoes a marked increase in expression.[32,33] At the molecular level, this transition is effected through a complex interaction of nuclear proteins with DNA sequences in the dynorphin promoter or even downstream within the gene itself.[18,35,38,39,45] The protein-DNA interaction(s) ultimately activates transcription via RNA polymerase II (see[9,42,48,49,50,53,64,78] for reviews). We examine the interaction of DNA binding proteins with a specific enhancer element in the prodynorphin promoter and the ability of second messenger systems to activate transcription via this enhancer element. The element has sequence homology with the consensus AP-1 element (12-O-tetradecanoyl phorbol-13-acetate (TPA) responsive element or TRE) which binds members of the Fos/Jun families of transcription factors[1-3,7,14,22,56,65,66,68,83] and the cAMP responsive element (CRE).[9,24,25,50,61,80] The dynorphin enhancer is located at -1545 base pairs (bp) upstream from the transcription start site and has the same 9 base sequence

(CTGCGTCAG) as the cAMP-responsive element or enhancer located at -92 in the proenkephalin promoter called the ENKCRE-2 element[15,16](see upper part of Figure 3 for diagram). We will mainly consider the heptamer core TGCGTCA sequence and refer to the element based on its location, as the -1545 enhancer, site or element.

Two sets of experimental data, both focused on the -1545 enhancer, will be discussed in the present paper. The first set of experiments examines the binding of proteins extracted from isolated brain cell nuclei to the -1545 site and uses the electrophoretic method of gel mobility shift analysis. The second set of experiments examines the ability of this DNA element to function as an enhancer and its sensitivity to stimulation by second messenger systems and uses the method of transient transfection with various promoter/reporter constructs. Because the -1545 sequence is also present in the promoter region of the enkephalin promoter, as noted above, and the tachykinin and c-fos promoters, our results may be applicable to these genes as well. However, it must be kept in mind that the enhancer elements in these genes have additional enhancers immediately adjacent to the target element which may modify the response of the target element.[10,15,16,36,69,70,76] Such a situation has not been fully explored for the sequences adjacent to the -1545 site.

MATERIALS AND METHODS

Gel mobility shift assay: These methods are presented in detail in ref. 34. Nuclei were isolated by a method adapted from Tata.[74] Briefly, rat brains were homogenized in 6 X wt to vol of ice cold 0.32 M sucrose, 3 mM $MgCl_2$, 1 mM Hepes, pH 6.8 (SMH buffer), the homogenate was filtered through mesh and spun at 2,500 x g for 20 min in a swinging bucket rotor at 4°C. The pellet was resuspended in 2.1 M sucrose, 1 mM $MgCl_2$, 1 mM Hepes pH 6.8, using the same volume as originally used for the first homogenization, mixed well and spun at 48,000 X g for 1.5 hr at 4°C. This pellet was recovered in SMH by brief centrifugation at 2,500 X g and homogenized in 420 mM NaCl, 20% glycerol, 0.2 mM EDTA, 0.25 mM dithiothreitol, 0.5 mM phenylmethylsulfonylfluoride, 1.5 mM $MgCl_2$ and 20 mM Hepes, pH 7.5 (C buffer (adapted from 17). The homogenate was cleared by centrifugation at 48,000

X g for 1 hr. The protein content of the supernatant was measured by the dye binding assay of Bradford[8] with the reagent supplied by BioRad and various concentrations of the supernatant were used in the gel shift assay.

The brain nuclear extract, at various protein concentrations, was added in a volume of 1 µl of 1 x C buffer, followed by 1 µl of 2.5 µg/µl poly(dl-dC) (sodium salt, Midland Certified Reagent Co) in H_2O. If indicated, the next addition was 1 µl of antibody solution in phosphate buffered saline or cold oligonucleotide in 50 mM NaCl, followed by 1µl of concentrated buffer (200 mM HEPES, pH 7.9, 20% glycerol, 2 mM EDTA, 5 mM phenylmethylsulphonylfluoride, 50 mM dithiothreitol, and 0.5% Tween 20), then 0.2 ng of labeled probe (20-50,000 cpm) in 1 µl of TE (10 mM Tris, 1 mM EDTA, pH 7.4) buffer and 5 ml of dye solution (0.05% xylene cyanol, 0.05% bromophenol blue and 30% glycerol). The final volume of the reaction was 10 µl. Reactions were incubated at room temperature for 20 min, and terminated by loading the entire sample on the gel while applying 100 V; further electrophoresis was at 160 V in a BRL V16 apparatus. Four percent polyacrylamide gels, (29:1 acrylamide monomer:bisacrylamide) were cast with a backing of gelbond (FMC Corp). Six percent gels (39:1) were purchased from Novex. In all cases, gel and running buffer were 0.5 x Tris-borate-EDTA pH 8.3 (1x TBE = 89 mM Tris, 89 mM boric acid, 2 mM EDTA). Upon completion of electrophoresis, the gel was removed, dried in a vacuum oven for ~2 hrs if run with gel bond, or onto paper in a gel dryer and autoradiograms obtained. Exposures were between 2 and 16 hours at -70ºC with intensifying screens.

Oligonucleotides and anti-Fos antibody: Preparation and properties of the anti-Fos antiserum have been described.[35,64] In brief, it is an antigen-affinity purified rabbit polyclonal anti-peptide antiserum directed against a Fos sequence, KVEQLSPEEEEKRRIRRERNKMAAA, that is conserved among the members of the Fos family including Fos-related antigen 1 (Fra 1),[14] Fra 2,[44] and Fos B.[83] Oligonucleotides were synthesised on an Applied Biosystems DNA synthesizer and purified by electrophoresis through 20% polyacrylamide, 8 M urea gels. The major band from each synthesis was located by UV shadowing and cut out. DNA was eluted at 50ºC overnight in TE buffer, lyophilised and urea removed by repeated washing (5X) with 100% ethanol. Oligonucleotides were annealed in 50 mM NaCl starting at 70ºC followed by slow cooling to room temperature.

The sequences of the double stranded probes used in this study are listed in Table I. There are two oligonucleotides used for the transient transfection experiments each containing 41 bp surrounding the -1545 site, one wild type and one mutated. Three shorter probes were used in the gel shift experiments: the dynorphin -1545 site and two probes containing the AP-1 consensus sequence (TGAGTCA), from the gibbon ape leukemia virus enhancer (GALV)[64] and SP-AP-1, from the pro-tachykinin promoter.[10] Most experiments were performed with probes that were 5' end-labeled with T4 polynucleotide kinase and [gamma-32P]ATP. In order to check whether gel shifts might be due to the presence of kinase-labeled single stranded material, gel shift assays were also performed for each probe labeled by filling in the recessed 3' end with the appropriate [alpha-32P]dNTPs and Klenow fragment.[35]

A) -1545 DYNORPHIN AP-1/CRE OLIGONUCLEOTIDES USED IN TRANSIENT TRANSFECTION:

Wild type:

HindIII   Pstl

AGCT   GTGCCAAGTGTGGCTGCTGCGTCAGAGCATGACTTCATCAC   CTGCA

A   CACGGTTCACACCGACGACGCAGTCTCGTACTGAAGTAGTG   G

Mutant:

HindIII   Pstl

AGCT   GTGCCAAGTGTGGCTGCCTCGTCAGAGCATGACTTCATCAC   CTGCA

A   CACGGTTCACACCGACGGAGCAGTCTCGTACTGAAGTAGTG   G

B) OLIGONUCLEOTIDES USED IN GEL SHIFT:

-1545:   TGTGGCTGCTGCGTCAGAGCATG

                        CCGACGACGCAGTCTCGTAC

GALV: CGAGAAATAGATGAGTCACAG

                 TCTTTATCTACTCAGTGTCGC

SP-AP-1   TTTCCGAAGCATGAGTCACTTCGCTCAG

                 GGCTTCGTACTCAGTGAAGCGAGTC

TABLE I. The oligonucleotides for the transient transfection were flanked by HindIII and Pstl linkers for subcloning into the DMP/pCAT BASIC vector (45). The oligonucleotides used for gel shift generally were labeled at the 5' ends with T4 polynucleotide kinase. However, all had at least one recessed 3' end for labeling with deoxynucleotide triphosphates and Klenow fragment of DNA polymerase. This allowed us to eliminate the possibility that gel shifts might be due to single stranded oligonucleotides (35). The 7 bases in the AP-1/CRE -1545 element and the AP-1 consensus oligonucleotides are underlined; the mutation is in bold.

Transient transfection assay: The methods are presented in detail in (45). The double stranded 41 bp oligonucleotide, (Table I) was sub-cloned into the pCAT basic plasmid (Promega) which had previously been engineered to contain the dynorphin minimal promoter (DMP) consisting of bases -135 to +65 which includes the TATA box.[18] A similar construct containing a 2 bp mutation in the -1545 heptamer element was made for comparison (Table I). After transformation of HB101 cells and subsequent amplification, recombinant plasmids were isolated and the presence of the oligonucleotide was confirmed by restriction digestion and DNA sequencing. Undifferentiated rat PC12 cells were grown in Dulbecco's modified Eagle's medium supplemented with 7.5% fetal bovine serum and 7.5% horse serum. Cells were plated at approximately 2 X 106 cells per 60 mm petri dish. After 16 to 20 hrs of incubation, media was removed and 8 µg of test plasmid, 0.5 µg of a luciferase expressing plasmid (to control for transfection efficiency), and 20 µl of lipofectin (Gibco/BRL) were added in 3 ml of Opti-MEM (Gibco/BRL). Following 6 hours of incubation at 37°C the serum free Opti-MEM medium was replaced with normal growth media. After 40 hrs the cells were washed, incubated for 5 min in TEN bufffer (40 mM Tris HCl, pH 7.4, 1 mM EDTA, 150 mM NaCl) and harvested. Following three freeze-thaw cycles, the cells were centrifuged at 18,000 x g and the supernatant assayed for CAT and luciferase enzyme activity. Cell extract, n-butyryl coenzyme A and 14C-chloramphenicol (50 mCi/mmol) were incubated for 2 hrs at 37°C. The butyrylated 14C-chloramphenicol products partition into xylene, and following extraction, the xylene phase was counted in a liquid scintillation counter. Cell extract (10 µl out of 50 µl) was added to 350 µl of luciferase buffer (25 mM glycylglycine, 25 mM $MgSO_4$, 2 mM ATP and 10 % glycerol). Using an automated luminometer (Analytical Luminescence Laboratory), luciferin substrate was added and light emission measured. Second messenger pathways were stimulated at 48 hrs after transfection. Media was replaced with fresh media containing either 20 µM forskolin or 200 nM TPA and incubated for an additional 6 hrs at which time cells were harvested and analyzed as described. The ratio of n-butryrylated 14C-chloramphenicol product to luciferase activity was determined for each sample and the average of triplicate samples determined. Experiments were repeated at least 3 times. A representative experiment is shown; data represent the mean ± standard error of the mean.

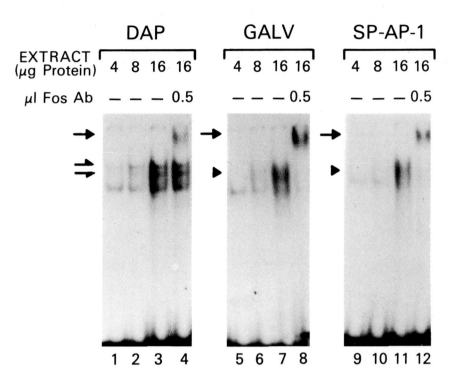

Figure 1. Protein DNA complex formation at the DAP site compared to the AP-1 consensus. The DAP element forms two complexes using nuclear extract from rat brain and analysis on a 6% non-denaturing polyacrylamide gel. The two AP-1 consensus containing elements, one from the gibbon ape leukemia virus enhancer (GALV), the other from the promoter of the tachykinin gene (SP-AP-1), formed one basal complex. The anti-*c-Fos* antiserum was directed against a peptide corresponding to a highly conserved region in the Fos protein families. Addition of *c-Fos* antiserum caused a complete super-shift (single arrow) of the basal AP-1 complex forming with the GALV and SP-AP-1 consensus sequences (arrowhead) but only a partial shift of the basal complexes forming with the DAP element (double arrows). The amount of the two complexes that remain in the basal shift is relatively unmodified by addition of the antibody suggesting that they do not contain Fos-immunoreactive proteins (figure adapted from 35).

RESULTS

The synthetic double stranded oligonucleotide centered on the -1545 site formed a protein-DNA complex when incubated with rat brain nuclear extract. Depending on the gel percentage, the basal gel shift was observed as two bands (with a 6% gel, Figure 1) or as one wide band (with a 4% gel, Figure 2). Binding of

Dynorphin AP-1-like

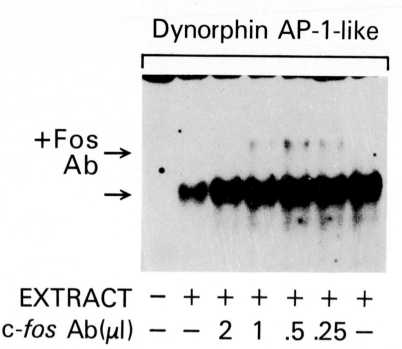

+Fos Ab →

→

EXTRACT − + + + + +

c-*fos* Ab(μl) − − 2 1 .5 .25 −

Figure 2. Titration of the super-shift. The Fos-immunoreactive complex seen by the supershift is highly dependent upon the amount of antiserum. The maximum amount of supershifted material is seen in with 0.5 μl of antiserum. At 1 and 2 μl of antiserum the complex is progressively disrupted suggesting that these concentrations of serum sequester Fos-immunoreactive proteins, making them unavailable for complex formation. The non-Fos nature of the basal complex is emphasized under these conditions since no apparent disruption of the basal gel shift occurs at the high Fos antibody concentrations.

the *c-Fos* antibodies to the -1545 element-protein complex caused a small amount of the specific gel shift band to become larger in molecular weight and migrate more slowly, yielding a "supershifted" band. However, the majority of the basal gel shift bands that formed with the -1545 site were resistant to being supershifted. We infer that the resistant portion of the gel shift does not contain Fos-immunoreactive proteins but rather some other set of proteins. In contrast, when AP-1 consensus-containing oligonucleotides were used as probes, the entire basal gel shift band was supershifted by the Fos antibody. These data indicate that essentially all of the protein/DNA complex(s) forming with AP-1 consensus probes contained Fos-immunoreactive proteins. Previous studies have shown that these complexes are specifically competed by excess unlabeled oligonucleotide corresponding to the probe, but not by an oligonucleotide of unrelated sequence.[35] The experiment also addresses an additional point regarding the influence of the sequences flanking the AP-1 consensus. The flanking sequences are different for both the GALV and SP-AP-1 oligonucleotides (see Table I) yet each displays a complete supershift. This result indicates that specificity resides in the AP-1 consensus and that the flanking bases have a minimal influence on composition of the protein complex.

The complexes forming with the -1545 site differed from an AP-1 consensus element in another, related characteristic: they were resistant to being disrupted by the *c-Fos* antibody. At the same time, the Fos-containing complex in the super-shifted band is susceptible to disruption. This is clearly demonstrated in Figure 2 where ascending concentrations of *c-Fos* antibody were added to the gel shift assay. The basal shift is not responsive at any concentration of antibody. For the super-shifted material, the concentration-response relationship is biphasic. Low amounts of antibody produce a partial super-shift. At higher concentrations of Fos antibody the supershifted band begins to become less intense and, upon addition of 2 µl antibody, disappears. In contrast, the basal shift is resistant to disruption and remains intact. This emphasizes the distinctiveness of the proteins in the basal complex from the super-shifted complex.[35]

Transient transfection studies show that the -1545 element supports constitutive and induced transcription in the rat PC12 pheochromocytoma cell line. We focused directly on the -1545 region of the dynorphin promoter by synthesizing a short oligonucleotide centered on the heptamer TGCGTCA sequence. The oligonucleotide was cloned 5' to a rat dynorphin minimal promoter (DMP) which had been previously ligated to the coding sequence of the chloramphenicol acetyl transferase (CAT) reporter gene. Measurement of CAT activity yields an indirect measure of the strength of the promoter: the greater the transcription rate of the gene, the more mRNA available for translation to CAT protein and the greater the enzyme activity in a cell extract. We also synthesized a similar oligonucleotide but with a 2 bp mutation in the -1545 element. The wild type -1545 element displayed constitutive activity that was greater in comparison to either the DMP alone or to the mutated -1545 oligonucleotide construct. Stimulation of second messenger systems highlighted the enhancer activity of the -1545 site.[45] Transcription driven by the wild type -1545 element was greatly augmented by treatment of the cells with forskolin which caused more than a 150-fold stimulation in some experiments. A typical experiment is shown in Figure 3 in which the effect of forskolin is compared to phorbol ester. Forskolin provided the most effective stimulation. We observed a 31-fold increase in CAT activity with the wild type -1545 oligonucleotide-containing construct in comparison to the dynorphin minimal promoter following 6 hrs of forskolin treatment. Phorbol ester was much less effective; activity did not exceed that obtained in the presence of vehicle alone. At best, with phorbol ester CAT activity increases approximately 2-fold if the wild type construct is compared to the dynorphin minimal promoter.

The -1545 oligonucleotide containing the 2 bp mutation was nearly incapable of supporting forskolin-induced transcription. The mutant displayed only 7.4% of the activity of the intact -1545 element following forskolin treatment. The same situation was obtained for constitutive activity: the mutant yielded approximately 32% of the activity seen with the wild type -1545 element. These data demonstrate that the effects of the mutation are accentuated under conditions of stimulation.

DISCUSSION

The in vitro binding and transient expression data provide several new insights into the possible molecular mechanisms governing dynorphin gene induction in vivo. In addition, new insights into pain processes may be obtained since the dynorphin-synthesizing neurons are within the pain-processing spinal laminae and receive direct nociceptive primary afferent input. Two main points are addressed by our experiments: (1) the connection between induction of immediate early genes and induction of dynorphin gene expression and (2) the potential second messenger signal transduction mechanisms that activate dynorphin gene expression. Both observations relate to transmission between nociceptive primary afferents and second order spinal cord neurons expressing the dynorphin gene. Regarding the first point, dynorphin mRNA has been co-localized in neurons that show an increase in Fos-immunoreactive proteins in their nuclei,[60] moreover, several other families of transcription factors are also found in the same spinal laminae.[26,78] Thus, dynorphin gene expression is likely to be co-localized with several sets of known cIEG transcription factors and we have examined the binding of some of these factors to

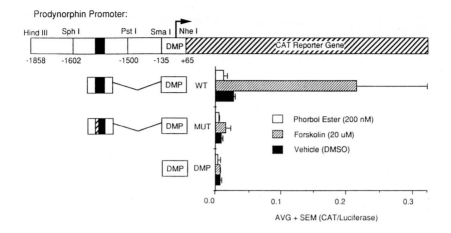

Figure 3. Transient transfection analysis of the -1545 enhancer. At the top is a diagram of the entire 1852 bp of promoter sequence fused to the chloramphenicol acetyltransferase reporter gene. The dynorphin minimal promoter is abbreviated DMP and the rightward directed arrow designates the transcription start site.. The DMP spans the start site and contains 65 bp of downstream exon I sequence and 135 bp of promoter sequence that includes the TATA box. The -1545 site is indicated by the black box. A synthetic 41 bp oligonucleotide centered on this site (wild type, WT) was ligated to the DMP as was a similar oligonucleotide containing a 2 bp mutation (MUT) in the -1545 element. These construct are compared to a construct driven by only the DMP. All transfections were preformed in undifferentiated rat PC12 cells. Note the marked (32-fold) stimulation produced by forskolin treatment of cells transfected with the intact -1545 element in comparison to cells transfected with the DMP alone. Mutation of the -1545 element nearly abolished forskolin-inducibility. The presence of the -1545 element also conferred a greater degree of constitutive expression in comparison to the DMP and the mutant. Relative to forskolin, all constructs were un-responsive to stimulation with phorbol ester (figure adapted from 45).

potential recognition sequences in the dynorphin promoter. Regarding the second point, because the spinal cord dynorphin neurons receive direct contacts from primary afferent terminals, it is tempting to hypothesize that the increases in expression of the dynorphin gene and cellular immediate early genes are triggered by transmitters or neuropeptides released from primary afferents. The transient transfection data functionally categorize the -1545 site as a cAMP responsive enhancer.[45] Interpreting this in regard to pain, it suggests that one of the primary afferent transmitters or neuropeptides activates a receptor coupled to adenylate cyclase in second order neurons.[55] We speculate that a series of acute and long-term modifications in second order pain processing neurons is set in motion and maintained by cAMP-dependent processes.

The linkage between regulation of genes such as dynorphin, the cIEGs and the gel shift and transient transfection data must be considered in the context of receptor-coupled second messenger systems and transcriptional regulation. The present transcription-derived data suggest that some degree of "cross-talk" between the Fos/Jun families and the cAMP response element binding protein/activating transcription factor (CREB/ATF) families of DNA-binding proteins occurs during regulation of the dynorphin promoter.[9,24,48] The two families had been thought to be discretely stimulated by the phosphatidylinositol/diacylglycerol (PI) second messenger system for Fos/Jun[2,22,65] and the cAMP second messenger pathway for CREB/ATF proteins.[25,50,80] However, binding studies with in vitro transcribed and translated proteins suggests that there is considerable cross-family heterodimerization between the Jun proteins and the CREB/ATF proteins.[24,40] Furthermore, transmembrane ion flux, particularly calcium, can stimulate cIEG expression[51,52,71,73] and the fact that c-fos gene expression can be stimulated by cAMP[4,69-71] further complicates the ability to define relevant molecular mechanisms. This situation, and multiple receptor-effector couplings,[55] tend to compromise hypotheses that segregate each family of transcriptional proteins to the control of a single precise DNA sequence.

The PI and cAMP systems are two of the best defined pathways for coupling extracellular stimuli to gene transcription, although others exist that are less extensively delineated such as the protein tyrosine kinases.[5,75] The PI pathway couples signal transduction to transcriptional activation starting with receptors linked to phospholipase C. This enzyme catalyzes the cleavage of phosphatidyl inositol in the plasma membrane to release inositol trisphosphate and diacylglycerol (DAG) (for review see 5). The latter compound activates protein kinase C (PKC) and thereby stimulates PKC-dependent phosphorylation processes. The PKC pathway typically is stimulated by treating cells with phorbol ester (e.g. TPA) which mimics the effects of diacylglycerol. An enhancer element, called a TRE for TPA-responsive element was identified that conferred sensitivity to TPA in transient transfection assays with promoter-reporter constructs.[2,7,22,65] Subsequently, Fos and Jun proteins were shown to be the nuclear protein factors responsible for activation of transcription of target genes via TRE sequences.[1,3,66,68] The palindromic DNA sequence, TGAGTCA, is also known as the AP-1 enhancer element and AP-1 complex formation refers to the protein complex that binds to the TRE or AP-1 DNA element. The complex usually is composed of a heterodimer of Fos and Jun proteins, although members of the Jun family can form homodimers at this site[1,56,68] and Fos can heterodimerize with other proteins.[6,62] Fos was implicated in the control of dynorphin gene expression mainly on circumstantial time course[20] and immunocytochemical evidence such as the co-localization of dynorphin mRNA and Fos proteins in the same cells.[60] The next logical step was to directly examine the dynorphin promoter for Fos binding sites (i.e. a TRE or AP-1 element). In the rat dynorphin promoter, no AP-1 consensus (i.e. exact match to the TGAGTCA sequence) was found in approximately 2,000 bases of 5' flanking sequence. However, many potential sequences that contained base deletions, insertions or substitutions were identified and several have been evaluated.[35,57] The most robust in our hands, in all tests, was the far upstream -1545 element.

The present binding studies show that this sequence is a recognition site for multiple protein complexes, some of which are definitely Fos-containing protein complexes (i.e. those in the supershifted band) and some which are definitely non-Fos-containing. We are fairly confident the lower band does not contain Fos proteins based on the broad specificity of the anti-Fos antibody. The Fos antiserum was raised against the basic DNA binding portion of the *c-Fos* protein which is highly conserved between *c-Fos*, Fos B, Fra 1 and Fra 2. Previous western blot studies of dorsal spinal cord nuclear extracts showed that 4 distinct proteins, ranging from 38 to 55 kDa, are induced in dorsal cord nuclear extracts during peripheral inflammation.[35,73] Immunocytochemical studies have shown that, in addition to *c-Fos*, dorsal spinal cord also stains for Fos B (26). Thus, because of the conserved nature of the epitope, any or all of the proteins seen in the western blot may be present in the Fos-immunoreactive portion of the gel shift. We know from previous studies using spinal nuclear extracts from animals with peripheral inflammation that, with a radiolabeled AP-1 consensus, all of the complex formed is supershifted by the Fos antibody. Thus, the portion of the -1545 complex that is not supershifted and not disrupted by excess antibody probably does not contain Fos-immunoreactive proteins. The composition of the non-Fos-containing portion of the basal gel shift is open to speculation. Binding studies have shown the -1545 core sequence (as represented in the ENKCRE-2 site) will form complexes with Jun/Jun homodimers and heterodimers of Jun/Creb or Jun/ATF 2 or ATF 2/CELF (a basic leucine zipper protein).[24,36,40,68,72] In spinal cord during peripheral inflammation, we have observed that the amount of the non-Fos-containing complex is elevated in nuclear extracts.[35] Competition studies show that the non-Fos-containing complex has a higher affinity for the -1545 element than the Fos-containing portion since the AP-1 consensus does not effectively compete for binding.[35] Thus, the non-Fos complex may be a major determinant of transcriptional activity at the -1545 element. Nevertheless, we know that high levels of Fos-immunoreactive proteins exist for days in these neurons and that Fos/Jun transient co-transfection increases transcription using the -1545 site or the ENKCRE-2 element as an enhancer.[45,72] These data suggest that the presence of Fos-immunoreactive protein also contribute to positive transcriptional activation of the -1545 element and that elevated Fos levels may signify a heightened state of transcription for the dynorphin gene. However, the latter conclusion must be viewed with caution since the positive transcriptional activity of Fos may be a function of the Jun protein with which it heterodimerizes. In some cases inhibition, rather than stimulation, of transcription has been observed as is discussed further on in ref. 40.

We have less direct protein-DNA binding data to support the role of CREB/ATF proteins in activation of the dynorphin gene expression. However, involvement of CREB is suggested by the transient transfection data and binding studies from the enkephalin gene.[15,16,29,45,72] Activation of the cAMP system has been shown to stimulate the expression of genes that contain a CRE, the prototypic gene being somatostatin which contains a CRE element at -41 in its promoter.[50] The sequence of the CRE consensus is TGACGTCA which is a perfect inverted repeat and is similar to both the AP-1 and -1545 elements. This sequence bound a 43 kDa protein (CREB) which was the first member of a larger family of CRE binding proteins identified and later found to be homologous to the ATF family of proteins (reviewed in 9). Like Fos, CREB is a phosphoprotein which is activated by phosphorylation at serine residue 133.[80] Unlike Fos, which requires transcription and translation into protein and translocation into the nucleus before it can affect gene expression, CREB is usually found to pre-exist in the cell. Thus, a transmitter whose receptor is linked to adenylate cyclase can activate CREB via phosphorylation by protein kinase A (PKA). Our transient transfection data suggest this pathway provides the most effective stimulus for dynorphin gene transcription. Indeed, the strongest case for the involvement of cAMP-dependent processes in dynorphin gene regulation comes from the transient transfection data. A direct comparison of supramaximal concentrations of phorbol ester (stimulation of the PI system) versus forskolin (stimulation of the cAMP system) shows that forskolin produced approximately 16-fold greater induction than the phorbol ester. This was also seen in HeLa cells (data not shown). The effect of forskolin was attributable to the -1545 region based on the lack of efficacy of the mutant -1545 clone to support forskolin induction. The efficacy of the cAMP system in stimulating dynorphin transcription is not limited to the PC12 cells but also occurs in primary zona glomerulosa cells upon stimulation with FSH or co-transfection with a PKA expression vector.[29,38,39] There may be additional sites on the dynorphin promoter that also possess enhancer activity.[18] However, we have examined nearly 2,000 bp of upstream sequence with various promoter-reporter constructs and transient transfection assays and the most robust constitutive activity is obtained with the clones that contain the -1545 element and only the -1545-containing clones display stimulation with forskolin. By comparison, the rest of the promoter is fairly inactive when tested in PC12 or Hela cells, including the region surrounding the non-canonical AP-1 site located at -249.[57]

It must be recognized that the results of the transient transfection assay are determined both by the promoter-reporter constructs as well as by the cells within which the constructs are evaluated. We used PC12 cells in the present experiments which clearly have their own peculiarities and are clearly not the same cells as those in the dorsal horn that express dynorphin. The PC12 cells probably do not have the same complement of transcription factors and receptors as the dorsal horn neurons. However, at least one report has suggested that PC12 cells can express dynorphin especially following treatment with NGF.[43] Also, in vivo, adrenal medullary cells express enkephalin, although the degree is highly species dependent.[81] Expression from the enkephalin promoter is enhanced through the tandem ENKCRE-1 and 2 elements, the ENKCRE-2 element has the identical sequence as the -1545 element. Thus, while these cells may not provide a totally accurate picture of in vivo regulation, they do have characteristics appropriate for opioid gene expression. Furthermore, the results are not unique to PC12 cells, since we have obtained identical results in HeLa cells[35,45] and others have demonstrated a cAMP-responsive transcription mediated by this region of the dynorphin promoter in primary ovarian granulosa cells.[38,39] These cells express dynorphin during the follicular phase of the estrus cycle. Co-transfection of granulosa cells with a 100 bp SphI-PstI fragment of the promoter, which contains the -1545 element, and an expression vector coding for the C-alpha catalytic subunit of adenylate cyclase shows a marked enhancement of expression (i.e. in the presence of excess cAMP). Thus, the cAMP dependency of enhancement is exhibited in several cell lines and primary cells. The present data, in combination with previous observations made with larger pieces of the promoter, pinpoint the -1545 sequence as a critical element mediating cAMP activation of the dynorphin promoter. By extrapolation from the PC12 cells to the spinal cord, we suggest that the cAMP pathway is activated by nociceptive afferents in vivo and stimulates dynorphin gene transcription. Furthermore, these data suggest an important role for cAMP-dependent phosphorylation of other proteins (e.g. ion channels) in relationship to spinal cord nociceptive processes.

The preceding discussion suggests that a complex regulatory apparatus involving Fos, Jun and CREB proteins is engaged during dynorphin gene up-regulation in spinal cord. Recombinantly expressed tachykinin receptor has been shown to couple to both phospholipase C and adenylate cyclase[55] Thus, in the dorsal horn it is possible that both the PI and cAMP second messenger pathways are activated simultaneously. One might therefore expect a concurrent activation of both Fos and CREB. In addition, CREB can bind to a CRE in the *c-fos* promoter which provides a direct link between cAMP activation and increased expression of the *c-fos* gene.[71] It is likely that some of these complex interactions reflect, at a molecular level, the evolving nature of the peripheral inflammation. As the peripheral inflammation persists and increases in severity, the concentration of factors and their phosphorylation state increases; also the variety of different factors or family members may increase.[26,73] There is a delay of several hours before clearly detectable increases in prodynorphin mRNA levels occur. During this period the spinal cord second order neurons integrate the afferent nociceptive stimulus. If the degree and duration of afferent input is sufficient, then the proper combination of nuclear transcription factors is achieved and a sustained increase in dynorphin gene transcription ensues. The exact details of this scenario still need to be delineated.

None of the above experiments address the role of prodynorphinderived peptides in spinal nociceptive processing. However, the recent molecular cloning of the kappa receptor (the receptor with which the larger dynorphin peptides preferentially interact) demonstrated that the kappa receptor, like the mu receptor, is negatively coupled to adenylate cyclase.[82]) This provides an interesting counterpoint to our suggestion of an important role for cAMP stimulation in transmitting nociceptive information. The dynorphin increase is parallels the time course of the inflammatory period.[32,33] It is quite possible that the increase in dynorphin gene expression and peptide content represents a sustained antinociceptive[27] response at the level of the dorsal horn. This hypothesis suggests that long-term activation of adenylate cyclase by nociceptive afferents during inflammation or injury is counteracted by activation of the dynorphin system. Inhibition of adenylate cyclase by dynorphin may modulate hyperexcitability in the system yet not produce complete analgesia of the inflamed or injured area. Electrophysiological experiments have indicated that dynorphin, or peptide fragments of dynorphin A 1-17, can produce excitation of spinal cord and hippocampal neurons.[11] Recent whole cell patch clamp studies of guinea pig hippocampal neurons indicate that low concentrations of dynorphin A-1-17 can increase N-methyl-D-aspartate (NMDA) mediated synaptic currents while higher concentrations inhibit the NMDA currents.[12] The dynorphin-induced increase in NMDA current was not reversed by naloxone suggesting it was a direct peptide effect on the NMDA receptor. The inhibitory effect was reversed by naloxone suggesting that it was mediated by opioid receptors.[12] Potential mechanisms appear to exist for dynorphin to both enhance and inhibit neuronal excitability.

In summary, the robustness of transcription enhancement by the -1545 site via cAMP in the PC12 cells suggests that the dynorphin gene may be regulated in vivo in the spinal cord via the same mechanism. Since primary afferent terminals make direct contact with dynorphin-synthesizing dorsal horn neurons it is tempting to hypothesize that a transmitter or neuropeptide in the primary afferents is linked to activation of adenylate cyclase. Recent data suggest that the tachykinins can fulfil this role.[55] Available evidence suggests that both the Fos/Jun and Creb/ATf families activate transcription from the -1545 site and we suggest that dynorphin gene expression is enhanced by both families of proteins in vivo. This may occur in a temporally distinct sequential fashion to avoid competition at the site or in some synergistic fashion if both occur together. Thus, multiple families of transcription factors may orchestrate the alterations in gene expression in the dorsal horn in response to a chronic pain input and the dynorphin gene is one upon which the cIEGs may act.

REFERENCES

1. ABATE, C., LUK, D., GAGNE, E., ROEDER R.G. AND CURRAN, T. (1990) Fos and jun cooperate in transcriptional regulation via heterologous activation domains. *Mol. Cell. Biol.* **10**, 5532-5535.
2. ANGEL, P., IMAGAWA, M., CHIU, R., STEIN, B., IMBRA, R.J., RAHMSDORF, H.J., JONAT C., HERRLICH, P. AND KARIN, M. (1987) Phorbol ester-inducible genes contain a common cis element recognized by a TPA-modulated trans-acting factor. *Cell* **49**, 729-739.
3. ANGEL, P., ALLEGRETTI, E.A., OKINO, S.T., HATTORI, K., BOYLE, W.J., HUNTER, T. AND KARIN M. (1988) Oncogene jun encodes a sequence specific trans-activator similar to AP-1. *Nature* **332**, 166-171.
4. BADING, H. AND GREENBERG, M.E. (1991) Stimulation of protein tyrosine phosphorylation by NMDA receptor activation. *Science* **253**, 912-914.
5. BERRIDGE, M.J. (1993) Inositol trisphosphate and calcium signalling. *Nature* **361**, 315-325.
6. BLANAR, M.A. AND RUTTER, W.J. (1992) Interaction cloning: identification of a helix-loop-helix zipper protein that interacts with *c-fos*. *Science* **256**, 1014-1018.
7. BOHMANN, D., BOS, T.J., ADMON, A., NISHIMURA, T., VOGT, P.K. AND TJIAN, R. (1987) Human proto-oncogene c-jun encodes a DNA binding protein with structural and functional properties of transcription factor AP-1. *Science* **238**, 1386-1392.
8. BRADFORD, M.M. (1976) A rapid and sensitive method for the quantitation of microgram quantities of protein utilizing the principle of protein-dye binding. *Anal. Biochem.* **72**, 248-254.
9. BRINDLE, P.K. AND MONTMINY, M.R. (1992) The CREB family of transcription activators. *Curr. Opinion Genet. Dev.* **2**, 199-204.
10. CARTER, M.S. AND KRAUSE, J.E. (1990) Structure, expression, and some regulatory mechanisms of the rat preprotachykinin gene encoding substance P, neurokinin A, neuropeptide K, and neuropeptide Y. *J. Neurosci.* **10**, 2203-2214.
11. CAUDLE, R.M. AND ISAAC, L. (1988) Influence of dynorphin (1-13) on spinal reflexes in the rat. *J. Pharmacol. Exp. Ther.* **246**, 508-513.
12. CAUDLE, R.M., CHAVKIN, C. AND DUBNER R. Kappa2 opioid receptors inhibit NMDA receptor-mediated synaptic currents in guinea pig CA3

pyramidal cells. (Submitted).

13. CIVELLI, O., DOUGLASS, J., GOLDSTEIN, A. AND HERBERT, E. (1985) Sequence and expression of the rat prodynorphin gene. *Proc. Natl. Acad. Sci. U.S.A.* **82**, 4291-4295.

14. COHEN, D. AND CURRAN, T. (1988) fra-1: a serum inducible, cellular immediate-early gene that encodes a fos-related antigen. *Mol. Cell. Biol.* **8**, 2063-2069.

15. COMB, M., BIRNBERG, N.C., SEASHOLTZ, A., HERBERT, E. AND GOODMAN, H.M. (1986) A cyclic AMP- and phorbol ester-inducible DNA element. *Nature* **323**, 353-356.

16. COMB, M., MERMOD, N., HYMAN S.E., PEARLBERG, J., ROSS, M.E. AND GOODMAN, H.M. (1988) Proteins bound at adjacent DNA elements act synergistically to regulate human proenkephalin cAMP inducible transcription. *EMBO J.* **7**, 3793-3805.

17. DIGNAM, J.D., LEBOVITZ, R.M. AND ROEDER, R.G. (1983) Accurate transcription initiation by RNA polymerase II in a soluble extract from isolated mammalian nuclei. *Nucleic Acids Res.* **11**, 1475-1489.

18. DOUGLASS J., MCMURRAY, C.T., GARRETT J.E., ADELMAN, J.P. AND CALAVETTA L. (1989) Characterization of the rat prodynorphin gene. *Mol. Endocrinol.* **13**, 2070-2078.

19. DRAISCI, G., KAJANDER, K.C., DUBNER, R., BENNETT, G.J. AND IADAROLA, M.J. (1991) Up-regulation of opioid gene expression in spinal cord evoked by experimental nerve injuries and inflammation. *Brain Res.* **560**, 186-192.

20. DRAISCI, G. AND IADAROLA, M.J. (1989) Temporal analysis of increases in *c-fos*, preprodynorphin and preproenkephalin mRNAs in rat spinal cord. *Molec. Brain Res.* **6**, 31-37.

21. DRAISCI, G. AND IADAROLA M.J. Evaluation of tachykinin, CGRP and cholecystokinin peptide and mRNA levels in dorsal root ganglion and spinal cord during peripheral inflammation. (Submitted).

22. FRANZA B.R. JR., RAUSCHER, F.J. III, JOSEPHS, S.F. AND CURRAN, T. (1988) The fos complex and fos-related antigens recognize sequence elements that contain AP-1 binding sites. *Science* **239**, 1150-1153.

23. GOLDSTEIN, A., FISHLI, W., LOWNEY, L.I., HUNKAPILLAR, M. AND HOOD, L.E. (1981) Porcine pituitary dynorphin: complete amino acid sequence of the biologically active heptadecapeptide. *Proc. Natl. Acad. Sci., U.S.A.* **78**, 7219-7223.

24. HAI, T. AND CURRAN, T. (1991) Cross-family dimerization of transcription factors fos/jun and ATF/CREB alters DNA binding specificity. *Proc. Natl. Acad. Sci. U.S.A.* **88**, 3720-3724.

25. HAI, T., LIU, F., COUKOS, W.J. AND GREEN, M.R. (1989) Transcription factor ATF cDNA clones: an extensive family of leucine zipper proteins able to selectively form DNA-binding heterodimers. *Genes Dev.* **3**, 2083-2090.

26. HERDEGEN, T., KOVARY, K., LEAH, J. AND BRAVO, R. (1991) Specific temporal and spatial distribution of JUN, FOS and KROX-24 proteins in

spinal neurons following noxious transsynaptic stimulation. *J. Comp. Neurol.* **313**, 178-191.

27. HERMAN, B.H. AND GOLDSTEIN, A. (1985) Antinociception and paralysis induced by intrathecal dynorphin A. *J. Pharmacol. Exp. Ther.* **232**, 27-32.

28. HOLLT, V., HAARMANN, I., MILLAN, M.J. AND HERZ, A. (1987) Prodynorphin gene expression is enhanced in the spinal cord of chronic arthritic rats. *Neurosci. Letts.* **73**, 90-94.

29. HUGGENVIK, J.I., COLLARD M.W., STOFKO, R.E., SEASHOLTZ, A.F. AND UHLER, M.D. (1991) Regulation of the human enkephalin promoter by two isoforms of the catalytic subunit of cyclic adenosine 3',5'-monophosphate-dependent protein kinase. *Mol. Endocrinol.* **5**, 921-930.

30. HYLDEN, J.L.K., NAHIN, R.L., TRAUB, R.L. AND DUBNER R. (1989) Expansion of receptive fields of spinal lamina I projection neurons in rats with unilateral adjuvant-induced inflammation: the contribution of central dorsal horn mechanisms. *Pain* **37**, 229-243.

31. IADAROLA M.J., CIVELLI, O., DOUGLASS, J. AND NARANJO, J.R. Increased spinal cord dynorphin mRNA during peripheral inflammation. In: J.W. Holaday, P.-Y. Law and A. Herz (Eds.), Progress in Opioid Research, NIDA Research Monograph, Vol. 75, 1986, pp. 406-409.

32. IADAROLA, M.J., BRADY, L.S., DRAISCI, G. AND DUBNER, R. Enhancement of dynorphin gene expression in spinal cord following experimental inflammation: Stimulus specificity, behavioral parameters and opioid receptor binding. Pain, 35 (1988) 313-326.

33. IADAROLA, M.J., DOUGLASS, J., CIVELLI, O. AND NARANJO, J.R. Differential activation of spinal cord dynorphin and enkephalin neurons during hyperalgesia: evidence using cDNA hybridization. Brain Res., 455 (1988) 205-212.

34. IADAROLA, M.J. AND DRAISCI G. (1988) Elevation of spinal cord dynorphin mRNA compared to dorsal root ganglion mRNAs during peripheral inflammation. In: *The Arthritic Rat as a Model for Chronic Pain.* eds. J.M. Besson and G. Guilbaud. Excerpta Medica, Amsterdam, pp. 173-184.

35. IADAROLA, M.J., MOJDEHI, G., GU, J. AND MESSERSMITH, D.J. A protein complex differing from the Fos/Jun complex binds at an AP-1 variant enhancer element in the dynorphin promoter and is induced in spinal cord by peripheral inflammation. (Submitted).

36. KAGEYAMA, R., SASAI, Y. AND NAKANISHI, S. (1991) Molecular characterization of transcription factors that bind to the cAMP responsive region of the substance P precursor gene. *J. Biol. Chem.* **266**, 15525-15531.

37. KAJANDER, K.C., SAHARA, Y., IADAROLA, M.J. AND BENNETT, G.J. (1990) Dynorphin increases in the dorsal spinal cord in rats with a painful peripheral neuropathy. *Peptides* **11**, 719-728.

38. KAYNARD A.H. AND MELNER M.H. (1992) Stimulation of prodynorphin gene expression requires a functional protein kinase A. *Molec. Cellular Neurosci.* **3**, 278-285.

39. KAYNARD A.H., MCMURRAY, C.T., DOUGLASS, J., CURRY, T.E. JR., AND MELNER M.H. Regulation of prodynorphin gene expression in the ovary: distal DNA regulatory elements confer gonadotropin regulation of promoter activity. Molec. Endocrinol. (in press).

40. KOBIERSKI, L.A., CHU, H.-M., TAN, Y. AND COMB, M.J. (1991) cAMP-dependent regulation of proenkephalin by jun D and jun B: positive and negative effects of AP-1 proteins. *Proc. Natl. Acad. Sci. U.S.A.* **88**, 10222-10226.

41. LUCAS, J.J., MELLSTROM, B., COLADO, M.I. AND NARANJO, J.R. (1993) Molecular mechanisms of pain: serotonin 1a receptor agonists trigger transactivation by *c-fos* of the prodynorphin gene in spinal cord neurons. *Neuron* **10**, 599-611.

42. MANIATIS T., GOODBOURN S. AND FISCHER J.A. (1987) Regulation of inducible and tissue-specific gene expression. *Science* **236**, 1237-1244.

43. MARGIORIS, A.N., MARKOGIANNAKIS E., MAKRIGIANNAKIS, A. AND GRAVANIS, A. (1992) PC12 rat pheochromocytoma cells synthesize dynorphin. Its secretion is modulated by nicotine and nerve growth factor. *Endocrinology* **131**, 703-709.

44. MATSUI, M., TOKUHARA, M., KONUMA, Y., NOMURA, N. AND ISHIZAKI, R. (1990) Isolation of human fos-related genes and their expression during monocyte-macrophage differentiation. *Oncogene* **5**, 249-255.

45. MESSERSMITH, D.J., GU, J., DUBNER, R., DOUGLASS, J. AND IADAROLA, M.J. Constitutive and inducible transcriptional activity of a far upstream AP-1/CRE element in the prodynorphin promoter. (Submitted).

46. MINAMI, M., KURAISHI, Y., KAWAMURA, M., YAMAGUCHI, T., MASU, Y., NAKANISHI, S. AND SATOH, M. (1989) Enhancement of preprotachykinin A gene expression by adjuvant-induced inflammation in the rat spinal cord: possible involvement of substance P-containing spinal neurons in nociception. *Neurosci. Lett.* **98**, 105-110.

47. MILLAN M.J. MILLAN, M.H., CZLONKOWSKI A., HOLLT, V., PILCHER, C.W.T., HERZ, A. AND COLPAERT, F.C. (1986) A model of chronic pain in the rat: response of multiple opioid systems to adjuvant-induced arthritis. *J. Neurosci.* **6**, 899-906.

48. MINER, J.N. AND YAMAMOTO, K.K. (1991) Regulatory crosstalk at composite response elements. *Trends Biochem. Sci.* **16**, 423-426.

49. MITCHELL, P.J. AND TJIAN, R. (1989) Transcriptional regulation in mammalian cells by sequence-specific DNA binding proteins. *Science* **245**, 371-378.

50. MONTMINY, M.R. AND BILEZIKJIAN, L.M. (1987) Binding of a nuclear protein to the cyclic-AMP response element of the somatostatin gene. *Nature* **328**, 175-178.

51. MORGAN, J.I., AND CURRAN T., (1986) Role of ion flux in the control of *c-fos*

expression. *Nature* **322**, 552-555.

52. MORGAN, J.I. AND CURRAN, T. (1988) Calcium as modulator of the immediate-early gene cascade in neurons. *Cell Calcium* **9**, 303-311.

53. MORGAN, J.I. AND CURRAN, T. (1991) Stimulus-transcription coupling in nervous system: involvement of the inducible proto-oncogenes fos and jun. *Ann. Rev. Neurosci.* **14**, 421-451.

54. NAHIN, R.L., HYLDEN J.L.K., IADAROLA, M.J. AND DUBNER, R. (1989) 2Peripheral inflammation is associated with increased dynorphin immunoreactivity in both projection and local circuit neurons in the superficial dorsal horn of the rat lumbar spinal cord. *Neurosci. Lett.* **96**, 47-252.

55. NAKAJIMA Y., TSUCHIDA, K., NEGISHI, M., ITO, S. AND NAKANISHI, S. (1992) Direct linkage of three tachykinin receptors to stimulation of both phosphatidyl inositol hydrolysis and cyclic AMP cascades in transfected chinese hamster ovary cells. *J. Biol. Chem.* **267**, 2437-2442.

56. NAKABEPPU, Y., RYDER, K. AND NATHANS, D. (1988) DNA binding activities of three murine Jun proteins: stimulation by Fos. *Cell* **55**, 907.

57. NARANJO, J.R., MELLSTROM, B., ACHAVAL, M. AND SASSONE-CORSI, P. (1991) Molecular pathways of pain: Fos/Jun-mediated activation of a non-canonical AP-1 site in the prodynorphin gene. *Neuron* **6**, 607-617.

58. NOGUCHI, K., MORITA, Y., KIYAMA, H., ONO, K. AND TOHYAMA, M. A (1988) Noxious stimulus induces the preprotachykinin-A gene expression in the rat dorsal root ganglion: a quantitative study using in situ hybridization histochemistry. *Mol. Brain Res.* **4**, 31-35.

59. NOGUCHI, K. AND RUDA, M.A. Gene regulation in an ascending nociceptive pathway: inflammation-induced increase in preprotachykinin mRNA in rat lamina I spinal projection neurons. *J. Neurosci.* **12**, (1992) 2563-2572.

60. NOGUCHI, K., KOWALSKI, K., TRAUB, R., SOLODKIN, A., IADAROLA, M.J. AND RUDA, M.A. (1991) Dynorphin expression and fos-like immunoreactivity following inflammation induced hyperalgesia are colocalized in spinal cord neurons. *Mol. Brain Res.* **10**, 227-233.

61. NOMURA N., ZU, Y.-L., MAEKAWA, T., TABATA, S., AKIYAMA, T. AND ISHII S. (1993) Isolation and characterization of a novel member of the gene family encoding the cAMP response element-binding protein CRE-BP1. *J. Biol Chem.* **268**, 4259-4266.

62. ONO, S.J., LIOU, H.-C., DAVIDON, R., STROMINGER, J.L. AND GLIMCHER, L.H. (1991) Human X-box-binding protein 1 is required for the transcription of a subset of human class II major histocompatibility genes and forms heterodimer with *c-fos*. *Proc. Natl. Acad. Sci. U.S.A.* **884**, 309-4312.

63. PTASHNE, M. (1986) Gene regulation by proteins acting nearby and at a distance. *Nature* **322**, 697-701.

64. QUINN, J.P., TAKIMOTO, M., IADAROLA, M.J., HOLBROOK, N. AND LEVENS, D. (1989) Distinct factors bind the AP-1 consensus sites in gibbon ape

leukemia virus and simian virus 40 enhancers. *J. Virol.* **63**, 1737-1742.

65. RAUSCHER F.J. III, SAMBUCETTI, L.C., CURRAN, T., DISTEL, R.J. AND SPIEGELMAN, B.M. (1988) Common DNA binding site for Fos protein complexes and transcription factor AP-1. *Cell* **52**, 471-480.

66. RAUSCHER, F.J. III, COHEN, D.R., CURRAN, T., BOS, T.J., VOGT, P.K., BOHMANN, D., TJIAN R. AND FRANZA, B.R. JR. (1988) Fos-associated protein p39 is the product of the jun proto-oncogene. *Science* **240**, 1010-1016.

67. RUDA, M.A., IADAROLA, M.J., COHEN, L.V. AND YOUNG, W.S. (1988) In situ hybridization histochemistry and immunocytochemistry reveal an increase in spinal dynorphin biosynthesis in a rat model of peripheral inflammation and hyperalgesia. *Proc. Natl. Acad. Sci. USA* **85**, 622-626.

68. RYSECK, R.-P. AND BRAVO, R. (1990) c-jun, jun B, and jun D differ in their binding affinities to AP-1 and CRE consensus sequences: effect of FOS proteins. *Oncogene* **6**, 533-542.

69. SASSONI-CORSI, P., VISVADER, J., FERLAND, L., MELLON, P.L. AND VERMA, I.M. (1988) Induction of proto-oncogene fos transcription through the adenylate cyclase pathway: characterization of a cAMP-responsive element. *Genes Dev.* **2**, 1529-1538.

70. SHENG, M., DOUGAN, S.T., MCFADDEN, G. AND GREENBERG, M.E. (1988) Calcium and growth factor pathways of *c-fos* transcriptional activation require distinct upstream regulatory sequences. *Mol. Cell. Biol.* **8**, 2787-2796.

71. SHENG, M., MCFADDEN, G. AND GREENBERG, M. (1990) Membrane depolarization and calcium induce *c-fos* transcription via phosphorylation of transcription factor CREB. *Neuron* **4**, 571-582.

72. SONNENBERG, J.L., RAUSCHER, F.J., III, MORGAN, J.I. AND CURRAN, T. (1989) Regulation of proenkephalin by Fos and Jun. *Science* 246, 1622-1625.

73. SONNENBERG, J.L., MACGREGOR-LEON, P.F., CURRAN, T. AND MORGAN, J.I. (1989) Dynamic alterations occur in the levels and composition of transcription factor AP-1 complexes after seizure. *Neuron* **3**, 359-365.

74. TATA, J.R. (1974) Isolation of nuclei from liver and other tissues. *Meth. Enzymol.* **31A**, 253-257.

75. VELAZQUEZ, L., FELLOUS, M., STARK, G.R. AND PELLEGRINI, S. (1992) A protein tyrosine kinase in the interferon a/B signaling pathway. *Cell* **70**, 313-322.

76. VELCICH, A. AND ZIFF, E.B. (1990) Functional analysis of an isolated promoter element with AP-1 site homology reveals cell type-specific transcriptional properties. *Mol. Cell. Biol.* **10**, 6273-6282.

77. VINSON, C.R., SIGLER, P.B. AND MCKNIGHT, S.L. (1989) Scissors-grip model for DNA recognition by a family of leucine zipper proteins. *Science* **246**, 911-916.

78. WISDEN, W., ERRINGTON, M.L., WILLIAMS, S., DUNNETT, S.B., WATERS, C.,

HITCHCOCK, D., EVAN, C., BLISS, T.V.P., AND HUNT, S.P. (1990) differential expression of immediate early genes in the hippocampal formation and spinal cord. *Neuron* **4**, 603-614.

79. WOOLF, C., AND WIESENFELD-HALLIN, Z. (1986) Substance P and calcitonin gene-related peptide synergistically modulate the gain of the nociceptive flexor withdrawal reflex in the rat, *Neurosci. Lett.* **66**, 226-230.

80. YAMAMATO, K.K., GONZALEZ, G.A., BIGGS, W.H., AND MONTMINY, M.R. (1988) Phosphorylation-induced binding and transcriptional efficacy of nuclear factor CREB. *Nature* **334**, 494-498.

81. YANG, H.-Y.T., HEXUM, T. AND COSTA, E. (1980) Opioid peptides in adrenal gland. *Life Sci.* **27**, 1119-1125.

82. YASUDA, K., RAYNOR, K., KONG, H., BREDER, C.D., TAKEDA, J., REISINE, T. AND BELL, G.I. (1993) Cloning and functional comparison of K and S opioid receptors from mouse brain. *Proc. Natl. Acad. Sci. U.S.A.* **90**, 6736-6740.

83. ZERIAL, M., TOSCHI, L., RYSECK, R.-P., SCHUERMANN, M., MILLER, R. AND BRAVO, R. (1989) The product of a novel growth factor activated gene, fos B, interacts with JUN proteins enhancing their DNA binding activity. *EMBO J.* **8**, 805-813.

REGULATION OF CELLULAR PHENOTYPE IN THE NOCICEPTIVE PATHWAY

Eberhard Weihe and Martin K.-H. Schafer
Dept. of Anatomy
Johannes Gutenberg-University
D-55O99 Mainz
Germany

INTRODUCTION

In order to understand the molecular and cellular mechanisms of primary sensory signalling in the CNS and periphery it is important to know:

l) Which primary afferent transmitters and targets are involved in central and peripheral nociceptive and non-nociceptive neuro-effector functions?

2) What regulates the primary afferent phenotype?

3) How are peripheral nociceptor endings activated or sensitized and which factors reduce their activation or induce sensitization?

4) How is primary afferent input modulated in the spinal cord?

5) What are the molecular and cellular reactions of spinal and peripheral neurons and of non-neural elements to peripheral inflammation?

It is beyond the scope of this resumee to address these questions in detail as they have been extensively reviewed by Levine et al.[29]. The main objectives are to highlight new aspects and possible controversies. These considerations are based on immuno-cytochemical and molecular biological studies in our laboratory dealing with the characterization and localization of basal and inflammation-induced expression of neuropeptides, neuropeptide receptors and neuropeptide processing enzymes in peripheral and spinal neurons and non-neural cells believed to be relevant for the initiation and continuation of inflammatory pain.

NATO ASI Series, Vol. H 79
Cellular Mechanisms of Sensory Processing
Edited by Laszlo Urban
© Springer-Verlag Berlin Heidelberg 1994

Evidence that the majority of primary sensory neurons are peptidergic

Chromogranin A (CGA) is involved in the packaging and storage of neuropeptides in vesicles. Thus, CGA could be a useful marker of primary sensory peptidergic neurons. Surprisingly, CGA was found to be expressed in all primary sensory neurons of spinal and trigeminal ganglia.[52] This may imply that all primary sensory neurons are peptidergic. In this line, but in contrast to common thinking, we have evidence that indeed CGRP is one example in support of this view because it was found to be expressed in virtually all ganglionic cells of rat spinal ganglia. Two CGRP phenotype levels can be seen. About 50% to 60% of rat DRG neurons express strong CGRP immunoreactivity, present in small, medium sized and large diameter neurons while the remaining neurons exhibit weak to moderate immunopositivity. This confirms observations of Hokfelt[21] in monkey sensory ganglia where the vast majority of sensory neurons were shown to contain CGRP mRNA. In this line, we have shown that CGRP immunoreactivty is contained in virtually all ganglionic cells of rhesus monkey dorsal root ganglia (unpublished data). Thus, CGRP is not only a transmitter candidate of C- and A-delta nociceptor afferents but clearly also of large diameter myelinated neurons. This may be of relevance in Aβ-fiber mediated hyperalgesia.

Underestimation of primary afferent tachykinin populations?

A similar underestimation may have been made with tachykininergic primary sensory neurons. We see tachykinin immunoreactivity not only in small and medium sized neurons but also in many large diameter neurons. This was the case in rat, guinea pig and monkey dorsal root ganglia. In fact NK1 receptor mRNA is expressed throughout the spinal grey matter with no specificity for second order nociceptive or wide dynamic range neurons.[51] In contrast, the NK1 receptor appears not to be expressed on primary sensory neurons suggesting that substance P has no presynaptic autoregulatory function in the primary afferent transmission.

Opioid expression in primary sensory neuron

It is still an unresolved question to what extent primary sensory neurons of various species express opioids. In guinea-pig sensory neurons, dynorphin immunoreactivity is co-contained with substance P and CGRP while pro-enkephalin (PENK) derived opioid-immunoreactivity is absent.[11] In contrast to previous reports we now see expression of PENK in a sub population of small and large diameter neurons of dorsal root and trigeminal ganglia of the rat, both on the mRNA and protein level (unpublished data). While pro-dynorphin (PDYN) mRNA and immunoreactivity appeared to be below or at marginal detection level, POMC derived β-endorphin immunoreactivity was found at homogeneously low levels in the majority of spinal and trigeminal primary sensory neurons of intact rats. Previously, we reported the presence of alpha-MSH-like immunoreactivity in large primary sensory neurons. Interestingly, the POMC gene was recently reported to be expressed in dorsal root ganglia after sciatic nerve crush in the rat.[43] Peripheral nerve transection may change peptide phenotypes dramatically and in an opposite manner to peripheral inflammation. Thus, NPY, galanin and VIP expression are markedly upregulated by sciatic transection.[21,39] Primary afferent responses to opioids during inflammation or nerve transection are unexplored. In any case, the precise cellular localization and the levels of POMC mRNA in normal rats remains to be shown before definite conclusions can be drawn that POMC opioid and non-opioid peptides could play a significant role in normal primary afferent function. As opioid receptors are present on central and peripheral endings of primary afferents[29] we suggest the possibility that the peripheral excitability of primary sensory neurons is under autoinhibitory opioid control. In addition, opioids may autoinhibit peripheral and central transmitter release. Alternatively, the sub population of PENK primary sensory opioid neurons may coincide with tyrosine hydroxylase positive catecholaminergic (dopaminergic?) neurons which exhibit similar numbers and distribution. These arguments need to be further corroborated by localizing the mRNA of the three cloned opioid receptors[6,12,28,69] to primary sensory neurons in conjunction with thorough analysis of the gene expression of the three opioid precursors.

GABA in primary sensory neurons ?

Classical transmitters, like glutamate and aspartate are present in all classes of primary afferents. Glutamate receptor expression seems not to be selective for a particular class of primary afferents.[29] The classical inhibitory transmitter GABA is contained in a major population of primary afferents and GABA receptors are expressed in primary sensory neurons too.[29,41] This raises the possibility of GABA mediated autoinhibition of primary afferent activity in possible interaction with an autoinhibitory primary afferent opioid system.

Multiplicity and abundance of primary afferent transmitter/modulator candidates: no evidence for modality specificity

In the view of their abundant presence, none of the primary afferent neuropeptides and classical transmitters can be correlated with the activity of a physiologically defined entity of primary afferents. The specificity of action must be regulated by other factors than chemical phenotypes per se. It may be that the relative levels of expression of excitatory and inhibitory non-peptide and peptide transmitters and their receptor subtypes determine the specific function of a given primary sensory neuron at a given time window. There may be a temporal factor in phenotype and functional plasticity of primary sensory neurons. In any case, the classical transmitter glutamate and the neuropeptides substance P (SP), neurokinin A (NKA) and CGRP appear to be the most important messenger candidates for nociceptive transmission in the spinal cord where they are believed to be co-released from small diameter afferents and to exert synergistic functions. These result in excitation and wind up of second order nociceptive neurons.[11,29,49]

Peripheral neuro-effector targets and neuropeptide receptors

Peripheral neuro-effector functions of small diameter sensory neurons are a domain of neuropeptides. There is no evidence that primary afferent-derived excitatory amino acids have a peripheral role. According to Dale's principle such a possibility is, however, conceivable. It may be worthwhile to search for the presence and function of glutamate receptors on peripheral target cells and on peripheral endings of primary afferents.

Specific peripheral neuro-effector functions require stimulus-specific release of primary afferent transmitters and the presence and function of corresponding receptors on nearby target cells. Therefore, it is reasonable to determine the spatial relationships between transmitter-identified peripheral nerve endings and the type of target cell in conjunction with receptor identification on particular target cell types. Synaptic contacts between endings and target are not present. It is unclear how close nerve endings have to be located to target cells so that effective concentrations of transmitters reach the target. As argued in the CNS, volume transmission mechanisms may be operational in the periphery, too.

Varicose nerve fibers co-containing SP and CGRP form close spatial relationships with somatic and visceral fenestrated postcapillary venules suggestive of a stereotyped target-selective function on this part of the microvasculature throughout the organism. In fact, SP mediates electrically and capsaicin-evoked plasma protein extravasation in postcapillary venules.[33] Calcitonin gene-related peptide (CGRP) is known to enhance this effect by inhibiting SP degradation without having an effect on its own. Neuropharmacology indicates that effects of SP on the peripheral microvasculature are mediated by NK1 receptors and can occur independent of histamine release from mast cells.[2] In accordance with this, we have evidence that NK1 receptor mRNA is expressed in subepidermal postcapillary venules. NK1 receptor was also localized in endothelial cells of arterial and venous blood vessels. (unpublished observation). This conforms to the common view that SP-induced vasodilatation is endothelium dependent.

Neuro-immune targets and neuropeptide receptors

Immunomodulatory effects of neuropeptides revealed *in vitro* and close spatial relationships of SP and CGRP containing varicose nerve fibers with macrophages, mast cells, plasma cells, dendritic cells, Langerhans cells, granulocytes, lymphocytes and reticulum cells suggest complex neuroimmune effector roles of sensory neuropeptides *in vivo*.[61,63] However, the relevance and mechanisms of sensory-immune effector functions in vivo are not yet well understood. The specific *in vivo* patterns of the expression of receptor subtypes for peptide and classical transmitters in the different classes of immune cells and antigen presenting cells are largely unknown but constitute a promising though difficult area of research. We have begun to address this issue by in situ hybridization of various lymphoid tissues and have obtained preliminary evidence that the NK1 receptor is expressed in resident macrophages. This is in accordance with SP-inducible cytokine release from macrophages.[29] There was no apparent evidence for an *in vivo* expression of NK1 receptors on T-cells which contrasts to reports indicating *in vitro* effects of SP on T-lymphocytes.

Relevance of target cell relationships for nociceptor activation/sensitization and peripheral antinociception?

Multiple mediators are involved in the activation and direct or indirect sensitization of peripheral nociceptor endings. In the case of inflammation or tissue injury, these mediators are produced by a variety of resident and infiltrating inflammatory cells (e.g. cytokines, prostaglandins, 5-HT, histamine etc) or they are cleaved from high molecular precursors leaving the blood stream and gaining access to the site of injury (bradykinin) (see Dray, this volume; Levine et al.[29]). Specific target cell relationships of nociceptor endings may be totally irrelevant when inflammation has fully developed and nociceptors are simply "bathing in the inflammatory soup".[16] On the other hand, the obvious target relations of SP and CGRP containing terminals with macrophages, granulocytes, mast cells, fibroblasts etc may have significance in the initiation, development and perpetuation of inflammatory pain.

In the following scenario of neuro-target cell cross-talk is conceivable. Tissue injury leads to parallel induction of inflammatory mediator release and activation of nociceptive terminals which then release neuropeptides. The neuropeptides function as chemo-attractans for inflammatory cells and enhance cytokine and growth factor release and synthesis in these cells and in a variety of juxtaterminal resident cells such as endothelial cells, fibroblasts, mast cells and, probably Schwann cells. Mediators released from these cells activate and sensitize nociceptors but also cause long term changes in primary afferents. NGF-induced and NGF-maintained upregulation of neuropeptide gene expression in nociceptor afferents may be mechanisms of the hyperalgesic actions of NGF[30] or there may be direct activation by NGF octapeptide.[56] The hyperalgesic actions of NGF occur without apparent signs of inflammation suggesting that NGF hyperalgesia is independent of neurogenic inflammation.[30] On the other hand, there may be very local mini-inflammation. Cytokines may be upregulated in a very localized area and in specific cells. With a highly sensitive in situ hybridization technique it may be possible to reveal kinetics of local cytokine production on the mRNA level.[5]

In vitro experiments have demonstrated cytokine-induced increase of substance P expression in sensory neurons. In cultured sympathetic neurons, interleukin-I caused an induction of SP expression, apparently by an indirect mechanism involving the leukemia inhibitory factor (LIF).[14,53] It is unresolved whether interleukin-1 has a similar effect *in vivo*. Interleukin-8 has a potent hyperalgesic action in vivo which depends on the sympathetic system.[9] Sensory-sympathetic interactions are poorly understood. In the periphery they are anatomically restricted to perivascular areas sparing intra-epidermal nociceptors and perhaps, also pericytic fenestrated venules. Janig reported recently sprouting of sympathetic fibers into the sensory ganglia.[23,33a] This could be a novel link for sympathetic-sensory maintained pain.

Interestingly, cutaneous sites of cytokine and NGF synthesis are partly overlapped. The epidermal keratinocytes are a major source of interleukin and NGF synthesis. NGF and cytokines are synthetized in macrophages and mast cells and probably in many more cell types. Nerve transection causes upregulation of cutaneous NGF production which was taken as evidence that peripheral NGF production is regulated by intact nerve supply.[34]

Opioid and non-opioid peptides in Merkel cells: paracrine action on nociceptors?

Opioids appear to be expressed in Merkel cells. Cutaneous Merkel cells in the guinea-pig contain met-enkephalin-like immunoreactivity. In rat Merkel cells dynorphin immunoreactive material is present.[66] Merkel cells are strategically situated in the vicinity of subepidermal postcapillary venules and SP/CGRP containing nerve fibers. Thus, Merkel cell-derived dynorphin-related opioids could be released in a paracrine fashion to reduce nociceptor excitability via peripheral kappa receptors. In support of this suggestion, peripherally acting kappa opioid receptors were shown to cause antinociception.[3,47] It is also noteworthy that CGRP is expressed in Merkel cells and that even SP is contained in a subpopulation of Merkel cells of some species.[62]

Inflammation-induced expression of opioid peptide in immune cells in vivo?

In spite of abundant evidence for the expression of PENK and POMC mRNA in stimulated immune cells, *in vitro,* PENK and POMC mRNAs have been reported to be present at high levels in immune cells of inflamed skin *in vivo*.[46,54] This issue in our opinion is incompletely resolved as our own *in situ* hybridization data indicate that inflammation-evoked signals, which are clearly above background, are limited to a few spots in both normal and inflamed skin. We have the impression that normal rats exhibited marginal signals for POMC mRNA in the epidermis and for PENK mRNA ,diffusely throughout the dermis. There was some tendency for a small increase in the levels of these mRNAs in inflamed skin. In support of our in situ hybridization experiments Northern blot analysis revealed no major upregulation of opioid mRNA levels in inflamed versus non-inflamed skin.

The question arises whether possible changes in cutaneous opioid gene expression are due to the invasion of additional cells expressing opioid mRNA or to increases of opioid expression in resident cells (macrophages, mast cells, granulocytes, fibroblasts, myofibroblast-like cells, endothelial cells, epidermal cells, smooth muscle cells and Schwann cells). We addressed this issue by using highly specific antisera against opioid sequences of the three opioid precursors. These antisera stained neurons and nerve fibers in the CNS and a variety of endocrine cells. We obtained no evidence for specific staining of immune cells in the inflammed tissue. This is in contrast to a previous report showing PENK and POMC opioid immunoreactivity in a variety of immune cells (T-cells, B-cells, macrophages and granulocytes), of inflamed skin.[46] The presence of DYN and CGRP immunoreactive material in inflammatory cells was also reported.[19] In our hands however, preabsorption controls revealed non-specificity of such staining.

Negative evidence for a lymphocyte-derived POMC system in human peripheral blood mononuclear cells was reported by van Woudenberg et al.[68] POMC gene expression was absent from rat splenic lymphocytes *in vivo* but was present in a small population of monocyte-macrophage-like cells, in the red pulp, but not in the marginal zone.[35] It is noteworthy, that there is widespread organ expression (including the skin but not the spleen) of rat pro-enkephalin gene during early postnatal development.[27] Furthermore, the proenkephalin gene, expressed in mesenchymal cells, gives rise to bone and cartilage.[48] In fact, have occasionally seen, opioid immunoreactivity in chondrocytes). Cutaneous inflammation and tissue repair upon injury may activate opioid gene expression in proliferating connective tissue cells (fibroblasts, myofibroblasts, endothelial cells) rather than in immune cells. In support of this view we see general upregulation of *c-fos* expression in inflammed tissue. In the inflamed skin, the prepropeptide processing enzyme PC2 was markedly expressed in myofibroblast-like cells but not in immune cells. CGA expression was generally upregulated in many cell types of the inflamed skin.

Mechanisms of peripheral opioid antinociception: Induction of peripheral opioid receptors on nociceptors and function of immune cell-derived opioids?

Peripheral antinociceptive actions of exogenous opioids, apparently mediated by all three opioid receptors, are seen in inflammed and absent in non-Inflamed tissue.[54] This induction of peripheral opioid analgesia was attributed to an effect on opioid receptors located on nociceptor endings. The concept of inflammation-induced peripheral antinociception mediated by endogenous opioids implicates synthesis and release from local immune cells, reducing excitability of nociceptor endings. Evidence for this tonic antinociception by locally released opioids was deduced from the effect of naloxone to lower nociceptive thresholds in inflamed but not in non-inflamed paws. We suggest alternative mechanisms. There is a source of stress-induced increase in plasma met-enkephalin.[4] Further, inactive opioid precursor fragments circulate in the plasma. Thus, the plasma reaching the inflamed tissue has to be considerd as a source of opioids. We hypothesize that a panoply of enzymes upregulated in the inflamed area could locally generate bioactive opioids from inactive circulating precursors. These bioactive forms may act on specific opioid receptors located on nociceptors.

Endogenous and exogeneous peripheral opioid analgesia may not only operate by reducing nociceptor excitability but also by an inhibitory action on inflammatory cells. There is *in vitro* evidence for the presence of functionally relevant opioid receptors on immune cells. We propose that a peripheral opioid action could be to block pro-algesic mediator release and expression in inflammatory and other cells, producing the "inflammatory soup", both in a short and long term fashion.

One could simply argue that the main difference between normal and inflamed tissue consists in the amount of inflammatory cells present and active. Thus, this could be the main reason for an early "lighting up" of peripheral opioid analgesia in the course of inflammation when increased receptor transport from the primary sensory cell body to the peripheral nociceptor cannot yet be operational. However, in prolonged periods of inflammation upregulation of opioid receptor expression in primary afferent nociceptors projecting into the inflamed tissue may well be effective. With the recent cloning of the opioid receptors.[6,12,28,69] It will be possible to find out whether primary sensory opioid receptor expression is upregulated by inflammation and the exact cellular sites of opioid receptor synthesis in the skin and their possible plasticity in inflammation will be determined.

Upregulation of NK1 receptor expression in inflamed skin

NK-I receptor gene expression was found to be upregulated in endothelial cells and a minor number of subepidermal and dermal connective tissue, probably macrophages. This suggests that the plasticity of pro-inflammatory receptor expression may be a pathophysiological factor in the periphery.

Spatio-temporal changes of peptidergic innervation in inflamed skin

In Freund's adjuvant-induced inflammation, we observed marked topographical and time-specific changes in CGRP, SP and NPY innervation. In the early phase of unilateral inflammation (4 h post-inoculation) image analysis revealed a moderate decrease in the area density of the number and total length of intraepidermal CGRP-ir nerve fibers in the inflamed paw as compared to the contralateral sham-injected paw or to the paw of untreated rats. In contrast, a significant 2-3 fold increase in the area density of intraepidermal CGRP-ir nerves was measured 6 days post-inoculation. A similar biphaasic change is displayed by intraepidermal SP-ir nerve fibers.

In the early phase of unilateral inflammation (4 h post-inoculation), the density of periarterial CGRP fibers was slightly reduced in the inflamed paw as compared to the contralateral or to control paws. In the prolonged phase (6 days) of unilateral inflammation, periarterial CGRP innervation was markedly reduced as compared to non-inflamed skin.

Prolonged inflammation also caused a marked reduction of periarterial NPY innervation while 4 h post-inoculation only a very moderate decrease of periarterial NPY was seen.

The early phase decrease in the number of intraepidermal and periarterial nerve CGRP and SP innervation may reflect an acute response characterised by increased release of neuropeptides from perivascular terminals and some preterminal region, too. In fact, there appeared to be no decrease in the number of CGRP-ir nerve fibers or in the intensity of their immunostaining further upstream supporting the view that the early events affect the very terminal portions of peripheral nerves. The same may apply to the early moderate decrease in NPY-ir innervation. While the intraepidermal CGRP/TK innervation represents primary sensory afferents of presumed nociceptive function, the origin of the periarterial CGRP, and perhaps that of the periarterial SP innervation, may be of dual origin, sensory and postganglionic sympathetic. The expression of the sensory prototype peptides SP and CGRP in postganglionic sympathetic neurons may be upregulated in chronic inflammatory pain condition.

The increase of intraepidermal SP and CGRP fibers is interpreted as local sprouting possibly maintained by increased production of NGF in epidermal keratinocytes of inflamed skin. In support of this view the density of intraepidermal fibers staining for the developmental sprouting marker GAP-43 and for the pan-neural marker PGP were similarly increased. GAP 43 and PGP are also characteristic of chronic inflammatory conditions in humans such as chronic pancreatitis and non-acute appendicitis probably involving sensory and autonomic (sympathetic, parasaympathetic) peptidergic neurons (unpublished data). Although our method is extremely sensitive we cannot exclude that the increased density of SP/CGRP fibers seen in the epidermis is due to the fact that more peptides are transported in the epidermal terminals of inflamed than in that of non-inflamed paw so that simply more positive profiles can be visualized in the inflamed as compared to non-inflamed epidermis. Nevertheless, real intraepidermal sprouting of presumed nociceptive fibers upon inflammatory challenge may be a simple explanation for the phenomenon of hyperalgesia as due to numerical changes of nociceptive endings. Indeed, peripheral sprouting of nociceptive fibers is discussed by dermatologists as an explanation of hypersensitive and itchy skin in UV erythema. On the other hand, changes in neuropeptide synthesis in peripheral neurons or sprouting of peripheral nerve fibers may not be causally related to nociception but rather to neurogenic mechanisms in the repair of damaged tissue.[66]

Herpes virus and primary afferent neuropeptides

Experimental viral infection may be another model for studying molecular mechanisms in primary sensory neurons and even central neurons which are relevant for inflammatory pain, and possibly neuropathic pain. Herpes virus infection causes recurrent local inflammation accompanied by pain suggesting an involvement of peptidergic nociceptive afferents. Interestingly, we observe a striking incidence of co-existence of herpes simplex virus (HSV) immunoreactivity and TK/CGRP immunoreactivity in trigeminal ganglionic cells of experimentally infected mice. This phenotype-specific preference of HSV neurotropism may be causally involved in the symptoms of pain and peripheral inflammation occurring in herpes infection. It is noteworthy that the expression of opioids in primary afferents was found to be upregulated in herpes-infected trigeminal ganglia. Inflammation in the ganglion may be causally related to the changes in transmitter expression. Changes in primary afferent neurotransmitter metabolism may be even important in exacerbation of silent herpes infection.

Steroid sensitivity of inflammation-induced and basal primary afferent CGRP gene expression

In contrast to Hanesch et al.[17] we have no evidence for an increase in the number of primary afferents expressing CGRP in inflammatory states as compared to controls. Using the model of collagen-induced arthritis[42] CGRP mRNA levels in spinal ganglia were found to be increased. Steroid treatment of arthritic rats downregulated the upregulated CGRP gene expression. There was also a slight corticosteroid-induced downregulation of CGRP mRNA levels in spinal ganglia of normal rats. We suggest that steroid treatment may not only influence primary afferent neuropeptide synthesis indirectly by reducing inflammatory mediators (e.g. cytokines) and peripheral growth factors but also by a direct effect on the primary sensory neurons.[25] Susceptibility of primary afferent neuropeptides to steroids has been reported before.[55] At least in the CNS, peptidergic neurons have been shown to be endowed with glucocorticoid receptors and there is evidence for glucocorticoid-induced regulation of neuropeptide expression.[8,11,36,64] Thus, dystrophic effects of chronic steroid treatment in the skin may be explained by a relative deficiency of positive trophic influences mediated by sensory neuropeptides.

Molecular anatomy of the spinal cord

There is an enormous amount of data on the molecular anatomy, neurophysiology and neuropharmacology of neuropeptides and classical transmitters in the spinal cord and the reader is referred to recent reviews and references therein.[8,11,36,64] Here we report on novel preliminary data concerning the distribution of mRNAs encoding CGA, processing enzymes, NKI receptor and PRO-ENK and the immediate early gene *c-fos*.

In contrast to the common view that CGA is expressed in specific subsets of CNS neurons[67] we have evidence that high levels of CGA mRNA are expressed in all dorsal and ventral horn neurons of rat spinal cord and also in preganglionic autonomic neurons. CGA-immunoreactivity was present in all categories of spinal cord neurons of rat and monkey.

Contary to the view that there is no relevant basal expression of *c-fos* in the spinal cord[1,10,15,20] our current in situ hybridization analysis reveals the presence of *c-fos* mRNA in many neurons.

The basal expression of PRO-ENK mRNA is much higher than that of PRO-DYN mRNA. Noteworthy, PRO-ENK mRNA was not only found at high levels in neurons throughout the dorsal horn and in preganglionic autonomic neurons but also at moderate levels in motoneurons. This is in agreement with our recent observations that rat motoneurons contain weak immunostaining for the PRO-ENK derivative ME-RGL.

We detected low levels of NKI receptor mRNA in neurons throughout the cervical, thoracic and lumbosacral grey matter, but not in white matter.[51] In any case, the data support the view that spinal NKI receptors have sensory, motor and autonomic functions and are not specific for nociception.

In situ hybridization and immunocytochemistry in rat and monkey revealed that the processing enzymes PC1 and PC2 were expressed in neurons throughout the grey matter with high abundance in the superficial and deep layers of the dorsal horn and in motoneurons. PC1 was less abundant and more restricted in its distribution than PC2.[50] Immunocytochemistry revealed PC1 and PC2 immunoreactive fibers throughout the grey matter. PC1-ir fibers and endings were concentrated in the superficial dorsal horn where they overlapped with TK-ir fibers and endings suggesting coexistence and major origin from primary afferents. In fact, the PC 1 and PC 2 appear to be pan-neural in the DRG. PAM mRNA was present throughout the grey matter but concentrated in the dorsal horn and in motoneurons indicating preferential spinal sites of peptide amidation. In addition, PAM was expressed in the ependyma and in endothelial cells. Carboxypeptidase E mRNA showed high levels of pan-neural expression. Furin mRNA exhibited pan-neural and pan-glial expression.

Molecular plasticity of the spinal cord in peripheral inflammation

In unilateral models of inflammation, changes in the expression of neuropeptides, neuropeptide receptors, and pre-pro-peptide processing enzymes were essentially ipsilateral and tended to increase with the duration of inflammation. As reported earlier, there was striking ipsilateral increase in the expression of DYN and ENK mRNAs and immunoreactivity for the respective peptides in the dorsal horn.[22,45,64] Some deep dorsal horn neurons exhibited co-upregulation of PRO-ENK and PRO-DYN mRNA and immunoreactivities. DYN and ENK was always co-upregulated with *c-fos*.[37,64] Serotonin-1A receptors were implicated as crucial activators of increased PRO-DYN expression[32] suggesting that descending pathways are needed for DYN-Fos co-upregulation while FOS-upregulation alone is 5HT-1A independent. There was a striking increase in the density of DYN-ir fibers throughout the ipsilateral dorsal horn. Many of these DYN-ir fibers co-stained for SP.[64] Some galanin-ir neurons were also observed in the deep dorsal horn.[64]

Unilateral inflammation caused a significant upregulation of PC1 and PC2 mRNA levels and immunostaining in a selective subpopulation of neurons in the ipsilateral superficial and deep dorsal horn. These neurons also exhibited increased opioid gene expression. The increased spinal expression of PC1 and PC2 following peripheral inflammation and the suggestive colocalization of the changes with upregulated opioid-genes point to a potentially important role of PCs in spinal processing of nociception. Unilateral inflammation also caused a 2-fold increase in NK1 receptor mRNA in a distinct subpopulation of neurons in the ipsilateral superficial and deep dorsal horn.[51] The distribution of such neurons coincided with that of neurons exhibiting increased levels of DYN mRNA in the superficial and deep dorsal horn. However direct evidence for coexistence of NK1 receptor and DYN expression is missing. NK1 receptor expression may even be upregulated in those lamina I projection neurons which exhibit an inflammation-induced increase in preprotachykinin mRNA.[38] Increased spinal release of SP and NKA, known to occur in adjuvant induced inflammation,[11] may cause downregulation of spinal TK receptors at the sites of increased release. Thus, it was surprising to find that the NK1 receptor expression was upregulated. The increased expression of spinal NK1 receptors in peripheral inflammation may reflect a fundamental spinal mechanism in hyperalgesia. Fleetwood-Walker's group provides evidence that inflammation-induced PRO-DYN upregulation can be suppressed by NK-2 receptor antagonist whereas the NK1 receptor is without effect.[40] Brief nociceptive inputs to lamina III/V were mediated by NK-2 receptors.[13] These NK receptor data lend further support to the crucial role of TKs and NK receptor subtypes in spinal nociception and antinociception and processing of inflammatory signals from the periphery.

Interestingly, there is also evidence for molecular plasticity in motoneurons.[57] CGRP-immunoreactivity and CGRP gene expression in motoneurons are downregulated by inflammation. Corticosteroid treatment of arthritic rats restores this downregulation. CCK and galanin may also be important in motoneuron function but it is not known whether their expression in motoneurons changes in inflammation.[24]

Various opioids downregulate inflammation-induced upregulation of spinal FOS expression.[1,8,44,59] Kappa agonists were found to downregulate carrageenin-induced spinal c-fos immunoreactivity and expression of c-fos and PRO-DYN genes. Whether downregulation of FOS expression leads to selective downregulation of the inflammation-induced upregulation of opioid and NK-receptor gene expression is an open question.

In rats subjected to collagen-induced arthritis (CIA), PRO-DYN gene expression and immunoreactivity in the dorsal horns was dramatically upregulated compared to the low basal expression in control animals. There was an enormous increase in the density of DYN-ir fibers in the superficial and deep dorsal horns and around the central canal. Corticosteroid treatment of arthritic rats caused a reduction of Inflammation-induced upregulation of PRO-DYN gene expression and immunoreactivity. Control rats treated with budesonide responded with a small upregulation of PRO-DYN gene expression and immunoreactivity. Changes in PRO-ENK gene expression and immunoreactivity were essentially similar, but started from a much higher basal level.

Thus, corticosteroids slightly upregulate basal and significantly downregulate inflammation-induced opioid gene expression. This suggests differential molecular mechanisms regulating the response of spinal opioid expression to corticosteroids that are not stereotyped but depend on the specific state of cellular activity. The spinal changes of dynorphin expression are nicely paralleled by synchronous changes in enzymatic activity of the dynorphin converting enzyme which is decreased in the CSF at the peak phase of collagen arthritis.[42] This finding has also been observed in monoarthritic rats. Interestingly, opposite changes of dynorphin converting enzyme activity were observed in spontaneously hypertensive rats subjected to long term voluntary running as compared to non-runners.[41] This may point to challenge specific plasticity of spinal dynorphin expression and dynorphin converting enzyme activity.

SUMMARY, CONCLUSIONS, AND FUTURE PERSPECTIVES

The expression of opioid and proto-type sensory neuropeptides SP/CGRP in primary afferents is much more widespread than currently believed. Peripheral target cell relations of peptidergic nociceptors are complex and include a wide range of cell types, namely keratinocytes, endothelial cells, smooth muscle cells, mast cells, plasma cells, dendritic cells, macrophages, fibroblasts, and Schwann cells. Multiple short and long term neuroeffector functions of primary afferent mediators on these target cells are conceivable. Neuropeptide receptor expression revealed at the cellular level (e.g. NK1 receptor on endothelial cells) by applying molecular biology techniques on intact tissues will provide further insight into the molecular specificity of neuro-target cell communication. The enormous potential of cytokines, growth factors and other substances which are produced by, and released from these target cells are likely to influence short and long term functions of primary afferents. The molecular events in inflamed tissues and mechanisms of nociceptor activation during acute and chronic phases of inflammation are extremely complex and involve multiple pro-inflammatory and pro-algesic mediators but probably an unrecognized panoply of anti-inflammatory and analgesic mediators too. Opioids may be among them but their precise cellular production site in the periphery remains to be defined. In any case, mutual influences between neural and non-neural elements can be envisaged as a regulating principle of physiological homeostasis. Pathophysiological reactions may be triggered and maintained by a disturbance of neuro-target cell cross-talk rather than by isolated dysfunction of neural elements or a particular target cell type. This applies to the CNS too. There is likely role of microglia- and astrocyte-derived cytokines, NO, prostaglandins etc in neuropathic pain with degeneration/regeneration events in the dorsal horn. These may effect neuronal peptide-gene expression in the spinal cord directly. Such mechanisms may be reponsible for pain in multiple sclerosis and HIV-infection. Experimental peripheral inflammation in the rat induces cytospecific, and spatially and temporally coordinated changes in the neuronal and non-neuronal expression of neuropeptides, neuropeptide receptors and pre-pro-peptide processing enzymes. In the periphery, the biphasic opposite response of intraepidermal CGRP-ergic and TK-ergic innervation may reflect increased release and depletion of neuropeptides from nociceptor endings in the early phase of inflammation, and sustained increase in the intraepidermal density of CGRP/TK containing fibers suggests sprouting phenomena during the prolonged phase of inflammation. Maintained reduction of peri-arterial NPY innervation may indicate downregulation of NPY synthesis in postganglionic sympathetic neurons supplying the inflamed target region or reflect sympathetic degeneration. Whether the various changes in the expression of messengers and receptors in non-neural cells may be epiphenomena of the inflammatory process or causally related to peripheral mechanism of nociception and neuroimmune interactions remains unclear.

Molecular changes in the spinal cord are a domain of sensory opioid and TK circuits in the dorsal horn but also concern motoneurons. Molecular responses of preganglionic sympathetic neurons such as upregulation of NK1 receptors and plasicity in the gene expression of postganglionic sympathetic neurons are a promising unexplored area.

The modulation of inflammation-induced FOS and opioid expression by receptor-selective opioid agonists and corticosteroids, respectively, suggests promising perspectives of the use of other selective neuromessenger agonists/antagonists and anti-inflammatory drugs. Using such strategies it may be possible to unravel the cybernetics of molecular plasticity of spinal nociceptive processing and antinociceptive drug action. Furthermore, it is timely to envisage intrathecal appplication of oncogene- and transmitter-selective anti-sense oligodeoxynucleotides[60] to further explore basic molecular mechanism of inflammatory pain and its pharmacotherapy.

ACKNOWLEDGEMENT

We thank T. Fink, D. Nohr, D. Knebel, H. Romeo, R. Stark from our laboratory for personal communication of unpublished data. Data of R. Stark and D. Knebel will be contained in their medical thesis. Work from our laboratory on the effect of kappa opioid agonists on carrageenan--induced inflammation was carried out in collaboration with and support by Merck, Darmstadt (Prof. Wolf, Dr. Bartoszyk, Dr. Seyfried, Dr. Haase). The study of the collagen-II induced arthritis is an ongoing collaboration with Prof. C. Post and Dr.G. Ekstrom (Astra Draco AB, Lund, Sweden) and Prof. F. Nyberg and Stefan Persson (Institute of Pharmaceutical Bioscience, Division of Pharmacology, University of Uppsala, Sweden). Data on prohormone processing enzymes (PC1 and PC2) are from collaborative work with Dr. R. Day and Dr. N. G. Seidah (J.A. DeSeve Laboratories of Biochemical Neuroendocrinology, Clinical Research Institute of Montreal, Canada). Data mentioned about Herpes-virus were obtained in collaboration with Prof. P. Falke (Dept. Virology, University of Mainz, F.R.G.). Chromogranin and monkey studies were done with Dr. L.E. Eiden (NIMH, Bethesda). We thank Prof. F. Nyberg for the donation of antisera against CGRP and Dynorphin A 1-17. We thank Prof. N. Yanaihara (Shizuoka, Japan) for supply of antisera against VIP, PHI, NPY, galanin and c-fos and Dr. M. Iadarola

(NIH, Bethesda) for donation of *c-fos* antisera. The study was supported by the Deutsche Forschungsgemeinschaft (DFG grants We 910/2-1/2-2/2-3), by the Stiftung Volkswagenwerk, BMFT and the Naturwissenschaftlich-Medizinisches Forschungszentrum (NMFZ) der Universitat Mainz.

REFERENCES

1. ABBADIE, C. AND BESSON, J. (1993) Effects of morphine and naloxone on basal and evoked Fos-like immunoreactivity in lumbar spinal cord neurons of arthritic rats. *Pain* **52**, 29-39.
2. BARANIUK, J.N., KOWALSKI, M.L., AND ALINER, M.A. (1990) Relationship between permeable vessels, nerves, and mast cells in rat cutaneous neurogenic inflammation. *J. Appl. Physiol.* **68**, 2305-2311.
3. BARBER, A. AND GOTTSCHLICH, R. (1992) Opioid agonists and antagonists: an evaluation of their peripheral actions in inflammation. *Med. Res. Rev.* **12**, (1992) 525-562.
4. BARRON, B.A., PIERZCHALA K. AND VAN LOON G.R. (1990) Source of stress-induced increase in plasma met-enkephalin in rats: contribution of adrenal medulla and/or sympathetic nerves. *J. Neuroendocrinol.* **2**, 381-388.
5. BETTE, M., SCHAFER, M.K.-H., VAN ROOIJEN, N. AND WEIHE, E. (1993) Distribution and kinetics of superantigen-induced cytokine gene expression in mouse spleen. (in press).
6. CHEN, Y., MESTEK, A., LIU, J., HURLEY, J.A. AND YU, L. (1993) Molecular cloning and functional expression of a u-opioid receptor from rat brain. *Mol. Pharmacol.* **44**, (in press).
7. CINTRA, A., FUXE, K., SOLFRINI, V., AGNATI, L.F., TINNER, B., WIKSTROM, A., STAINES, W., OKRET, S. AND GUSTAFSSON, J. (1991) Central peptidergie neurons as targets for glucocorticoid action. Evidence for the presence of glucocorticoid receptor immunoreactivity in various types of classes of peptidergic neurons, J. Steroid Biochem. *Mol. Biol.* **40**, 93-103.
8. CODERRE, T.J., KATZ, J., VACCARINO, A.L. AND MELZACK, R. (1993) Contribution of central neuroplasticity to pathological pain: review of clinical and experimental evidence. *Pain* **52**, 259-285.
9. CUNHA, F.Q., LORENZETTI, B.B., POOLE, S. AND FERREIRA, S.H., Interleukin-8 as a mediator of sympathetic pain. *Br. J. Pharmacol.* **104**, 765-767.
10. DUBNER, R. AND RUDA, M. A. (1992) Activity-dependent neuronal plasticity following tissue injury and inflammation. *Trends Neurosci.* **15**, 96-103.
11. DUGGAN, A.W. AND WEIHE, E. (1991) Central transmission of impulses in

nociceptors: events in the superficial dorsal horn. In: *Towards a new pharmacotherapy of pain.* eds. A. I. Basbaum and J. Besson. John Wiley & Sons Ltd, Chichester, pp. 35-67.

12. EVANS, C. J., KEITH, JR., D. E., MORRISON, H., MAGENDZO, K. AND EDWARDS. R. H. (1992) Cloning of a delta opioid receptor by functional expression. *Science* **258**, 1952-1955.

13. FLEETWOOD-WALKER, S.M., PARKER, R.M.C., MUNRO, F.E., YOUNG, M.R., HOPE, P.J. AND MITCHELL, R. (1993) Evidence for a role of NK-2 receptors in mediating brief nociceptive inputs to rat dorsal horn (laminae II-V) neurons, *Eur. J. Pharmacol.* (in press).

14. FREIDIN, M. AND KESSLER, J. A. (1991) Cytokine regulation of substance P expression in sympathetic neurons. *Proc. Natl. Acad. Sci. USA* **88**, 3200-3203.

15. GOGAS, K. R., PRESLEY, R. W., LEVINE, J. D. AND BASBAUM, A. I. (1991) The antinociceptive action of supraspinal opioids results from an increase in descending inhibitory control; correlation of nociceptive behavior and c-fos expression. *Neuroscience* **42**, 617-628.

16. HANDWERKER, H. 0. (1991) What peripheral mechanisms contribute to nociceptive transmission and hyperalgesia? In: *Towards a new pharmacotherapy of pain.* eds.: A.I. Basbaum and J.-M. Besson. John Wiley & Sons Ltd, Chichester, pp.5-19.

17. HANESCH, U., HEPPELMANN, B. AND SCHMIDT, R. F. (1991) Substance P- and calcitonin gene-related peptide immunoreactivity in primary afferent neurons of the cat's knee joint. *Neuroscience* **45**, l85-193.

18. HARLAN, R. E. (1988) Regulation of neuropeptide gene expression by steroid hormones. *Mol. Neurobiol.* **2**, 183-200.

19. HASSAN, A. H. S., PRZEWLOCKI,R., HERZ, A. AND STEIN, C. (1992) Dynorphin, a preferential ligand for k-opioid receptors, is present in nerve fibers and immune cells within inflamed tissue of the rat. *Neurosci. Lett.* (in press).

20. HERDEGEN, T., KOVARY, K., LEAH, J. AND BRAVO, R. (1991) Specific temporal and spatial distribution of JUN, FOS, and KROX-24 proteins in spinal neurons following noxious transsynaptic stimulation. *J. Comp. Neurol.* **313**, 178-91.

21. HOKFELT, T., Neuropeptides in perspective: The last ten years, Neuron, 7 (1991) 867-879.

22. IADAROLA, M. J., BRADY, L. S., DRAISCI, G. AND DUBNER, R. (1988) Enhancement of dynorphin gene expression in spinal cord following experimental inflammation: stimulus specificlty, behavioral parameters and opioid receptor binding. *Pain* **35**, 313-326.

23. JANIG, W. AND McLACHLAN, E.M. (1992) Characteristics of function-specific pathways in the sympathetic nervous system. *Trends in Neurosci.* **15**, 478-481.

24. JOHNSON, H., HOKFELT, T. AND ULFHAKE, B. (1992) Galanin and CGRP-like immunoreactivity coexist in rat spinal motoneurons, *NeuroReport* **3**, 303-306.

25. JONAT, C., RAHMSDORF, H.J., PARK, K.-K., CARO, A.C.B., GEBEL, S., PONTA, H. AND HERRLICH, P. (1990) Antitumor promotion and antiinflammation: down-modulation of AP-1 (Fos/Jun) activity by glucocorticoid hormone. *Cell* **62**, 1189-1204.

26. KAR, S., GIBSON, S. J., REES, R. G., JURA, W. G., BREWERTON, D. A. AND POLAK, J. M. (1991) Increased calcitonin gene-related peptide (CGRP), substance P, and enkephalin immunoreactivities in dorsal spinal cord and loss of CGRP-immunoreactive motoneurons in arthritic rats depend on intact peripheral nerve supply. *J. Mol. Neurosci.* **3**, 7-18.

27. KEW, D. AND KILPATRICK, D.L. (1990) Widespread organ expression of the rat proenkephalin gene during early postnatal development. *Mol. Endocrinol.* **4**, 337-340.

28. KIEFFER, B. L., BEFORT, K., GAVBRIAUX-RUFF, C. AND HIRTH, C. G. (1992) The d-opioid receptor: Isolation of a cDNA by ex The d-opioid receptor and pharmacological characterization. *Proc. Natl. Acad. Sci. USA* **89**, 12048-12052.

29. LEVINE, D.J., FIELDS H.L. SAND BASBAUM, A.I. (1993)Peptides and the primary afferent nociceptor. *J. Neurosci.* **13**, 2273-2286.

30. LEWINE, G.R. AND MENDELL, L.M. (1993) Nerve growth factor and nociception. *Trends Neurosci* **16**, 353-359.

31. LU, J., HATHAWAY, C.B.,. AND BEREITER, D.A.,. (1993) Adrenalectomy enhances fos-like immunoreactivity within the spinal trigeminal nucleus induced by noxious thermal stimulation of the cornea. *Neuroscience* **54**, 809-818.

32. LUCAS, J.J., MELLSTROM, B., COLADO, M.I. AND NARANJO, J.R. (1993) Molecular mechanisms of pain: Serotonin 1A receptor agonists trigger transactivation by c-fos of the prodynorphin gene in spinal cord neurons. *Neuron* **10**, 599-611.

33. MAGGI, C. A. (1991) The pharmacology of the efferent function of sensory nerves. *J. Auton. Pharmac.* **11**, 173-208.

33a. McLACHLAN, E.M., JANIG, W., DEVOR, M. AND MICHAELIS, M. PERIPHERAL NERVE INJURY TRIGGERS NORADRENERGIC SPROUTING WITHIN DORSAL ROOT GANGLIA. *Nature* **363**, 543-546.

34. MEAROW, K.M., KRIL, Y. AND DIAMOND, J. (1993) Increased NGF mRNA expression in denervated rat skin. *NeuroReport* **4**, 351-354.

35. MECHANIK, J.I., LEVIN, N., ROBERTS, J.L. AND AUTELITATNO, D.J. (1992) Proopiomelanocortin gene expression in a distinct population of rat spleen and lung leukocytes. *Endocrinology* **131**, 518-525.

36. MILLAN, M. J., Multiple opioid systems and chronic pain. In: *The opioids.* ed.: A. Herz. Springer, Heidelberg, (in press).

37. NOGUCHI, K., KOWALSKI, K., TRAUB, R., SOLODKIN, A., IADAROLA, M. J. AND RUDA, M. A. (1991) Dynorphin expression and Fos-like immunoreactivity following inflammation induced hyperalgesia are colocalized in spinal cord neurons. *Mol Brain Res.*. **10**, 227-233.

38. NOGUCHI, K. AND RUDA, M.A. (1992) Gene regulation in an ascending

nociceptive pathway: inflammation-induced increase in preprotachykinin mRNA in rat lamina I projection neurons. *J. Neurosci.* **12**, 2563-2572.

39. NOGUCHI, K., DE LEON, R.L., NAHIN, E., SENBA, E. AND RUDA, M.A. (1993) Quantification of axotomy-induced alteration of neuropeptide mRNAs in dorsal root ganglion neurons with special reference to neuropetide Y mRNA and the effects of neonatal capsaicin treatment. *J. Neurosci. Res.* **35**, 54-66.

40. PARKER, R.M.C., FLEETWOOD-WALKER, S.M., ROSIE, R., MUNRO, F.E. AND MITCHELL, R. (1993) Inhibition by NK-2 but not NK1 antagonists of carrageenan-induced preprodynorphin expression in rat dorsal horn lamina I. *Neuropeptides* (In press).

41. PERSONN, E., MALHERBE, P. AND RICHARDS, J. G., In situ hybridization histochemistry reveals a diversity of GABA receptor subunit mRNAs in neurons of the rat spinal cord and dorsal root ganglia, Neuroscience, 42 (1991) 497-507.

42. PERSSON, S., POST, C., HOLMDAHL, R. AND NYBERG, F. (1992) Decreased neuropeptide-converting enzyme activities in cerebrospinal fluid during acute but not chronic phases of collagen induced arthritis in rats. *Brain Res.* **581**, 273-282.

43. PLANTINGA, L.C., VERHAAGEN, J., EDWARDS, P.M., SCHRAMA, L.H., BURBACH J.P.H., AND GISPEN, W.H., Expression of the pro-opiomelanocortin

44. PRESLEY, R. W., MENETREY, D., LEVINE, J. D. AND BASBAUM, A. I. (1990) Systemic morphine suppresses noxious stimulus-evoked Fos protein-like immunoreactivity in the rat spinal cord. *J. Neurosci.* **10**, 323-335.

45. PRZEWLOCKA, B., LASON, W. AND PRZEWLOCKI, R. (1992) Time-dependent changes in the activity of opioid systems in the rat spinal cord of monoarthritic rats - a release and in situ hybridization study. *Neuroscience* **46**, 209-216.

46. PRZEWLOCKI, R., HASSAN. A. H. S., LASON, W., EPPLEN, C., HERZ, A. AND STEIN, C. (1992) Gene expression and localization of opioid peptides in immune cells of inflamed tissue: functional role in antinociception. *Neuroscience* **48**, 491-500.

47. ROGERS, H., BIRCH, P.J., HARRISON, S.M., PALMER, E., MANCHEE, G.R., JUDD, D.B., NAYLOR, A., SCOPES, D.I.C. AND HAYES, A.G. (1992) GR94839, a kappa-opioid agonist with limited access to the central nervous system, has antinociceptive activity. *Br. J. Pharmacol.* **106**, 783-789.

48. ROSEN, H., POLAKIEWICZ, R.D., BENZAKINE, S. AND BAR-SHAVIT, Z. (1991) Proenkephalin A in bone-derived cells. *Proc. Natl. Acad. Sci. USA* **88**, 3705-3709.

49. RUSIN, K. I., RYU, P. D. AND RANDIC, M. (1992) Modulation of excitatory amino acid responses in rat dorsal horn neurons by tachykinins. *J. Neurophysiol.* **68**, 265-286.

50. SCHAFER, M. K.-H., DAY, R., SEIDAH, N., CHRETIEN, M. AND WEIHE, E. (1992) Gene expression of novel prohormone convertases in the rat spinal cord. *Neuropeptides* **22**, 59-60.

51. SCHAFER, M. K.-H., NOHR, D., KRAUSE, J. E. AND WEIHE, E. (1993) Unilateral peripheral inflammation upregulates tachykinin receptor gene expression in the ipsilateral dorsal horn of rat spinal cord. *NeuroReport* **4**, 1007-1010.

52. SCHAFER, M.K.-H., NOHR, D., ROMEO, H., EIDEN, L.E. AND WEIHE, E. (1993) Pan-neuronal expression of chromogranin A in rat nervous system. *Peptides* (in press).

53. SHADIACK , A.M., HART, R.P., CARLSON, C.D. AND MILLER JONAKEIT, G. (1993) Interleukin-1 induces substance P in sympathetic ganglia through the induction of leukemia inhibitor factor (LIF). *J. Neurosci.* **13**, 2601-2609.

54. STEIN, C., GRAMSCH, C. AND HERZ, A. (1990) Intrinsic mechanisms of antinociception in inflammation: local opioid receptors and β-endorphin. *J. Neurosci.* **10**, 1292-1298.

55. SMITH, G.D., SECKL, J.R., SHEWARD, W.J., BENNIE, J.G., CARROLL S.M., DICK, H. AND HARMAR, A.J. (1991) Effect of adrenalectomy and dexamethasone on neuropeptide content of dorsal root ganglia in the rat. *Brain Res.* **564**, 27-30.

56. TAIWO, Y. O., LEVINE, J. D., BURCH, R. M., WOO, J. E. AND MOBLEY, W. C. (1991) Hyperalgesia induced in the rat by the amino-terminal octapeptide of nerve growth factor. *Proc. Natl. Acad. Sci. USA* **88**, 5144-5148.

57. TAQUUET, H., PLACHOT, J.J. POHL, M., COLLIN, E., BENOLIEL, J.J., BOURGOIN, S., MAUBORGNE, A., MEUNIER, J.C., CESSELIN, F. AND HAMON, M. (1992) Increased calcitonin gene-related peptide- and cholecystokinin-like immunoreactivities in spinal motoneurones after dorsal rhizotomy. *J. Neur. Transmiss.* **88**, 127-141.

58. THAI, L., LEE, P. H. K., HO, J., SUH, H. AND HONG, J. S. (1992) Regulation of prodynorphin gene expression in the hippocampus by glucocorticoids. *Mol. Brain Res.* **16**, 150-157.

59. TOLLE, T. R., CASTRO-LOPES, J. M. AND ZIEGLGANSBERGER, W. (1991) C-fos induction in the spinal cord following noxious stimulation: prevention by opiates but not by NMDA antagonists. In: *Proceedings of the VIth World Congress on Pain.* eds: M. R. Bond, J. E. Charlton, and C. J. Woolf. Elsevier Science Publishers, Amsterdam, pp. 299-305.

60. WAHLESTEDT, C., PICH, E.M., KOOB, G.F., YEE, F. AND HEILIG (1993) Modulation of anxiety and neuropeptide Y-Y1 receptors by antisense oligodeoxynucleotides. *Science* **259**, 528-531.

61. WEIHE, E., NOHR, D., MICHEL, S., MULLER, S., ZENTEL, H., FINK, T. AND KREKEL, J. (1991) Molecular anatomy of the neuro-immune connection. *Intern. J. Neurosci.* **59**, 1-23.

62. WEIHE, E., HARTSCHUH, W. AND NOHR, D. (1991) Light microscopic immunoenzyme and electron microscopic immunogold cytochemistry reveal tachykinin immuno-reactivity in Merkel cells of pig skin. *Neurosci. Lett.* **124**, 260-263.

63. WEIHE, E., MULLER, S., BUCHLER, M., FRIESS, H. AND NOHR, D. (1991) The tachykinin neuroimmune connection in inflammatory pain. In: *Substance P*

and related peptides: cellular and molecular physiology. eds.: S. E. Leeman, J. E. Krause, and Lembeck, F. New York Academy of Sciences, New York, pp. 283-295.

64. WEIHE, E. (1992) Neurochemical anatomy of the mammalian spinal cord: functional implications. *Annals of Anatomy* **174**, 89-118.

65. WEIHE, E., SCHAFER, M-K.-H., PERSSON, S., NOHR, D., POST, C., EKSTROM, G. AND NYBERG, F. (1993) Glucocorticoids modulate basal and inflammation-induced opioid gene expression in rat spinal cord. *Br. J. Pharmacol.* (in press).

66. WEIHE, E., SCHAFER, M.K.-H., NOHR, D. AND PERSSON, S. (1993) Expression of neuropeptides, neuropeptide receptors and neuropeptide processing enzymes in spinal neurons and peripheral non-neural cells and plasticity in model of inflammatory pain, In: *Neuropeptides, nociception and pain.* eds.: Schmidt, R.F. and Schaible, H.G. V.C.H. Weinheim, (In press).

67. WINKLER, H. AND FISCHER-COLBRIE, R. (1992) The chromogranins A and B: the first 25 years and future perspestives, **49**, 497-528.

68. VAN WOUDENBERG, A.D., METZELAAR, M.J., VAN DER KLEIJ, A. A. M., DE WIED, D., BURBACH, J.P.H. AND WIEGANT, V.M.(1993) Analysis of pro-opiomelanocortin (POMC) mRNA and POMC-derived peptides in human peripheral blood mononuclear cells: no evidence for a lymphocyte-derived POMC system, *Endocrinology* (in press).

69. YASUDA, K., RAYNOR, K., KONG, H., BREDER, C.D., TAKEDA, J., REISINE, T. AND BELL, G.I. (1993) Cloning and functional comparison of kappa and delta opioid receptors from mouse brain. *Proc. Natl. Acad. Sci. USA* **90**, 6736-6740.

ALTERED FUNCTIONS OF NEUROPEPTIDES AND NITRIC OXIDE IN SOMATOSENSORY AFFERENTS AND SPINAL CORD AFTER PERIPHERAL NERVE LESIONS IN THE RAT

Zsuzsanna Wiesenfeld-Hallin and Xiao-Jun Xu
Department of Clinical Physiology, Section of Clinical Neurophysiology
Karolinska Institute, Huddinge University Hospital
S-141 86 Huddinge
Sweden

EFFECTS OF PERIPHERAL NERVE INJURY ON THE EXPRESSION OF NEUROPEPTIDES AND NITRIC OXIDE IN PRIMARY SENSORY AFFERENTS

Peripheral nerve injury causes complex physiological and biochemical changes in sensory neurons and the spinal cord, including dramatic alteration of peptide synthesis. Thus, a few days after axotomy of the peripheral branch of sensory nerves, there is a significant decrease in the number of substance P (SP) and somatostatin (SOM) containing dorsal root ganglion (DRG) cells and SP and SOM content in afferent terminals in the spinal cord,[8,32,46] which was recently demonstrated to be due to decreased synthesis in sensory neurons.[41] Similar, but less profound and slower reduction of calcitonin gene-related peptide (CGRP) level has also been reported[52]. In contrast, the levels of vasoactive intestinal peptide (VIP), galanin (GAL), neuropeptide Y (NPY) and cholecystokinin (CCK) are dramatically increased in sensory neurons,[26,36,46,48,54,73] which is also due to upregulated peptide synthesis.[41,42,48,51]

NATO ASI Series, Vol. H 79
Cellular Mechanisms of Sensory Processing
Edited by Laszlo Urban
© Springer-Verlag Berlin Heidelberg 1994

Nitric oxide (NO) is a recently identified messenger in the nervous system and may have a variety of functions.[11,19,39] NO may mediate mechanical, chemical and thermal nociceptive input in the somatosensory system at spinal level[22,33,38]. NO is synthesised from L-arginine by the enzyme NO synthase (NOS)[10]. Due to its high lipophilicity, NO can diffuse through cell membranes and influence adjacent cells[11] and in rat dorsal root ganglia NO has been suggested to function as a signalling system between sensory and satellite cells[40]. It was recently found that there is a marked increase in NOS mRNA in rat DRG within two days after peripheral nerve section, which was maintained for at least two months,[50] and was paralleled by increase in NOS protein.[78] The increase in NOS mRNA in axotomized ganglion cells was similar to the increased levels of several neuropeptides and NOS mRNA was found to partially co-exist with the mRNA for these neuropeptides after axotomy.[50]

The functional significance of these changes in levels of peptides and NO after peripheral axotomy has been unclear, although it has been proposed that peptides like VIP may have trophic functions to promote neuronal regeneration[35]. Physiologically, peripheral nerve injury leads to a number of changes in primary afferents and spinal cord, including the development of ongoing discharges in both myelinated and unmyelinated afferents,[12,21,56,58] the appearance of spontaneous discharges and altered receptive fields in deafferented dorsal horn neurons,[4,14,30,34] as well as a decrease of the dorsal root potential and of primary afferent depolarization.[55] However, there was no change in the effect of C-fiber input onto dorsal horn neurons, neither was the facilitation of the flexor reflex induced by sural nerve conditioning stimuli (CS) influenced by peripheral nerve section.[60]

Peripheral nerve injury can lead to the development of chronic painful states in some patients which can be difficult to treat.[47] There have been numerous animal models developed for neuropathic pain, including autotomy, a behavior where an animal inflicts damage to the deafferented limb after transection of a peripheral nerve or dorsal roots.[13,57] Autotomy may reflect painful or abnormal sensations referred to the deafferentated body region.[13]

In recent years, our laboratory has been engaged in examining the involvement of peptidergic systems and NO in studies of plasticity in primary afferent and spinal cord functions after peripheral nerve injury and some of the results have reviewed.[63,67,69,70,75,77] We have employed an electro-physiological preparation in which the spinal nociceptive flexor reflex was recorded in decerebrate, spinalized, unanesthetized rats with intact peripheral nerves or after unilateral section of the sciatic nerve.[59] The reflex is exquisitely sensitive to either intrathecally (i.t.) or systemically applied drugs, with increased excitability following the application of hyperalgesic and decreased reflex magnitude after analgesic substances. We have used the autotomy model to examine the involvement of some peptides in altering this behavioral sign of neuropathic pain. Finally, in the study with NO we have used a preparation in which the spontaneous acitivity originating from DRG after peripheral nerve injury was recorded.

ON THE INVOLVEMENT OF SP AND VIP IN THE MEDIATION OF SPINAL HYPEREXCITABILITY IN RATS WITH INTACT AND SECTIONED SCIATIC NERVES

A transient CS train of 20 shocks at 1 Hz applied to unmyelinated afferents elicits a pronounced increase in spinal cord excitability, lasting from a few minutes following cutaneous nerve stimulation to about an hour after activation of muscle afferents, as indicated by a prolonged facilitation of the flexor reflex[59]. This phenomenon, known as central sensitization, may reflect the hyperalgesia that occurs after tissue injury. We have observed that the reflex facilitation caused by cutaneous nerve CS in rat was blocked by peptide and non-peptide SP antagonists,[66,72] indicating that central sensitization can be mediated by the release of SP from C-afferents in rats with intact sciatic nerves. This conclusion seems, however, to be contradictory to the fact that there is severe depletion of SP from primary sensory afferents after nerve transection[8,32] and yet the central sensitization remained in axotomized rats.[60] In addition to SP, a number of sensory peptides were capable of inducing spinal hyperexcitability upon i.t. injection. Some of these, such as VIP[63] are upregulated after nerve section. It is therefore possible that the inconsistency between the level of SP in axotomized afferents and the ability of C-fibers to induce central sensitization may reflect the substitution of SP's function by VIP. To test this hypothesis, we have studied and compared the effect of the potent and non-toxic tachykinin antagonist spantide II[66] and a selective antagonist of

VIP, (Ac-Tyr[1], D-Phe[2])-GRF (1-29)[53], on the facilitation of the flexor reflex induced by cutaneous C-fiber CS in rats with intact and sectioned sciatic nerves. I.t. spantide II blocked the reflex facilitatory effect of i.t. SP and neurokinin A (NKA), but not other sensory peptides, such as VIP, SOM and CGRP, indicating the effect of spantide II was selective towards tachykinin receptors.[66] Similar selective blocking effect of VIP-induced reflex facilitation was observed with the VIP receptor antagonist.[74] In rats with intact sciatic nerves, pretreatment with spantide II effectively blocked reflex facilitation by the sural afferent CS with potency and duration similar to its blocking effect of i.t. SP[66] whereas no effect was found with the VIP antagonist.[74]

Ten to 14 days post axotomy, i.t. spantide II and the VIP-antagonist maintained their ability to block the reflex facilitation caused by i.t. SP and VIP respectively, just as in rats with intact sciatic nerves.[67] Furthermore, the sural CS caused comparable facilitation of the flexor reflex in rats with intact and sectioned sciatic nerves. However, the VIP-antagonist, but not spantide II, blocked the sural CS-induced reflex facilitation at 10-14 days post-axotomy.[67] Experiments performed at various times after nerve section revealed a linear decrease in the effectiveness of spantide II to block sural CS-induced reflex facilitation, which had the same time course as the decrease of SP synthesis in DRG after axotomy[41]. These results suggested that the normal role of tachykinins in inducing spinal hyperexcitability was taken over by VIP after peripheral nerve section. This was recently confirmed, as a coexpression of VIP and SP mRNA was observed in some DRG neurons a few days after axotomy, indicating that VIP is produced in the same neurons after axotomy that previously produced SP.[25]

ENDOGENOUS INHIBITORY CONTROL BY GALANIN ON SPINAL REFLEX EXCITABILITY AND AUTOTOMY BEHAVIOR AFTER PERIPHERAL NERVE SECTION

Galanin (GAL), a neuropeptide consisting of 29 amino acids, has been shown to occur in a relatively small population of DRG cells, primarily with small somata.[64] Previous studies in this and other laboratories have indicated that

GAL may have inhibitory actions upon nociceptive transmission at spinal level.[44,64,65,77,80] An increase in GAL synthesis and levels in primary sensory neurons and afferent terminals was demonstrated after peripheral nerve axotomy.[26,51] Correspondingly, there was increased outward-transport of newly synthesised GAL in both central and peripheral branches of primary sensory neurons.[52] These findings suggested that GAL may have a particularly important role in modulating sensory input in axotomized rats. Intrathecal (i..t.) GAL elicited three types of effects on the flexor reflex in rats with intact sciatic nerves: facilitation, facilitation followed by depression and in a few cases pure depression, in a dose-dependent manne.r[65] I.t. GAL in rats with sectioned nerves also evoked these three types of responses.[70] There was no significant difference in the magnitude of the facilitation by GAL on the flexor reflex between rats with intact and sectioned nerves, as judged by the peak response and duration of facilitation. However, after nerve section the depressive effect of GAL was significantly increased.[70] Inhibition occurred more often and at much lower doses. The depressive effect of GAL in axotomized rats was stronger and had more rapid onset than in rats with intact nerves. Coadministration of various doses of GAL with the sural nerve CS dose-dependently suppressed reflex facilitation induced by the sural CS in animals with intact, as well as sectioned, nerves.[65,77] There was no significant difference in the ability of GAL to antagonise the facilitatory effect of sural CS before and after nerve section.[77] The antagonistic effect of GAL on sural CS induced spinal hyperexcitability in rats with intact peripheral nerve was attributed, at least partly, to a post-synaptic antagonism of the facilitatory effect of i.t. SP and CGRP, peptides that normally coexist with GAL. After nerve section, GAL blocked the reflex facilitation induced by VIP and CGRP, but not by SP. Meanwhile, a strong coexistence between GAL and VIP emerged in deafferented DRG cells.

With the help of a series of chimeric peptides that are high affinitiy GAL antagonists,[9] we have examined the role of endogenous GAL in the mediation of spinal cord hyperexcitability and autotomy behavior. I.t. M35, GAL (1-12)-Pro-bradykinin (2-9)-amide, one of these GAL antagonists, potentiated the facilitation of the flexor reflex induced by sural nerve CS, an effect that was significantly enhanced in rats with sectioned sciatic nerves and after up-regulation of GAL in sensory neurons.[69] Similarly, chronic i.t. infusion of M35 through an osmotic minipump significantly exaggerated the autotomy behavior in rats after unilateral sciatic transection compared to saline treatment, without noticeably influencing the level of GAL mRNA in corresponding DRG and the dorsal horn.[49] These results strongly suggested that GAL plays an endogenous inhibitory role in somatosensory transmission and along with an increase in GAL level in sensory neurons, this role was enhanced after peripheral nerve injury. Thus, GAL may possess an inhibitory control upon the expression of neuropathic pain related symptoms.

The endogenous inhibitory function of GAL in the somatosensory system described in our studies supports a general inhibitory action of this peptide in the central and peripheral nervous systems.[23] An inhibitory action of GAL was further supported by studies at the molecular level in which it was found that the GAL receptor is coupled to an inhibitory guanine nucleotide binding protein and activation of the GAL receptor may lead to closure of a voltage-dependent Ca^{2+} channel, opening of an ATP-sensitive K^+ channel, inhibition of adenylate cyclase activity, and inhibition of inositol trisphosphate production, events associated with inhibition of neuronal function.

UP-REGULATION OF CHOLECYSTOKININ IN SENSORY NEURONS AND MORPHINE INSENSITIVITY ON NEUROPATHIC PAIN-RELATED BEHAVIOR IN RATS

Ever since the publication of the clinical study by Arnér and Meyerson[5] indicating that neuropathic pain is not relieved by morphine, the subject of morphine as a therapeutic agent for neuropathic pain has been fiercely contested.[43] Although no definite conclusion has been reached, it seems clear from the impression of many clinicians and from the literature that morphine and possibly other opioids are indeed relatively ineffective in treating pain originating from nervous system injury. We have previously reported that chronic i.t. infusion of morphine suppressed autotomy behavior.[62] However, this effect may be related to a preventive, rather than analgesic, effect of morphine upon the development of autotomy. We have recently found that a single i.t. injection of morphine 60 min before nerve transection effectively reduced the incidence of autotomy in axotomized rats during the following three weeks.[45] However, if i.t. injection commenced 24 h after nerve section, morphine applied twice daily had no beneficial effect upon autotomy.[45] Thus, this experimental study seems to support the clinical observation that morphine has a poor effect on neuropathic pain. We have suggested that this phenomenon may be derived from reduced sensitivity of the spinal cord to the antinociceptive effect of morphine in autotomizing rats.[75]

The mechanism(s) for a lack, or reduced effect of morphine on neuropathic pain is unclear, but this phenomenon is similar to the appearance of morphine tolerance, i.e., under both circumstances morphine failed to elicit the expected analgesic effect. CCK, being an endogenous peptide and well documented physiological opioid antagonist,[6,18,31,68] has been convincingly implicated in the development of morphine tolerance.[6,17,61,76,79] CCK normally exists in spinal cord interneurons, but not primary sensory neurons, in rat.[24,71] It was recently demonstrated that peripheral nerve injury caused a marked increase in CCK synthesis in rat DRG cells primarily with small somata.[48] We have conducted a study to determine whether endogenous CCK is involved in controlling the development of autotomy, as well as morphine insensitivity, after peripheral nerve section with CI 988, a highly selective and potent antagonist of the CCK-B receptor.[29,68] Autotomy behavior was not influenced by chronic i.t. injection of saline or morphine, nor by subcutaneous (s.c.) saline or CI988 alone. However, the combination of s.c. CI988 plus i.t. morphine significantly suppressed autotomy behavior.[73] This finding suggested that a possibly increased release of CCK from the terminals of primary sensory afferents antagonised the analgesic actions of opioid released either endogenously or applied exogenously. This resulted in the development of neuropathic pain-related behavior in rats. Another source of CCK in the spinal cord is from the terminals of descending tracts and spinal interneurons, but there was no evidence for increased CCK synthesis in these areas after peripheral nerve injury (Verge et al., unpublished observation). Thus, the clinical use of CCK receptor antagonists alone or in combination with opioid analgesics may provide a promising alternative in the pharmacological management of chronic neuropathic pain.

INVOLVEMENT OF NITRIC OXIDE IN SENSORY TRANSMISSION AFTER NERVE INJURY IN DORSAL ROOT GANGLIA AND SPINAL CORD

Ever increasing evidence indicates that nitric oxide (NO) may be an intra- and intercellular signal substance in the central and peripheral nervous system[11,19,39] and may be involved in the mediation of nociceptive input at the spinal level.[22,33,37,38] A marked increase in nitric oxide synthase (NOS) mRNA was observed in rat DRG within two days after peripheral nerve section, which was maintained for at least two months,[50] and was paralleled by increase in NOS protein[78]. We have conducted functional studies to examine the possible role of NO in somatosensory transmission in rats after peripheral nerve injury.

Two types of experiments have been performed. First, we have examined the involvement of NO in the spinal cord and DRG in the mediation of spinal cord hyperexcitability after CS of C-afferents. The NOS inhibitor nitro-L-arginine methyl ester (L-NAME) applied i.t. blocked with similar efficacy the facilitation of the flexor reflex induced by C-afferent CS in rats with intact and sectioned sciatic nerves.[50] Since i.t. L-NAME blocked spinal hyperexcitability similarly in normal and axotomized rats, we concluded, in agreement with previously reported antinociceptive effect of NOS inhibitors, that NO may have a role in some aspect of nociceptive transmission at the spinal level. This was not influenced by peripheral nerve section, also in agreement with the finding that the level of NOS mRNA in the dorsal horn interneurons was unchanged after axotomy (Zhang et al., unpublished observation). In contrast, L-NAME applied intravenously was much more effective in blocking C-fiber CS-induced reflex facilitation in axotomized than in normal rats, suggesting that L-NAME may have a peripheral action involving C-fiber activation which was enhanced by axotomy and may be related to the upregulation of NOS in DRG.[50]

Peripheral nerve injury can promote the development of ongoing discharges in both myelinated and unmyelinated afferents originating in the neuroma at the proximal stump of the axotomized nerve,[21,56,58] as well as in the DRG at associated segments.[12,56] We have conducted experiments to examine whether NO was involved in abnormal neural activity in axotomized rats. Spontaneously ongoing discharges were recorded in dorsal rootlets L4-5 which were responsive to electrical stimulation of the proximal end of the sectioned sciatic nerves. The latency of the evoked response indicated that the activity originated from afferents with myelinated axons with conduction velocities between 13 and 50 m/s. In order to identify the site of the effect of L-NAME on ongoing discharges, i.e. the DRG and/or the neuroma, the sciatic nerve was sectioned in some rats proximal to the neuroma after the sciatic origin of the ongoing activity in the rootlets was established by electrical stimulation. The nerve section induced a brief, intense discharge, followed by a stable ongoing discharge in all cases, which was not appreciably different from that recorded prior to cutting the nerve, suggesting that the ongoing activity recorded from the dorsal rootlets arose mainly, if not exclusively, from DRG. In rootlets activated by sciatic nerve stimulation, 100 µmol/kg i.v. L-NAME caused a reduction of ongoing activity by 55 % and 200 µmol/kg L-NAME reduced ongoing discharges by 81 %. In 3 out of 6 preparations, 200 µmol/kg L-NAME totally abolished the ongoing activity. L-arginine, the precursor of NO synthesis, briefly reversed the effect of L-NAME.

Increased NOS mRNA has been observed in axotomized DRG cells with widely ranging diameters and only the largest cells seemed to be devoid of NOS mRNA.[50] The block of ongoing activity in axotomized myelinated afferents by L-NAME, as well as the greater effectiveness of this NOS inhibitor in blocking C-fiber CS-induced reflex facilitation after axotomy, may indicate that NO may have a role in the function of both A and C-afferents after axotomy.

Ongoing activity was also recorded from more caudal or rostral rootlets in axotomized rats which were not influenced by sciatic stimulation, as well as from dorsal rootlets in normal rats that could be influenced by flexion or extension of the hind limb, presumably reflecting activity in proprioceptor afferents. Ongoing activity in rootlets that were not responsive to stimulation of the sciatic nerve or in rats with intact sciatic nerves was not influenced by 200 or 400 µmol/kg L-NAME. The lack of effect of L-NAME in normal rootlets may be correlated to the low level of NOS enzyme[2] and NOS mRNA in normal DRG[50] and indicated that the depressive effect of L-NAME on activity originating in axotomized DRG was not due to unspecific effects, such as changes in vasomotor tone.

Results from our physiological studies indicated that NO may act as an intra- and intercellular messenger within DRG cells after axotomy. A transmitter-like function has been assigned to NO. Activation of the N-methyl-D-aspartate (NMDA) receptor subtype for glutamate triggers NO formation, which activates soluble guanylate cyclase, leading to the formation of intracellular cGMP.[20] A role for NO in synaptic transmission involving the NMDA receptor at spinal cord has also been suggested.[37] NMDA receptor mRNA has been observed in rat sensory ganglion cells.[46a] It is possible that after peripheral nerve section activation of these receptors may lead to the production of NO. However, at the present time there is little evidence that receptors on DRG cell bodies are activated synaptically. Moreover, DRG neurons are not sensitive to NMDA[1] and DRG exposed to NMDA *in vitro* exhibit no change in basal cGMP levels.[40] Thus, it is unclear if this mechanism is involved in the generation of ongoing discharges in axotomized DRG cells.

Ongoing activity in DRG has been associated with the accumulation of K^+ in the extracellular space. NO, acting as an intracellular second messenger,[11] may be involved in generation of ongoing activity. Another possible mechanism for initiating ongoing discharges is the presence of cross-excitation among injured nerve fibers[3] and DRG cells.[15] It has been suggested that the cross-excitation among DRG neurons may be mediated by non-synaptic release of neuroactive compounds.[15] Due to the unusual features of NO, such as its ability to diffuse between neurons and to increase cellular cGMP, it may represent a good candidate for a neuroactive compound involving the interaction between DRG neurons. Although the triggering of NO synthesis in DRG cells is not likely to be through an interaction with NMDA receptors, there are many other neurotransmitters that may be candidates, as NO synthesis can be induced by an increase in intracellular calcium.[11] Neurotransmitters, such as substance P, have been collected from superfused DRG[27] and DRG neurons contain a wide range of membrane-associated neurotransmitter receptors.[7,16]

CONCLUSIONS

Our physiological and behavioral studies, in association with morphological studies, have established a complex plasticity of the role of peptides and NO in the mediation of somatosensory transmission at spinal level after peripheral axotomy, including a substitution of VIP in some of the functions of tachykinins, an enhanced role for GAL as an endogenous inhibitor, a role for CCK as an endogenous antagonist of opioids and a role for NO. Some of these functional changes may reflect abnormal sensory processing in the spinal cord after peripheral nerve injury. It is possible that drugs which can manipulate the function of peptidergic and NO systems, such as antagonists of VIP and CCK, GAL agonists and NOS inhibitors may be useful in treating neuropathic pain.

ACKNOWLEDGEMENTS: These studies have been supported by the Swedish MRC (project no. 07913), the Bank of Sweden Tercentenary Foundation, Astra Pain Control AB, Marcus och Amalia Wallenbergs Minnesfond, the Wenner-Gren Centre Foundation and research funds of the Karolinska Institute.

REFERENCES

1. AGRAWA,L S.G. AND EVANS, R.H. (1986) The primary afferent depolarizing action of kainate in the rat. *Br. J. Pharmacol.* **87**, 345-355.
2. AIMI, Y., FUJIMURA, S.R., VINCENT, S.R. AND KIMURA, H. (1991) Localization of NADPH-diaphorase-containing neurons in sensory ganglia of the rat. *J. Comp. Neurol.* **306**, 382-392.
3. AMIR, R. AND DEVOR, M. (1992) Axonal cross-excitation in nerve-end neuromas: Comparison of A- and C-fibers. J. Neurophysiol. **68**, 1160-1166.
4. ANDERSON, L.S., BLACK, R.G., ABRAHAM, J. AND WARD, A.A. (1971) Neuronal hyperactivity in experimental trigeminal deafferentation. *J. Neurosurg.* **35**, 444-452.
5. ARNÉR, S. AND MEYERSON, B. (1988) Lack of analgesic effect of opioids on neuropathic and idiopathic forms of pain. *Pain* **33**, 11-23.
6. BABER, N.S., DOURISH, C.T. AND HILL, D.R. (1989) The role of CCK, caerulein, and CCK antagonists in nociception. *Pain* **39**, 307-328.
7. BACCAGLINI, P.I. AND HOGAN, P.G. (1983) Some rat sensory neurons in culture express characteristics of differentiated pain sensory cells. *Proc. Natl. Acad. Sci. U.S.A.* **80**, 594-598.
8. BARBUT, D., POLAK, J.M. AND WALL, P.D. (1981) Substance P in spinal cord dorsal horn decreases following peripheral nerve injury. *Brain Res.* **205**, 289-298.

9. BARTFAI, T., FISONE, G. AND LANGEL, Ü. (1992) Galanin and galanin antagonists: molecular and biochemical perspectives. *Trends Pharmacol. Sci.* **13**, 312-317.

10. BREDT, D.S. AND SNYDER, S.H. (1990) Isolation of nitric oxide synthetase, a calmodulin-requiring enzyme. *Proc. Natl. Acad. Sci. U.S.A.* **87**, 682-285

11. BREDT, D.S., AND SYNDER, S.H. (1992) Nitric oxide, a novel neuronal messenger. *Neuron* **8**, 3-11.

12. BURCHIEL, K.J. (1984) Spontaneous impulse generation in normal and denervated dorsal root ganglia: Sensitivity to alpha-adrenergic stimulation and hypoxia. *Exp. Neurol.* **85**, 257-272.

13. CODERRE, T.J., GRIMES, R.W. AND MELZACK, R. (1986) Deafferentation and chronic pain in animals: an evaluation of evidence suggesting autotomy is related to pain. *Pain* **26**, 61-84.

14. DEVOR, M. AND WALL, P.D. (1981) Plasticity in the spinal cord sensory map following peripheral nerve injury in rats. *J. Neurosci.* **1**, 679-684.

15. DEVOR, M. AND WALL, P.D. (1990) Cross-excitation in dorsal root ganglia of nerve-injured and intact rats. *J. Neurophysiol.* **64**, 1733-1746.

16. DUNLAP, K. AND FISCHBACH, G.D. (1978) Neurotransmitters decrease the calcium conductance of sensory neurone action potentials. *Nature* **276**, 839-839.

17. DOURISH, C.T., O'NEILL, M.F., COUGHLAN, J., KITCHENER, S.J., HAWLEY, D. AND IVERSEN, S.D. (1990) The selective CCK-B receptor antagonist L-365,260 enhances morphine analgesia and prevents morphine tolerance in the rat. *Eur. J. Pharmacol.* **176**, 35-44.

18. FARIS, P.L., KOMISARUK, B.R., WATKINS, L.R. AND MAYER, D.J. (1983) Evidence for the neuropeptide cholecystokinin as an antagonist of opiate analgesia. *Science* **219**, 310-312.

19. GARTHWAITE, J. (1991) Glutamate, nitric oxide and cell-cell signalling in the nervous system. *Trends Neurosci.* **14**, 60-67

20. GARTHWAITE, J., CHARLES, S.L. AND CHESS-WILLIAMS, R. (1988) Endothelium-derived relaxing factor release on activation of NMDA receptors suggest a role as intracellular messenger in the brain. *Nature* **326**, 385-387.

21. GOVRIN-LIPPMANN, R. AND DEVOR, M. (1978) Ongoing activity in severed nerves: Source and variation with time. *Brain Res.* **159**, 406-410

22. HALEY, J.E., DICKENSON, A.H., AND SCHACHTER, M. (1992) Electrophysiological evidence for a role of nitric oxide in prolonged chemical nociception in the rat. *Neuroscience* **31**, 251-258

23. HÖKFELT, T., BARTFAI, T., JACOBOWITZ, D. AND OTTOSON, D. (eds) (1991) Galanin, A New Multifunctional Peptide in the Neuroendocrine System, Wenner-Gren Center Internaitonal Symposium Series, Vol. 58, Macmillan Press, Basingstoke.

24. HÖKFELT, T., HERRERA-MARSCHITZ, M., SEROOGY, K., JU G., STAINES, W.A., HOLETS, V., SCHALLING, M., UNGERSTEDT, U.,

POST, C., REHFELD, J.F., FREY, P., FISCHER, J., DOCKRAY, G., HAMAOKA, T., WALSH, J.H. AND GOLDSTEIN M. (1988) Immunohistochemical studies on cholecystokinin (CCK)-immunoreactive neurons in the rat using sequence specific antisera and with specific reference to the caudate nucleus and primary sensory neurons. *J. Chem. Neuroanat.* **1**, 11-52.

25. HÖKFELT, T., VERGE, V.M.K., WIESENFELD-HALLIN, Z. AND ERIKSSON, M. (1991) Upregulation of vasoactive intestinal peptide in substance P expressing primary sensory neurons after injury. *Soc. Neurosci. Abstr.* **17**, 439.

26. HÖKFELT, T., WIESENFELD-HALLIN, Z., VILLAR, M.J. AND MELANDER, T. (1987) Increase of galanin-like immunoreactivity in rat dorsal root ganglion cells after peripheral axotomy. *Neurosci. Lett.* **83**, 217-220.

27. HOLZ, G.G., IV, DUNLAP, K. AND KREAM, R.M. (1988) Characterization of the electrically evoked release of substance P from dorsal root ganglion neurons: methods and dihydropyridine sensitivity. *J. Neurosci.* **8**, 463-471.

28. HUETTNER, J.E. (1990) Glutamate receptor channels in rat DRG neurons: activation by kainate and quisqualate and blockade of desensitization by Con A. *Neuron* **5**, 255-266.

29. HUGHES, J., BODEN, P., COSTALL, B., DOMENEY, A., KELLY, E., HORWELL, D.C., HUNTER, J.C., PINNOCK, R.D. AND WOODRUFF, G.N. (1990) Development of a class of selective cholecystokinin type B receptor antagonists having potent anxiolytic activity. *Proc. Natl. Acad. Sci. U.S.A.* **87**, 6728-6732.

30. HYLDEN, J.L.K., NAHIN, R.L. AND DUBNER, R. (1987) Altered responses of nociceptive cat lamina I spinal dorsal horn neurons after chronic sciatic neuroma formation. *Brain Res.* **411**, 341-350.

31. ITOH, S., KATSUURA, G. AND MAEDA, Y. (1982) Caerulein and cholecystokinin suppress b-endorphin-induced analgesia in the rat. *Eur. J. Pharmacol.* **80**, 421-425.

32. JESSELL, T., TSUNOO, A., KANAZAWA, I. AND OTSUKA, M. (1979) Substance P: depletion in the dorsal horn of rat spinal cord after section of the peripheral processes of primary sensory neurons. *Brain Res.*, **168**, 247-259.

33. LEE, J.-H., WILCOX, G.L. AND BEITZ, A.J. (1992) Nitric oxide mediates Fos expression in the spinal cord induced by mechanical noxious stimulation. *Neuroreport* **3**, 841-844.

34. LOMBARD, M.-C. AND BESSON, J.-M. (1989) Attemps to gauge the relative importance of pre- and postsynaptic effects of morphine on the transmission of noxious messages in the dorsal horn of the rat spinal cord. *Pain* **37**, 335-346.

35. MAGISTRETTI, P.J., MORRISON, J.H., SHOEMAKER, W.J., SAPIN, V. AND BLOOM, F.E. (1981) Vasoactive intestinal polypeptide induced glycogenolysis in mouse cortical slices: A possible regulatory mechanism for the local control of energy metabolism. *Proc. Natl. Acad. Sci. U.S.A.* **78**, 6535-6539.

36. MCGREGOR, G.P., GIBSON, S.J., SABATE, I.M., BLANK, M.A., CHRISTOFIDES, N.D., WALL, P.D., POLAK, J.M. AND BLOOM, S.R. (1984) Effect of peripheral nerve section and nerve crush on spinal cord neuropeptides in the rat: increased VIP and PHI in the dorsal horn. *Neuroscience* **13**, 207-216.

37. MELLER, S.T., DYKSTRA, C. AND GEBHART, G.F. (1992) Production of endogenous nitric oxide and activation of soluble guanylate cyclase are required for N-methyl-D-aspartate-produced facilitation of the nociceptive tail-flick reflex. *Eur. J. Pharmacol.* **214**, 93-96.

38. MELLER S.T., PECHMAN, P.S., GEBHART, G.F. AND MAVES, T.J. (1992) Nitric oxide mediates the thermal hyperalgesia produced in a model of neuropathic pain in the rat. *Neuroscience* **50**, 7-10.

39. MONCADA, S. (1992) The L-arginine:nitric oxide pathway. The 1991 von Euler Lecture. *Acta Physiol. Scand.* **145**, 201-227.

40. MORRIS,, R., SOUTHAM, E., BRAID, D.J. AND GARTHWAITE, J. (1992) Nitric oxide may act as a messenger between dorsal root ganglion neurones and their satellite cells. *Neurosci. Lett.* **137**, 29-32.

41. NIELSCH, U. AND KEEN, P. (1989) Reciprocal regulation of tachykinin- and vasoactive intestinal peptide-gene expression in rat sensory neurones following cut and crush injury. *Brain Res.* 481, 25-30.

42. NOGUCHI, K., SENBA, E., MORITA, Y., SATO, M. AND TOHYAMA M. (1989) Prepro-VIP and preprotachykinin mRNAs in the rat dorsal root ganglion cells following peripheral axotomy. *Mol. Brain Res.* **6**, 327-330.

43. PORTENOY, R.K., FOLEY, K.M AND INTURRISI, C.E. (1991) The nature of opioid responsiveness and its implications for neuropathic pain: new hypothesis derived from studies of opioid infusions. *Pain.* **43**, 273-286.

44. POST, C., ALARI, L. AND HÖKFELT, T. (1988) Intrathecal galanin increases the latency in the tail flick and hot plate tests in mouse. *Acta Physiol. Scand.* **132**, 583-584.

45. PUKE, M.J.C. AND WIESENFELD-HALLIN, Z. (1993) The differential effects of morphine and the α_2 agonists clonidine and dexmedetomidine on the prevention and treatment of experimental neuropathic pain. *Anesth. Analg.* (in press).

46. SHEHAB, S.A.S. AND ATKINSON, M.E. (1986) Vasoactive intestinal polypeptide (VIP) increases in the spinal cord after peripheral axotomy of the sciatic nerve originates from primary afferent neurons. *Brain Res.* **372**, 37-44.

46a. SHIGEMOTO, R., OHISHI, H., NAKANISHI, S. AND MIZUNO, N. (1992) Expression of the mRNA for the rat NMDA receptor (NMDAR1) in the sensory and autonomic ganglion neurons. *Neurosci. Lett.* **144**, 229-232.

47. SUNDERLAND S. (1978) Nerves and Nerve Injuries, Churchill-Livingston, London.

48. VERGE, V.M.K., WIESENFELD-HALLIN, Z. AND HÖKFELT, T. (1993) Cholecystokinin in mammalian primary sensory neurons and spinal

cord: In situ hybridization studies on rat and monkey spinal ganglia. *Eur. J. Neurosci.* (in press).

49. VERGE V.M.K., XU, X.-J., LANGEL, Ü., HÖKFELT, T., WIESENFELD-HALLIN, Z. AND BARTFAI T. (1993) Evidence for endogenous inhibition of autotomy by galanin in the rat after sciatic nerve section: demonstrated by chronic intrathecal infusion of a high affinity galanin receptor antagonist. *Neurosci. Lett.* **149**, 193-197.

50. VERGE, V.M.K., XU, Z., XU, X.-J., WIESENFELD-HALLIN, Z. AND HÖKFELT, T. (1992) Marked increase in nitric oxide synthase mRNA in rat dorsal root ganglia after peripheral axotomy: In situ hybridization and functional studies. *Proc. Natl. Acad. Sci. U.S.A.* **89**, 11617-11621.

51. VILLAR, M.J., CORTÉS, R., THEODORSSON, E., WIESENFELD-HALLIN, Z., SCHALLING, M., FAHRENKRUG, J., EMSON, P.C. AND HÖKFELT, T. (1989) Neuropeptide expression in rat dorsal root ganglion cells and spinal cord after peripheral nerve injury with special reference to galanin. *Neuroscience* **33**, 587-604.

52. VILLAR, M.J., WIESENFELD-HALLIN, Z., XU X.-J., THEODORSSON, E., EMSON, P. AND HÖKFELT, T. (1991) Further studies on galanin-, substance P-, and CGRP-like immunoreactivities in primary sensory neurons and spinal cord: effects of dorsal rhizotomies and sciatic nerve lesions. *Exp. Neurol.* **112**, 29-39.

53. WAELBROECK, M., ROBBERECHT, P., COY, D.H., CAMUS, J.C., DE NEEF, P. AND CHRISTOPHE, J. (1985) Interaction of growth hormone-releasing factor (GRF) and 14 GRF analogs with vasoactive intestinal peptide (VIP) receptors of rat pancreas. Discovery of (N-Ac-Tyr1, D-Phe2)-GRF-(1-29)-NH2 as a VIP antagonist. *Endocrinology* **116**, 2643-2649.

54. WAKISAKA, S., KAJANDER, K.C. AND BENNETT G.J. (1991) Increased neuropeptide Y (NPY)-like immunoreactivity in rat sensory neurons following peripheral axotomy. *Neurosci. Lett.* **124**, 200-203.

55. WALL P.D. AND DEVOR, M. (1981) The effect of peripheral nerve injury on dorsal root potentials and on transmission of afferent signals into the spinal cord. Brain Res. **209**, 95-111.

56. WALL P.D. AND DEVOR M. (1983) Sensory afferent impulse originate from dorsal root ganglia as well as from the periphery in normal and nerve injured rats. *Pain* **17**, 321-339.

57. WALL, P.D., DEVOR, M., INBAL, R., SCADDING, J.W., SCHONFIELD D., SELTZER, Z. AND TOMKIEWICZ, M.M. (1979) Autotomy following peripheral nerve lesions: experimental anaesthesia dolorosa. *Pain* **7**, 103-113.

58. WALL, P.D. AND GUTNICK, K. (1974) Ongoing activity in peripheral nerves: the physiology and pharmacology of impluses originating from a neuroma. *Exp. Neurol.* **43**, 580-593.

59. WALL, P.D. AND WOOLF, C.J. (1984) Muscle but not cutaneous C-afferent input produces prolonged increases in the excitability of the flexion reflex in the rat. *J. Physiol.* **356**, 443-458.

60. WALL, P.D. AND WOOLF, C.J. (1986) The brief and prolonged facilitatory effects of unmyelianted afferent input on the rat spinal cord are independently influenced by peripheral nerve section. *Neuroscience* **17**, 1199-1205.

61. WATKINS, L.R., KINSCHECK, I.B. AND MAYER, D.J. (1984) Potentiation of opiate analgesia and apparent reversal of morphine tolerance by proglumide. *Science* **224**, 395-396.

62. WIESENFELD-HALLIN, Z. (1984) The effect of intrathecal morphine and natrexone on autotomy in sciatic nerve sectioned rats. *Pain* **18**, 267-278.

63. WIESENFELD-HALLIN, Z. (1989) Nerve section alters the interaction between C-fibre activity and intrathecal neuropeptides on the flexor reflex in rat. *Brain Res.* **489**, 129-136.

64. WIESENFELD-HALLIN, Z., BARTFAI, T. AND HÖKFELT T,. (1992). Galanin in sensory neurons in the spinal cord. *Frontiers Neuroendocrinol.* **13**, 319-343.

65. WIESENFELD-HALLIN, Z., VILLAR, M.J. AND HÖKFELT, T. (1989). The effect of intrathecal galanin and C-fiber stimulation on the flexor reflex in the rat. *Brain Res.* **486**, 205-213.

66. WIESENFELD-HALLIN, Z., XU, X-J., HÅKANSON, R., FENG, D.M. AND FOLKERS, K. (1990) The specific antagonistic effect of intrathecally injected spantide II on substance P- and C-fiber conditioning stimulation- induced facilitation of the nociceptive flexor reflex in rat. *Brain Res.* **526**, 284-290.

67. WIESENFELD-HALLIN, Z., XU X.-J., HÅKANSON, R., FENG, D-M. AND FOLKERS, K. (1990) Plasticity of the peptidergic mediation of spinal reflex facilitation. Neurosci. Lett. **116**, 293-298.

68. WIESENFELD-HALLIN, Z., XU, X.-J., HUGHES, J., HORWELL, D.C. AND HÖKFELT, T. (1990) PD134308, a selective antagonist of cholecystokinin type-B receptor, enhances the analgesic effect of morphine and synergistically interacts with intrathecal galanin to depress spinal nociceptive reflexes. *Proc. Natl. Acad. Sci. U.S.A.* **87**, 7105-7109.

69. WIESENFELD-HALLIN, Z., XU, X.-J., LANGEL, Ü., BEDECS, K., HÖKFELT, T. AND BARTFAI, T. (1992). Galanin mediated control of pain: enhanced role after nerve injury. *Proc. Natl. Acad. Sci. U.S.A.* **89**, 3334-3337.

70. WIESENFELD-HALLIN, Z., XU, X.-J., VILLAR, M.J. AND HÖKFELT, T. (1989). The effect of intrathecal galanin on the flexor reflex in rat: increased depression after sciatic nerve section. *Neurosci. Lett.* **105**, 149-154.

71. WILLIAMS, R.G., DIMALINE, R., VARRO, A., ISETTA, A.N., TRIZIO, D. AND DOCKRAY, G.J. (1987) Cholecystokinin octapeptide in rat central nervous system: immunocytochemical studies using a monoclonal antibody that does not react with CGRP. *Neurochem. Int.* **11**, 433-442.

72. XU, X.-J., DALSGAARD, C.-J. AND WIESENFELD-HALLIN, Z. (1992) Intrathecal CP-96,345 blocks reflex facilitation induced in rats by substance P and C-fiber-conditioning stimulation. *Eur. J. Pharmacol.* **216**, 337-344.

73. XU, X.-J., PUKE, M.J.C., VERGE, V.M.K., WIESENFELD-HALLIN, Z. HUGHES, J. AND HÖKFELT T. (1993) Up-regulation of cholecystokinin in primary sensory neurons is associated with morphine insensitivity in experimental neuropathic pain. *Neurosci. Lett.* 1993. (in press).

74. XU, X-J. AND WIESENFELD-HALLIN, Z. (1991) An analogue of growth hormone releasing factor (GRF), (Ac-Tyr1 , D-Phe2)-GRF-(1-29), specifically antagonizes the facilitation of the flexor reflex induced by intrathecal vasoactive intestinal peptide in rat spinal cord. *Neuropeptides* **18**, 129-135.

75. XU, X.-J., WIESENFELD-HALLIN, Z. (1991) The threshold for the depressive effect of intrathecal morphine on the spinal nociceptive flexor reflex is increased during autotomy after sciatic nerve section in rats. *Pain* **46**, 223-229.

76. XU, X.-J., WIESENFELD-HALLIN, Z., HUGHES, J., HORWELL, D.C. AND HÖKFELT, T. (1992) CI988, a selective antagonist of cholecystokinin B receptors, prevents morphine tolerance in the rat. *Br. J. Pharmacol.* **105**, 591-596.

77. XU, X.-J., WIESENFELD-HALLIN, Z., VILLAR, M.J., FAHRENKRUG, J. AND HÖKFELT, T. (1990) On the role of galanin, substance P and other neuropeptides in primary sensory neurons of rat: studies on spinal reflex excitability and peripheral axotomy. *Eur. J. Neurosci.* **2**, 733-743.

78. Zhang, X., Verge, V., Wiesenfeld-Hallin, Z., Ju, G., Bred,t D., Snyder, S.H. and Hökfelt, T. (1993) Nitric oxide synthase-like immunoreactivity in lumbar dorsal root ganglia and spinal cord of rat and monkey and effect of peripheral axotomy. *J. Comp. Neurol.* (in press).

79. Zhou, Y., Sun, Y.-H., Zhang, Z.-W. and Han, J.-S. (1992) Accelerated expression of cholecystokinin gene in the brain of rats rendered tolerant to morphine. *Neuroreport* **3**, 1121-1123.

80. Yanagisawa, M., Yag,i N., Otsuka, M., Yanaihara, C. and Yanaihara, N. (1986) Inhibitory effects of galanin on the isolated spinal cord of the newborn rat. *Neurosci. Lett.* **70**, 278-282.

HYPEREXCITABILTY IN THE SPINAL DORSAL HORN: COOPERATION OF NEUROPEPTIDES AND EXCITATORY AMINO ACIDS

Laszlo Urban, Stephen W. N. Thompson, Istvan Nagy* and Andy Dray
Department of Pharmacology, Sandoz Institute for Medical Research
5 Gower Place, London WC1E 6BN
United Kingdom

INTRODUCTION

There is a large body of evidence showing that during hyperalgesia both nociceptive specific (NS) and wide dynamic range neurons (WDR) in the spinal dorsal horn become hyperexcitable (see Coggeshall and Willis[73]). Increased spike discharge and/or sustained membrane depolarization evoked by peripheral stimulation have been used as the measure of this hyperexcitability and this has been described following acute complete Freund's adjuvant (CFA)-induced arthritis or skin inflammation[59,63] and in chemically evoked inflammation.[14,27]

Similar persistent hyperexcitability has also been reproduced by repetitive electrical stimulation of primary afferent C-fibers. Such a stimulation paradigm evokes a sustained membrane depolarization and an increased firing of dorsal horn neurons termed "wind up"[46,66] and is considered to be involved in the development and maintenance of hyperalgesia. During and following the period of "wind up" an activity-dependent increase of synaptic strength was observed.[34,67]

The unique feature of "wind up" is that it requires C-fiber activation.[46] The underlying mechanisms have been studied extensively and at present most groups agree that NMDA receptors are activated during the period of hyperexcitability.[14,17,77] This was further supported by the finding that slow postsynaptic depolarization, evoked by C fiber stimulation,[69,85] could be attenuated

---

* Dept. Anat., Univ. Med. School of Debrecen, Hungary

NATO ASI Series, Vol. H 79
Cellular Mechanisms of Sensory Processing
Edited by Laszlo Urban
© Springer-Verlag Berlin Heidelberg 1994

by the NMDA antagonist AP5.[23,24,66] The role of NMDA receptors in pathologic conditions involving hyperalgesia and pain is well established (Table I).

STIMULANT	MODEL	SOURCE
ACUTE (CFA) ARTHRITIS	CAT	SCHAIBLE et al., (1991)
CFA-INDUCED INFLAMMATION	RAT	REN et al., (1992)
TISSUE INJURY	RAT	HEADLEY & GRILLNER (1991)
FORMALIN	RAT	HALEY et al., (1990) CODERRE & MELZACK (1992)
ISCHEMIC AND POSTOPERATIVE PAIN	HUMAN	MAURSET et al., (1989)

Table I. Evidence for the role of NMDA receptors in nociception.

WHY IS IT NECESSARY TO EXCITE C-FIBERS TO EVOKE SUSTAINED HYPEREXCITABILITY?

One major difference between A- and C-fibers is that the terminals of small calibre fibers contain neuropeptides (CGRP, substance P and neurokinin A[25,30,35]) in addition to excitatory amino acids.[11] In particular the simultaneous release of neurokinins from C-fibers could alter both post- and presynaptic mechanisms, which may lead to enhanced excitability in the dorsal horn (Figure 1). Indeed the co-localization of substance P with excitatory amino acids in primary afferent terminals and in small dark DRG neurons has been confirmed by immunohistochemistry.[3,11] Furthermore CGRP is also co-localised with SP in capsaicin sensitive fibers.[21]

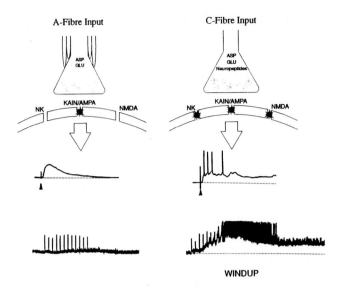

Figure 1. Comparison of the synaptic activation of dorsal horn neurons by A- and C-fiber stimulation. A-fibers contain excitatory amino acid transmitters and their stimulation activates predominantly non-NMDA receptors and evokes a brief excitatory postsynaptic potential. (Arrow points to stimulus artefact). Repetitive stimulation of the A-fibers does not produce persistent changes in the resting membrane potential (bottom trace).
C-fibers contain excitatory amino acid and neuropeptide transmitters which once released would activate postsynaptic neuropeptide, non-NMDA and NMDA receptors. This would evoke long lasting postsynaptic activity (top trace) and if the stimulation is repeated the resting membrane potential depolarises and "wind up" develops (bottom trace). See text for more details.

Release of excitatory amino acids (EAA) and neuropeptides (neurokinins and CGRP) from capsaicin sensitive small primary afferent terminals was measured in organotypic DRG cell cultures and in guinea-pig spinal cord.[32,33] Moreover SP and NK-A are released in the dorsal horn after noxious cutaneous stimuli[18,19] and during acute arthritis.[62] Furthermore there is evidence that CGRP and neurokinins (SP, NKA) enhance endogenous glutamate and aspartate release.[36] Although both neurokinins and CGRP are present in C-fiber terminals, there is little evidence for the involvement of CGRP in nociception. However the role of CGRP may differ from that of SP. Thus CGRP has been shown to enhance excitatory amino acid release in the spinal cord[36] and facilitate SP-induced spinal hyperactivity and nociceptive reflexes.[5,65] Furthermore Schaible et al.[64], have described the spread of SP immunohistochemical staining following the co-administration of CGRP in the dorsal horn. Inspite of the ongoing debate concerning the significance of neuropeptides in nociception[22] it is generally accepted at present that tachykinins, together with EAAs, are of major importance (Table II).

As both NMDA and neurokinin receptors appear to participate in spinal hyperexcitability it is important to ask whether some interaction between the two receptor types occurs. Thus A-fiber stimulation in which only EAA release occurs, generates brief EPSPs due to non-NMDA receptor activation. However C-fiber stimulation may in addition enhance NMDA-receptor activation with prolonged postsynaptic membrane potential changes.[23,54,67,68,70] As the same excitatory amino acid transmitter is released following both A- and C-fiber stimulation, but the postsynaptic receptor populations are different, it is reasonable to assume that co-release of neuropeptides make the difference (see Figure 1).

C-fiber evoked slow postsynaptic depolarization[57,69,85] and ventral root depolarization was attenuated by both EAA and NK antagonists.[6,55,58,68,81] In addition capsaicin induced hyperexcitability in the dorsal horn due to specific C-fiber activation was inhibited by both NK-2 receptor antagonists and NMDA receptor antagonists[54] while Brügger et al.[6] reported that AP5 depressed SP and capsaicin evoked contralateral VR depolarization in the immature spinal cord. However spantide did not antagonise capsaicin evoked responses in this preparation. Woodley and Kendig[74] presented evidence for both NK and NMDA components in the electrically evoked VR response in the rat hemisected spinal cord. However in a recent paper[24] the SP component was described to be age-related and after 11 days postnatal period it disappeared. More recent studies using more specific NK-1 antagonists, CP96 345 and RP67 580 have shown that these compounds were ineffective on the acute C-fiber evoked VRP in the spinal cord of young rats.[54,68]

Collectively these findings point towards the conclusion that neurokinin release and receptor activation is necessary to evoke sustained hyperexcitability in the spinal cord. This may occur by enhanced activity of C-fibers during inflammation when nociceptors are sensitised and silent C-fibers activated.[28,41] In addition such pathological conditions increase SP content in peripheral nerves[15] and in spinal terminals.[43]

STIMULANT	MODEL	SOURCE
FORMALIN	RAT	KANTNER et al., (1986)
CAPSAICIN	RAT	YAKSH et al., (1980)
METHYLENE-CHLORIDE	CAT	DUGGAN et al., (1988)
NOXIOUS THERMAL AND MECHANICAL	CAT	DUGGAN et al., (1990)
PINCH	RABBIT	KURAISHI et al., (1989)
ACUTE (CFA) ARTHRITIS	CAT	SCHAIBLE et al., (1990)

Table II. Evidence for the role of neurokinin receptors in nociception

Evidence for interaction between NK and NMDA receptors

Evidence for the interaction of neurokinin and excitatory amino acid receptors has been derived indirectly from work carried out *in vivo* and directly from studies *in vitro*. Xu et al.[79] have reported that MK 801 the selective NMDA antagonist, and the NK-1 receptor antagonist, CP96 345, synergistically attenuated the facilitation of the flexor reflex in the decerebrate spinal rat. These findings were complemented by other studies which showed that the hyperalgesia evoked by a peripheral heat injury[9] was reproduced by intrathecal coadministration of SP and NMDA but not after coapplication of CGRP and NKB, or kainate and AMPA. In addition SP receptor antagonists and the NMDA receptor antagonist AP5, reversed the hyperalgesia evoked by the intrathecal coapplication of SP and NMDA. Co-administration of

NMDA and SP also synergistically enhanced noxious behavioural responses in mice.[48] In this study SP and non-NMDA receptor ligands produced a similar effect.

METHOD	COND.	EAA RESPONSE FACILITATED	ANTAGONIST
ISOLATED DORSAL HORN CELLS[60]	NKA/SP	NMDA/AMPA	SPANTIDE II
MOUSE BEHAVIOR[42]	SP/N-TERM. FRAGMENT	KAIN	NO EFFECT
MONKEY IN VIVO SPINAL CORD[16]	C-FIBER STIMULUS	NMDA/AMPA/KAIN	NOT USED
RAT IN VITRO SPINAL CORD[71]	NKA/SP SPOMe	NMDA/QUIS	MEN10 376 CP96,3454

Table III. Evidence for interaction between excitatory amino acid and neurokinin receptors in the spinal cord.

Yashpal et al.[83] examined the effects of AP5 on the tail flick reflex in mice. This NMDA receptor antagonist did not have any effect on the baseline reflex, however after i.t. application of SP the reflex was facilitated and this facilitation was blocked by AP5. This finding indicates that NMDA receptors are not normally involved in the withdrawal response, but following an interaction with SP they regulate the efficacy of spinal signal transmission.

Direct evidence for cooperation between neurokinins and excitatory amino acid receptors at single cell level has been provided by Randic and colleagues.[60] Whole cell voltage clamp analysis of modulation of non-NMDA and NMDA receptor activated currents by neurokinins suggests that single dorsal horn neurons express both excitatory amino acid and neurokinin receptors. Both substance P and NKA (endogenous ligands released from C-fiber terminals) modulated NMDA and quisqualate/AMPA but not kainate activated currents. Augmentation of EAA currents was most commonly seen but in a substantial proportion of cells attenuation of the EAA evoked response was also recorded. Furthermore different components of the NMDA activated currents were differently affected and the time course of the effect was dependent on the application period of the neurokinin ligand. Spantide II, the non-selective neurokinin antagonist, blocked the enhancement of NMDA-induced current produced by both SP and NKA. This finding is important in view of other results[42] suggesting that excitatory amino acid (kainate, NMDA) induced behavioural effects in mice could be facilitated by the N-terminal fragment of SP (1-7) and by SP but not by the C-terminal fragment of SP. This type of facilitation does not appear to require neurokinin receptor binding (see table III for summary). At present we do not

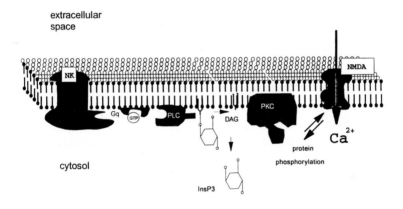

Figure 2. Possible model for neurokinin and NMDA receptor interaction. Activation of G-protein coupled neurokinin receptors (NK) leads to DAG and inositol trisphosphate (InsP3) production with a consequent activation of PKC. Phosphorylation of the NMDA receptor site by PKC will change the kinetics of Mg^{2+} binding and leads to Ca^{2+} influx through the activated NMDA receptor-channel complex. The increase in intracellular Ca^{2+} will then further enhance PKC activation. (See text for further details.)

know whether this interaction occurs at single cell level or whether it is selective for a particular NK receptor or for other sensory neuropeptides (NK-B, CGRP, opiates).[17,23,36]

Powerful modulation of NMDA receptor activity can also be achieved through the glycine and the magnesium binding sites.[2] In addition NMDA receptor activation is dependent on protein kinase C (PKC) activation.[8] Indeed both glutamate and NK receptors belong to the G-protein coupled receptor family which when activated gives rise to an intracellular cascade leading to diacylglycerol (DAG) and $InsP_3$ formation. Through this system PKC is activated and phosphorylates both cytosolic and membrane proteins, including the NMDA receptor (Figure 2). It has been further suggested that PKC reduces the Mg^{2+} block of the NMDA receptor via a change in the kinetics of Mg^{2+} binding, thus modulating channel activity.[8] Under this condition membrane depolarization would not be required to activate the NMDA receptor. Similar mechanisms could explain the neurokinin/NMDA receptor interaction seen in spinal dorsal horn cells.[60] Hence the enhancement of the NMDA response by tachykinins could be blocked by the PKC-inhibitor staurosporine.[60] However these data need further confirmation as PKC is also localised in non-neuronal elements in the dorsal horn[49] suggesting glia-neuron interactions. In this context it may be interesting that spinal microglia produce IL-1 in response to SP.[44]

We have recently confirmed that PKC participates in the enhancement of EAA responses in the isolated spinal cord of neonatal rats. Indeed staurosporine completely blocked the depolarization evoked by NKA (NK-2 receptor ligand) while both SPOMe- (NK-1 receptor ligand) and NMDA-evoked responses were unaffected (Figure 3). Interestingly both substance P methyl ester (SPOMe) and NKA enhanced NMDA and quisqualate responses but did not alter kainate evoked depolarization.[71] The enhancement of responses to excitatory amino acids by neurokinins was also blocked by staurosporine. The different effects of staurosporine on SPOMe and NKA evoked responses suggest different mechanisms for NK-1 and NK-2 receptor operation.

Other kinases may also be involved in regulating NMDA receptors. Thus Cerne et al.[7] found that the membrane permeable 8Br-cyclic AMP enhanced NMDA and non-NMDA evoked responses in the dorsal horn and the synaptic potentials evoked by electrical stimulation were facilitated as well. However there is little evidence that this mechanism plays any role in the interaction between NK and EAA-receptors.

Site of interaction of neurokinin and excitatory amino acids

It has been difficult to overcome the scepticism that an interaction between neurokinin and excitatory amino acid receptors may occur at the single cell level. Mechanisms involving polysynaptic activation of a network of neurons with either excitatory amino acid or neurokinin receptors was favoured. The major argument against the interaction at a single cell level was based on a mismatch between the distribution of substance P containing terminals[30] and the location of deep dorsal horn neurons with NMDA-related responses.[38] However It has been suggested that substance P and NK-A released from primary afferent terminals, particularly in pathologic conditions might spread ventrally from the dorsal horn and participate in volume transmission at deeper levels.[64] This hypothesis was supported by showing extrasynaptic leakage of macromolecules from primary afferent terminals during peripheral inflammation.[72]

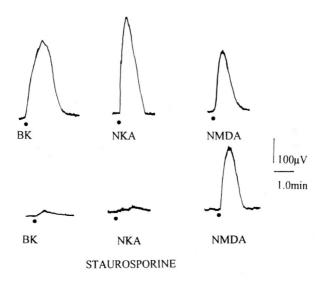

Figure 3. The effect of staurosporine (a protein kinase C inhibitor) on bradykinin- (BK), neurokinin A- (NKA) and NMDA- induced ventral root depolarization in the rat spinal cord in vitro preparation. While ventral root responses evoked by BK and NKA were blocked by staurosporine (1.0μM), NMDA-evoked depolarization was unaffected.

Immunohistochemical and autoradiographic localization of the transmitters and receptors show that NMDA receptor binding is very high in the superficial dorsal horn, particularly in lamina I-II.[47,50,56] Overall however there are few detailed descriptions of the spinal distribution of NMDA receptors. We have therefore used a new method based on cobalt uptake[56] to study the distribution of neurons expressing excitatory amino acid receptors in the spinal cord.[53] The largest proportion of stained cells are in lamina I and the outer layer of lamina II, while the inner layer contains fewer stained perykaria. However there are also strong indications that nerve processes rather than somata express NMDA receptors (Figure 4) in keeping with other studies showing NMDA receptors on the dendritic tree of dorsal horn cells.[1] The superficial laminae, which show the highest density of NMDA receptor sites are also the regions where small calibre neurokinin containing C-fibers terminate.[31] However a paradox appears to exist between the anatomical and physiological data. The synaptic input to substantia gelatinosa activates receptors mainly of the non-NMDA type.[84] Furthermore "wind up" which may involve an interaction between NMDA and neurokinin receptors occurs predominantly in deeper laminae[14,66,67,68] and there is no evidence that SG cells exhibit use-dependent excitability increases.[84,85]

Substance P induces a response in about 50% of cells in laminae III-VI,[69] which is a much higher percentage than expected from the number of primary afferent profiles observed in the deep dorsal horn showing SP-LI.[52] At least some of the deep dorsal horn cells which were sensitive to SP showed strong nociceptive input with slow postsynaptic depolarization, received direct connections from SP-LI positive fibers.[12,13] On the other hand Yoshimura et al.[86] reported that substantia gelatinosa cells are not excited by SP. Taken into account that these cells overwhelmingly express non-NMDA receptors they are unlikely targets for C-fiber afferents. Therefore the most probable site for interaction of NMDA/NK receptors would be the dendritic area of the deep dorsal horn cells, where there is extensive dendritic arborization (Figure 5). Obviously this does not exclude interaction between these two and other receptor types "downstream" in deeper laminae.

Identification of the NK receptor type involved in the interaction

Recent studies[26] have suggested that the NK-1 and NK-3 receptor sites are present in the cord but there was no evidence for the NK-2 receptor site. In situ hybridization experiments have also failed to show NK-2 receptor sites in the rat cord[39]. However Yashpal[82] reported differential distribution of all the three NK receptor subtypes in the rat spinal cord with selective radiolabelled ligands.

On the other hand physiological and pharmacological experiments have repeatedly shown that both NK-1 and NK-2 receptor ligands, highly selective for their respective postsynaptic sites, are active in the spinal cord.[20,51,54,55,71,78,79] NKA, the natural ligand for NK-2 receptors is present in the small calibre primary afferent terminals and released upon noxious stimulation[19] and by capsaicin.[32]

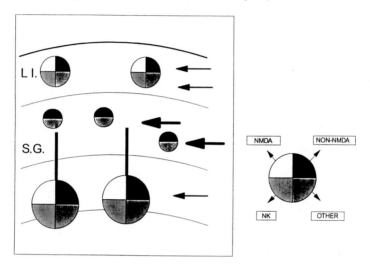

Figure 4. Structural and pharmacological considerations of the function of the spinal dorsal horn. Lamina I (Lam. I) and deep dorsal horn cells could be excited by non-NMDA, NMDA and neurokinin ligands, while substantia gelatinosa (SG) cells have low sensitivity for NMDA and neurokinins. Arrows represent peptide containing C-fiber input to different dorsal laminae. The thickness of the arrows show the relative strength of the C-fiber input to a particular lamina. The discrepancy between the sensitivity of deep dorsal horn cells towards neurokinins and NMDA and the neurokininergic primary afferent input is obvious. This can be resolved if we presume that the interaction between C-fibers and deep dorsal horn neurons takes place predominantly in superficial laminae. (For details see text.)

Selective NK-2 receptor antagonists have also been shown to block various components of postsynaptic activation of spinal cord neurones *in vitro*[54,68,71] whilst an NK1 receptor antagonist was ineffective.[54] *In vivo* NK-2 antagonists block the evoked activity of WDR cells[20] and the enhancement of the flexor reflex evoked following C-fiber stimulation.[78] Evidence is accumulating that during acute nociception NK-2 receptors are activated and the contribution of NK-1 receptors is small.

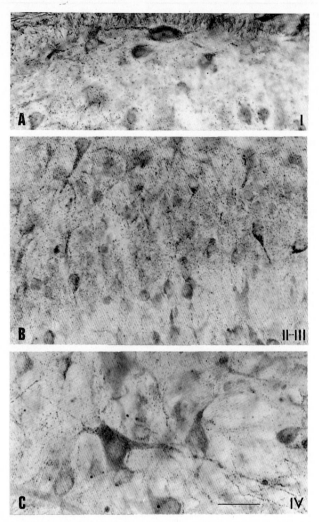

Figure 5. Cobalt labelling of spinal dorsal horn cells after exposure to NMDA. Black profiles represent neuronal elements expressing NMDA receptors. Note the relatively low density of positive cell bodies and the heavily "dotted" background in lamina II. A=lamina I; B= lamina II-s III; C= lamina IV. Calibration bar: 20μm.

PLASTICITY OF DORSAL HORN TRANSMISSION DURING HYPERALGESIA

The mechanisms involved in chronic nociception are different from those in acute pain (see: Woolf et al.[75]; Dubner and Ruda[17]; Bennett[4]). A variety of changes have been documented including novel receptor expression,[17] upregulation of receptor populations,[61] increase in neuropeptide production[15] and structural

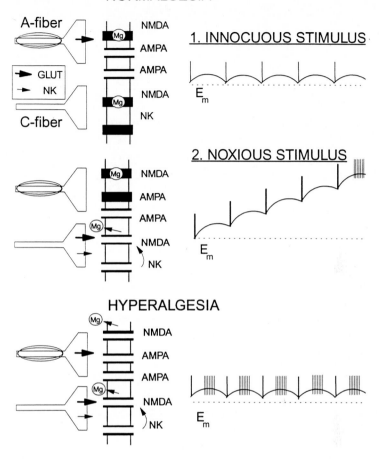

Figure 6. The mechanism of synaptic transmission between primary afferent fibers and secondary sensory neurons in the spinal dorsal horn during normalgesia and hyperalgesia.

NORMALGESIA: 1. Innocuous stimuli evoke A-fiber activation and excitatory amino acid release, which activates mostly non-NMDA receptors (AMPA) while the majority of NMDA receptors remains blocked by Mg^{2+}. This activation results in graded epsps, without progressive or sustained membrane depolarization.

2. During noxious peripheral stimulation, C-fibers release glutamate and neurokinins, which, via NK-1 and NK-2 receptors, enhance NMDA receptor activity. The activation of NMDA receptors is essential for the induction of activity dependent excitability increase ("wind up").

HYPERALGESIA: During hyperalgesia C-fibers become spontaneously active and release larger amount of neurokinins and amino acids. The previously described interaction between EAA and neurokinin receptors could maintain a high accessibility of the NMDA receptor population. Under this circumstances A-fiber stimulation can produce "wind up".

(See text for further details).

changes, including sprouting of spinal afferents[76] and cell death in the dorsal horn.[4] In addition there are qualitative and quantitative changes in the physiology and pharmacology of nociceptive processing within the spinal cord. These changes have now been well documented and contribute to the phenomenon of central sensitisation.[10,75,77] Recent observations of the plasticity of neurokinin receptor activation may relate to the central sensitisation observed following peripheral injury. Thus when small diameter primary afferent fibers were acutely stimulated only NK-2 but not NK-1 receptor antagonists were effective in attenuating the synaptic response evoked in the spinal dorsal and ventral horn.[54,68] Following the induction of a UV-induced hyperalgesia however both NK-2 and NK-1 sensitive components to the C-fiber evoked synaptic response were observed.[68] The introduction of the NK-1 sensitive component could be due to several mechanisms: (1) increased presynaptic SP content coupled with an increased release,[15] (2) postsynaptic upregulation of NK-1 receptor sites[61] and (3) a supression or exhaustion of endopeptidase activity which regulates synaptic overflow of neurokinins or CGRP.[64] Evidence for the latter possibility has recently been obtained[71]. Hence in a rat spinal cord preparation maintained *in vitro,* substance P did not enhance NMDA evoked ventral root responses, whilst the metabolically more stable SP analogue SPOMe had a significant effect. In the presence of endopeptidase inhibitors SP was also able to enhance NMDA responses.[71]

Further evidence for the involvement of novel neurokinin receptor activation following the induction of central sensitization has been recently demonstrated[68]. Under normal circumstances in the absence of peripheral injury, repeated A-fiber stimulation does not evoke "wind up" or any activity dependent increase in spinal cord excitability[66]. Following UV-induced hyperalgesia however low frequency repeated A-fiber afferent inputs may induce a substantial windup of spinal cord synaptic activity.[68] This response may be partially antagonised by NMDA and by both NK-1 and NK-2 receptor antagonists. A spinal neurokinin/NMDA receptor maintained mechanism which develops during hyperalgesia is therefore responsible for this phenomenon (Figure 6).

In summary there is accumulating evidence that neurokinin and excitatory amino acid receptor interaction in the spinal cord may play an important role in the development and maintenance of hyperalgesia and contribute to the central component of chronic pain conditions. It is likely that both NK-1 and NK-2 receptor sites are involved in these interactions which most likely takes place within the neuropil of the deep dorsal horn.

ACKNOWLEDGEMENT: We thank Mr S. Naeem and Mr I. A. Patel for assistance in some of the experiments presented in this paper. We are grateful to Miss A. Noble for helping with the manuscript.

REFERENCES

1. ARANCIO, O.M., YOSHIMURA, K.M. AND MacDERMOTT, A.B. (1993) The distribution of excitatory amino acid receptors on acutely dissociated dorsal horn neurons from postnatal rats. *Neuroscience* **52**, 159-167.

2. ASCHER, P. AND NOWAK, L. (1988) The role of N-methyl-D-aspartate responses of mouse central neurones in culture. *J. Physiol.* **399**, 247-266.

3. BATTAGLIA, G. AND RUSTIONI, A. (1988) Coexistence of glutamate and substance P in dorsal root ganglion neurons of the rat and monkey. *J. Comp. Neurol.* **277**, 302-312.

4. BENNETT, G.J. (1990) Experimental models of painful peripheral neuropathies. *News in Physiol. Sci.* **5**, 128-133.

5. BIELLA, G., PANARA, C., PECILE, A. AND SOTGIU, M.L. (1991) Facilitatory role of calcitonin gene-related peptide (CGRP) on excitation induced by substance P (SP) and noxious stimuli in the rat spinal dorsal horn neurons. An iontophoretic study *in vivo*. *Brain Res.* **559**, 352-356.

6. BRUGGER, F., EVANS, R.H. AND HAWKINS, N.S. (1990) Effects of N-Methyl-D-Aspartate antagonists and spantide on spinal reflexes and responses to substance P and capsaicin in isolated spinal cord preparations from mouse and rat. *Neuroscience* **36**, 611-622.

7. CERNE, R., JIANG, M. AND RANDIC, M. (1992) Cyclic adenosine 3' 5' - monophoshate potentiates excitatory amino acid and synaptic responses of rat spinal dorsal horn neurons. *Brain Res.* **596**, 111-123.

8. CHEN, L. AND MAE HUANG, L.-Y. (1992) Protein kinase C reduces Mg^{++} block of NMDA-receptor channels as a mechanism of modulation. *Nature* **356**, 521-523.

9. CODERRE, T.J. AND MELZACK, R. (1991) Central neural mediators of secondary hyperalgesia following heat injury in rats: neuropeptides and excitatory amino acids. *Neurosci. lett.* **131**, 71-74.

10. CODERRE, T.J. AND MELZACK, R. (1992) The contribution of excitatory amino acids to central sensitization and persistent nociception after formalin-induced tissue injury. *J. Neurosci.* **12**, 3665-36670.

11. DE BIASI, S. AND RUSTIONI, A. (1988) Glutamate and substance P coexist in primary afferent terminals in the superficial laminae of spinal cord. *Proc. Natl. Acad. Sci. USA* **85**, 7820-7824.

12. DE KONINCK, Y. AND HENRY, J.L. (1991) Substance P-mediated slow excitatory postsynaptic potential elicited in dorsal horn neurons *in vivo* by noxious stimulation. *Proc. Natl. Acad. Sci. USA* **88**, 11344-11348.

13. DE KONINCK, Y., RIBEIRO-DA-SILVA, A., HENRY, J.L. AND CUELLO, A.C. (1992) Spinal neurons exhibiting a specific nociceptive response receive abundant substance P-containing synaptic contacts. *Proc. Natl. Acad. Sci. USA* **89**, 5073-5077.

14. DICKENSON, A.H. AND SULLIVAN, A.F. (1987) Evidence for a role of the NMDA receptor in the frequency dependent potentiation of deep dorsal horn nociceptive neurons following C-fibre stimulation. *Neuropharm.* **26**, 1235-1238.

15. DONNERER, J., SCHUIGOI, R. AND STEIN, C. (1992) Increased content and transport of substance P and calcitonin gene-related peptide in sensory nerves innervating inflamed tissue: evidence for a regulatory function of nerve growth factor *in vivo*. *Neuroscience.* **49**, 693-698.

16. DOUGHERTY, P.M. AND WILLIS, W.D. (1991) Enhancement of spinaothalamic neuron responses to chemical and mechanical stimuli following combined microiontophoretic application of N-methyl-D-aspartic acid and substance P *pain* **47**, 85-93.

17. DUBNER, R. AND RUDA, M.A. (1992) Activity-dependent neuronal plasticity following tissue injury and inflammation. *Trends in Neurosci.* **15**, 96-103.

18. DUGGAN, A.W., HENDRY, I.A., MORTON, C.R., HUTCHISON, W.D. AND ZHAO, Z.Q. (1988) Cutaneous stimuli releasing immunoreactive substance P in the dorsal horn of the cat. *Brain Res.* **451**, 261-273.

19. DUGGAN, A.W., HOPE, P.J., JARROTT, B., SCHAIBLE, H.-G. AND FLEETWOOD-WALKER, S.M. (1990) Release, spread and persistence of immunoreactive neurokinin A in the dorsal horn of the cat following cutaneous stimulation. Studies with antibody microprobes. *Neuroscience* **35**, 195-202.

20. FLEETWOOD-WALKER, S.M., MITCHELL, R., HOPE, P.J., EL-YASSIR, N., MOLONY, V. AND BLADON, C.M. (1990) The involvement of neurokinin receptor subtypes in somatosensory processing in the superficial dorsal horn of the cat. *Brain Res.* **519**, 169-182.

21. FRANCO-CERECEDA, A., HENKE, H., LUNDBERG, J.M., PETERMANN, J.B., HOKFELT, T. AND FISCHER, J.A. (1987) Calcitonin gene-related peptide (CGRP) in capsaicin-snesitive substance P-immunoreactive sensory neurons in animals and man: distribution and release by capsaicin. *Peptides*, **8**, 399-410.

22. FRENK, H., BOSSUT, D., URCA, G. AND MEYER, D.J. (1988) Is substance P a primary afferent neurotransmitter for nociceptive input? Analysis of pain-related behaviours resulting from intrathecal administration of substance P and 6 excitatory compounds. *Brain Res.* **455**, 223-231.

23. GERBER, G., CERNE, R. AND RANDIC, M. (1991) Participation of excitatory amino acid receptors in the slow excitatory synaptic transmission in rat spinal dorsal horn. *Brain Res.* **561**, 236-251.

24. GIBBS, L.M. AND KENDIG, J.J. (1992) Substance P and NMDA receptor-mediated slow potentials in neonatal rat spinal cord: age-related changes. *Brain Res.* **595**, 230-241.

15. GIBSON, S.J., BLOOM, S.R. AND POLAK, J.M. (1984) A novel substance P pathway linking the dorsal and ventral horn in the upper lumbar segments of the rat spinal cord. *Brain Res.* **301**, 243-251.

26. HAGAN, R.M., BERESFORD, I.J.M., STABLES, J., DUPERE, J., STUBBS, C.M., ELLIOTT, P.J., SHELDRICK, R.L.G., CHOLLET, A., KAWASHIMA, E., McELROY, A.B. AND WARD, P. (1993) Characterisation, CNS distribution and function of NK-2 receptors studied using potent NK-2 receptor antagonists. *Reg. Peptides* **46**, 9-20.

27. HALEY, J.E., SULLIVAN, A.F. AND DICKENSON, A.H. (1990) Evidence for spinal N-methyl-D-aspartate receptor involvement in prolonged chemical noiciception in the rat. *Brain Res.* **518**, 218-226.

28. HANDWERKER, H.O., KILO, S. AND REEH, P.W. (1991) Unresponsive afferent nerve fibres in the sural nerve of the rat. *J. Physiol.* **435**, 229-242.

29. HEADLEY, P.M. AND GRILLNER, S. (1991) Excitatory amino acids and synaptic transmission: evidence for a physiological function. *Trends Pharmacol. Sci.* **11**, 205-211.

30. HOKFELT, T., KELLERTH, J.O., NILSSON, C. AND PERNOW,B. (1975) Experimental immunohistochemical studies on localisation and distribution of substance P in cat primary sensory neurons. *Brain Res.* **100**, 235-252.

31. HOKFELT, T., LJUNGDAHL, A., TERENIUS, L., ELDE, R. AND NILSSON, G. (1977) Immunohistochemical analysis of peptide pathways possibly related to pain and analgesia: enkephalin and substance P. *Proc. Natl. Acad. Sci. USA* **74**, 3081-3085.

32. HUA, X.-Y., SARIA, A., GAMSE, R., THEODORSSON-NORHEIM, E., BRODIN, E. AND LUNDBERG, J. (1986) Capsaicin induced release of multiple tachykinins (substance P, neurokinin-A and eledoisin-like material) from guinea-pig spinal cord and ureter. *Neuroscience* **19**, 313-319.

33. JEFTINIJA, S., JEFTINIJA, K., LIU, F., SKILLING, S.R., SMULLIN, D.H. AND LARSON, A.A. (1991) Excitatory amino acids are released from rat primary afferent neurons *in vitro*. *Neurosci. lett.* **125**, 191-194.

34. JEFTINIJA, S., KOJIC, L., CHEN, T.-H. AND URBAN. L. (1992) Analysis of primary afferent input to rat dorsal horn. *Soc. Neurosci. Abstr.* **18.**

35. KANAZAWA, I., OGAWA, T., KIMURA, S. AND MUNEKATA, E. (1984) Regional distribution of substance P, Neurokinin α and neurokinin β in rat central nervous system. *Neurosci. Res.* **2**, 111-120.

36. KANGRAGA, I. AND RANDIC, M. (1990) Tachykinins and calcitonin gene-related peptide enhance release of endogenous glutamate and aspartate from the rat spinal dorsal horn slice. *J. Neurosci.* **10**, 2026-2038.

37. KANTNER, R.M., GOLDSTEIN, B.D. AND KYRBY, M.L. (1986) Regulatory mechanisms for substance P in the dorsal horn during a nociceptive stimulus: Axoplasmic transport vs electrical activity. *Brain Res.* **385**, 282-290.

38. KING, A.E., THOMPSON, S.W.N., URBAN, L. AND WOOLF, C.J. (1988) An intracellular analysis of amino acid induced excitations of deep dorsal horn neurons in the rat spinal cord slice. *Neurosci. lett.* **89**, 286-292.

39. KIYAMA, H., MAENO, H. AND TOHYYAMA, M. (1993) Substance P receptors

(NK-1) in the central nervous system: possible functions from a morphological aspect. *Regul. Pept.* **46**, 114-123.

40. KURAISHI, Y., HIROTA, N., SATO, Y., HANASHIMA, N., TAKAGI, H. AND SATOH, M. (1989) Stimulus specificity of peripherally evoked substance P release from the rabbit dorsal horn in situ. *Neuroscience* **30**, 241-250.

41. LANG, E., NOVAK, A., REEH, W. AND HANDWERKER, H.O. (1990) Chemosensitivity of fine afferents from rat skin *in vitro*. *J. Neurophysiol.* **63**, 887-901.

42. LARSON, A.A., AND SUN, X. (1992) Amino terminus of substance P potentiates kainic acid-induced activity in the mouse spinal cord. *J. Neurosci.* **12**, 4905-4910.

43. MARLIER, L., POULAT, P., RAJAOFETRA, N. AND PRIVAT, A. (1991) Modifications of serotonin-, substance P- and calcitonin gene-related peptide-like immunoreactivities in the dorsal horn of the spinal cord of arthritc rats: a quantitative immunocytochemical study. *Exp. Brain Res.* **85**, 482-490.

44. MARTIN, F.C., ANTON, P.A., GORNBEIN, J.A., SHANAHAN, F. AND MERRILL,J.E. (1993) Production of interleukin-1 by microglia in response to substance P: role for a non-classical NK-1 receptor. *J. Neuroimmunol.* **42**, 53-60.

45. MAURSET, A.M., SKOGLUND, R.A. HUSTVEIT, O. AND OYE, I. (1989) Comparison of ketamine and pethidine in experimental and postoperative pain. *Pain* **36**, 37-41.

46. MENDELL, L. (1966) Physiological properties of nonmyelinated fiber projection to the spinal cord. *Exp. Neurol.* **16**, 316-332.

47. MITCHELL, J.J. AND ANDERSON, K.J. (1991) Quantitative autoradiographic analysis of excitatory amino acid receptors in the spinal cord. *Neurosci. lett.* **124**, 269-272.

48. MJELLEM-JOLY, N., LUND, A., BERGE, O.-G. AND HOLE, K. (1991) Potentiation of a behavioural response in mice by spinal coadministration of substance P and excitatory amino acid agonists. *Neurosci. Lett.* **133**, 121-124.

49. MOCHLY-ROSEN, D., BASBAUM, A.I. AND KOSHLAND, D.E. JR. (1987) Distinct cellular and regional localization of immunereactive protein kinase C in rat brain. *Proc. Natl. Acad. Sci. USA* **84**, 4660-4664.

50. MONAGHAN, D.T. AND COTMAN, C.W. (1985) Distribution of N-Methyl-D-aspartate-sensitve L-[^{3}H]Glutamate-binding sites in rat brain. *J. Neurosci.* **5**, 2909-2919.

51. MURASE, K., RYU, P.D. AND RANDIC, M. (1989) Excitatory and inhibitory amino acids and peptide-induced responses in acutely isolated rat spinal dorsal horn neurons. *Neurosci. lett.* **103**, 56-63.

52. NAGY, J.I. AND HUNT , S.P. (1983) The termination of primary afferents within the rat dorsal horn: Evidence for rearrangement following capsaicin treatment. *J. Comp Neurol.* **218**, 145-158.

53. NAGY, I., WINTER, J. AND WOOLF, C.J. (1993) Distribution of neurones expressing different excitatory amino acid receptors in the rat isolated spinal cord. *J. Physiol.* **459**, P162.

54. NAGY, I., MAGGI, C.A., DRAY, A., WOOLF, C.J. AND URBAN, L. (1993) The role of neurokinin and N-Methyl-D-Aspartate receptors in synaptic

transmission from capsaicin-sensitive primary afferents in the rat spinal cord *in vitro. Neuroscience* **52**, 1029-1037.

55. OTSUKA, M. AND YANAGISAWA, M. (1988) Effect of a tachykinin antagonist on a nociceptive reflex in the isolated spinal cord tail preparation of the newborn rat. *J. Physiol.(Lond.)* **395**, 255-270.

56. PRUSS, R.M., AKESON, R.L., RACKE, M.M. AND WILBURN, J.L. (1991) Agonist-activated cobalt uptake identifies divalent cation-permeable kainate receptors on neurons and glial cells. *Neuron* **7**, 5509-518.

57. RANDIC, M., JEFTINIJA, S., URBAN, L., RASPANTINI, C. AND FOLKERS, K. (1988) Effects of substance P analogues on spinal dorsal horn neurons. *Peptides* **9**, 651-660.

58. RANDIC, M., RYU, P.D. AND URBAN, L. (1986) Effects of monoclonal and polyclonal antibodies to substance P on slow excitatory transmission in the rat spinal dorsal horn. *Brain Res.* **383**, 15-27.

59. REN, K., HYLDEN,J.L.K., WILLIAMS, G.M., RUDA, M.A. AND DUBNER, R. (1993) The effects of a non-competitive NMDA receptor antagonist, MK-801, on behavioral hyperalgesia and dorsal horn neuronal activity with unilateral inflammation. *Pain* **50**, 331-344.

60. RUSIN, K.I., RYU, P.D. AND RANDIC, M. (1992) Modulation of excitatory amino acid responses in rat dorsal horn neurons by tachykinins. *J. Neurophysiol.* **68**, 265-286.

61. SCHAFER, M. K.-H., NOHR, D., KRAUSE, J.E. AND WEIHE, E. (1993) Selective upregulation in unilateral peripheral inflammation. *Neuropeptides* **24(4)**, P83.

62. SCHAIBLE, H.-G., JARROTT, B., HOPE, P.J. AND DUGGAN, A.W. (1990) Release of immunoreactive substance P in the spinal cord during development of acute arthritis in the knee joint of the cat: a study with antibody microprobes. *Brain Res.* **529**, 214-223.

63. SCHAIBLE, H.-G., GRUBB, B.D., NEUGEBAUER, V. AND OPPMANN, M. (1991) The effects of NMDA antagonists on neuronal activity in cat spinal cord evoked by acute inflammatiion in the knee joint. *Eur. J. Neurosci.* **3**, 981-991.

64. SCHAIBLE, H.-G., HOPE, P.J., LANG, C.W. AND DUGGAN, A.W. (1992) Calcitonin gene-related peptide causes intraspinal spreading of substance P released by peripheral stimulation. *Eur. J. Neurosci.* **4**, 750-757.

65. SMULLIN, D.H., SKILLING, R. AND LARSON A.A. (1990) Interactions between substance P, calcitonin gene-related peptide, taurine and excitatory amino acids in the spinal cord. *Pain* **42**, 93-101.

66. THOMPSON, S.W.N., KING, A.E. AND WOOLF, C.J. (1990) Activity-dependent changes in rat ventral horn neurons in vitro; summation of prolonged afferent evoked postsynaptic depolarizations produce a D-2-amino-5-phosphonovaleric acid sensitive windup. *Eur. J. Neurosci.* **2**, 638-649.

67. THOMPSON, S.W.N., WOOLF, C.J. AND SIVILOTTI, L.G. (1993) Small-caliber afferent inputs produce a heterosynaptic facilitation of the synaptic responses evoked by primary afferent A-fibres in the neonatal rat spinal cord *in vitro. J. Neurophysiol.* **69**, 1-13.

68. THOMPSON, S.W.N., URBAN, L. AND DRAY, A. (1993) NMDA and tachykinin receptor-mediated contributions to the C-fibre-evoked response in the

neonatal rat spinal cord in vitro are enhanced following peripheral inflammation. *Brit. J. Pharmacol.* **108**, 22P.

69. URBAN, L. AND RANDIC, M. (1984) Slow excitatory transmission in rat dorsal horn: possible mediation by peptides. *Brain Res.* **290**, 336-341.

70. URBAN, L. AND DRAY, A. (1992) Synaptic activation of dorsal horn neurons by selective C-fibre excitation with capsaicin in the mouse spinal cord *in vitro. Neuroscience* **47**, 693-702.

71. URBAN, NAEEM, S. AND DRAY, A. (1993) Effects of neurokinins on excitatory amino acid-induced activation in the neonatal rat spinal cord in vitro.*Br. J. Pharmacol.* **108**, 23P.

72. VALTSCHANOFF, J.G., WEINBERG, R.J. AND RUSTIONI, A. (1992) Peripheral injury and anterograde transport of wheat germ agglutin-horse radish peroxidase to the spinal cord. *Neuroscience* **50**, 685-696.

73. WILLIS, W.D.JR. AND COGGESHALL, R.E. (1991) Sensory mechanisms of the spinal cord. *Plenum Press.* (Second Ed.)

74. WOODLEY, S.J. AND KENDIG, J.J. (1991) Substance P and NMDA receptors mediates a slow nociceptive ventral root potential in the neonatal rat spinal cord. *Brain Res.* **559**, 17-21.

75. WOOLF, C.J. (1983) Evidence for a central component of post-injury pain hypersensitivitty. *Nature* **306**, 686-688.

76. WOOLF, C.J., SHORTLAND, P. AND COGGESHALL, R.E. (1993) Peripheral nerve injury triggers central sprouting of myelinated afferents. *Nature* **355**, 75-78.

77. WOOLF, C.J. AND THOMPSON, S.W.N. (1991) The induction and maintenance of central sensitization is dependent upon N-Methyl-D-Aspartate acid receptor activation; implications for the treatment of post-injury pain hpersensitivity states. *Pain* **44**, 293-299.

78. XU, X.-J., MAGGI, C.A. AND WIESENFELD-HALLIN, Z. (1991) On the role of NK-2 tachykinin receptors in the mediation of spinal reflex excitability in the rat. *Neuroscience*, **44**, 483-490.

79. XU, X.-J., DALSGAARD, C.J. AND WIESENFELD-HALLIN, Z. (1992) Spinal substance P and N-Methyl-D-Aspartate receptors are coactivated in the induction of central sensitzation of the nociceptive flexor reflex. *Neuroscience* **51**, 641-648.

80. YAKSH, T.L., JESSELL, T.M., GAMSE, R., MUDGE, A.W. AND LEEMAN, S.F. (1980) Intrathecal morphine inhibits substance P release from mammalian spinal cord in vivo. *Nature* **286**, 155-156.

81. YANAGISAWA, M., OTSUKA, M., KONISHI, S., AKAGI, H., FOLKERS, K. AND ROSTELL, S. (1982) A substance P antagonist inhibits a slow reflex response in the spinal cord of the newborn rat. *Acta. Physiol. Scand.* **116**, 109-112.

82. YASHPAL, K., DAM, T. AND QUIRION, R. (1990) Quantitative autoradioigraphic distribution of multiple neurokinin binding sites in rat spinal cord. *Brain Res.* **506**, 259-266.

83. YASHPAL, K., RADHAKRISHNAN, V. AND HENRY, J.L. (1991) NMDA receptor antagonist blocks the facilitation of the tail flick reflex in the rat induced by intrathecal administration of substance P and by noxious cutaneous stimulation. *Neurosci. Lett.* **128**, 269-272.

84. YOSHIMURA, M. AND JESSELL, T. (1990) Amino acid-mediated EPSPs at primary afferent synapses with substantia gelatinosa neurones in the rat spinal cord. *J. Physiol.* **430**, 315-335.
85. YOSHIMURA, M. AND JESSELL, T.M. (1989) Primary afferent evoked synaptic responses and slow potential generation in rat substantia geltinosa neurons *in vitro*. *J. Neurophysiol.* **62**, 96-108.
86. YOSHIMURA, M., SHIMIZU, T., YAJIRI, Y., INOKUCHI, H. AND NISHI, S. (1993) Primary afferent-evoked slow EPSPs and responses to substance P of dorsal horn neurons in the adult rat spinal cord slices. *Reg. Peptides* **46**, 407-409.

THE ROLE OF NITRIC OXIDE IN HYPERALGESIA

Stephen T. Meller and G.F. Gebhart
Department of Pharmacology, University of Iowa
Iowa City, Iowa, 52242
USA

INTRODUCTION

There is now a great deal of evidence that nitric oxide (NO) plays a role in synaptic transmission in both the central and peripheral nervous systems. NO is a small, reactive, gaseous molecule with a short half-life that is, under most circumstances, produced on demand. In the CNS, the enzyme NO synthase (NOS) requires activation of a calmodulin-sensitive site on the enzyme by intracellular Ca^{2+} in the presence of NADPH, tetrahydorbiopterin, FAD and FMN to produce NO and L-citrulline from free L-arginine and molecular oxygen.[13]

While there has been renewed interest and investigations into mechanisms of hyperalgesia associated with chronic pain,[36] it has become clear that glutamate acting at the NMDA receptor subtype in the spinal cord is involved in mechanisms that result in long-term, use-dependent changes in neuronal excitability, synaptic connectivity and synaptic plasticity.[27] Given that there appears to be a considerable amount of evidence to implicate NMDA receptors in spinal mechanisms of hyperalgesia, and as many of the effects of NMDA receptor activation appear to be mediated through production of NO, we have previously proposed that NO plays a significant role in the development and maintenance of thermal hyperalgesia.[25-27] In contrast, little is known about the mechanisms underlying mechanical hyperalgesia. This chapter deals with the evidence on NO that has been reported to date and attempts to suggest some unifying mechanisms for excitatory amino acid- and NO-produced hyperalgesia. Portions of these data have previously been reported.[25-29]

NATO ASI Series, Vol. H 79
Cellular Mechanisms of Sensory Processing
Edited by Laszlo Urban
© Springer-Verlag Berlin Heidelberg 1994

METHODS

Animals and Surgery

Male Sprague-Dawley rats included in the results summarised here were housed in a room maintained at a constant temperature of 22°C on a 12/12 hr light/dark cycle with food and water available *ad libitum*. Rats were deeply anesthetized with an intraperitoneal injection of sodium pentobarbital (45 mg/kg, NembutalR, Abbott Labs., North Chicago, IL) and an intrathecal (i.t.) catheter (8.5 cm; PE-10) was introduced into the lumbar i.t. space through an incision in the dura over the atlanto-occipital joint. All rats were allowed 3-7 days to recover from surgery before testing. There was no difference in the responses of rats when tested at 3 days or 7 days.[25,29]

Nociceptive testing

Experiments consisted of two types: acute and persistent. In the first experiment, the role of NO was examined in rats where acute thermal or mechanical hyperalgesia was produced by i.t. administration of NMDA or AMPA + trans-ACPD, respectively.[25,29] In the second experiment, the role of NO was examined in the persistent hyperalgesia produced by the intraplantar injection of carrageenan (thermal and mechanical) or by loose ligation of the sciatic nerve with chromic gut sutures (thermal only).

Thermal testing

In the first experiment, rats were allowed to crawl inside a canvas garden glove and changes in thermal withdrawal latencies were determined using a tail-flick (TF) device where heat was applied at one of 5 sites on the underside of the tail, 1 cm apart, with the most distal site at least 3 cm from the tip of the tail. Latencies for withdrawal were measured to the nearest 0.1 s using a feed-back controlled timer. A cut-off latency of 7 sec was used to avoid tissue damage.

In the second experiment, rats were placed under an inverted clear plexiglass cage (18 x 28 x 13 cm) on a piece of heat-tempered glass 3 mm thick and allowed 10 min to acclimatise. Radiant heat from a 50 W projector lamp was focused on the plantar surface of the hind paw with the beam (15 mm diameter) encompassing the glabrous skin including the toe pads. Withdrawal latencies were measured to the nearest 0.1 sec with a feedback-controlled timer as the time from onset of heating to the time of withdrawal of the hind paw from the beam. A cut-off latency of 20 sec was used to avoid tissue damage. Four trials, at least 4 min apart, were conducted on each hind paw; the last three trials were averaged to give a mean latency for each hind paw.

Mechanical testing

In the first experiment, rats were allowed to crawl inside a canvas garden glove and changes in mechanical nociceptive thresholds were determined using nylon (von Frey-like) monofilaments requiring different pressures to bow the filament. Mechanical stimulation was increased in a graded manner on the dorsal surface of the tail using successively greater diameter filaments until the tail was withdrawn. Thresholds were checked at least twice for each trial.

In the second set of experiments, changes in mechanical nociceptive thresholds were also measured using calibrated nylon monofilaments. For these experiments, rats were allowed to crawl freely into a large rumpled piece of cloth. Once the rat had settled, the tip of the nylon monofilaments were applied to the lateral edge of the hind paw. Mechanical stimulation was increased in a graded manner using successively greater diameter filaments until the hind paw was withdrawn. For successive tests, the placement of these stimuli was varied slightly from one trial to the next to avoid sensitization of the skin of the hind paw. Threshold was checked several times.

Experimental protocol

In the first experiment, rats were injected with doses of either NMDA (1 pmol) or a 1:1 combination of AMPA + trans-ACPD (total dose, 20 pmol) that we have shown produces acute thermal or mechanical hyperalgesia, respectively.[25,29]

Thermal withdrawal latencies or mechanical withdrawal thresholds were tested at 0.5, 1, 2, 5 and 10 min post-drug. Latency and threshold measurements were continued at 5 min intervals until they returned to the latency or withdrawal threshold established pre-drug. After the magnitude of the thermal or mechanical hyperalgesia was determined, the effect of L-NAME (1 nmol) was examined; testing with excitatory amino acid agonists continued every 10 min after i.t. administration of L-NAME until complete recovery of the agonist-produced hyperalgesia.

For rats in the second set of experiments, the effect of saline, L-NAME or D-NAME was examined on the persistent hyperalgesia produced either 3 hours after the intraplantar injection of carrageenan (2 mg in 100 µl) (200 nmol L-NAME or D-NAME) or 3 days after 4 loose 4-0 chromic gut ligatures were placed around the left sciatic nerve[24,26] (20 nmol L-NAME or D-NAME). Paw withdrawal latencies (PWL) to thermal stimulation and paw withdrawal thresholds (PWT) to mechanical stimulation were tested at time 0 and at 3 hrs post-carrageenan to establish that they were hyperalgesic; rats were then tested 10 min, 1, 3, 5 and 7 hr after i.t. administration of L-NAME, D-NAME or saline in the same rats. In the sciatic nerve ligation model of persistent hyperalgesia, PWL to thermal stimulation were examined at day 0 (prior to surgery) and at day 3 (day of maximal hyperalgesia);[24,26] rats were then tested 10 min, 1, 2, 3 and 4 hr after i.t. administration of L-NAME, D-NAME or saline.

Drugs

NMDA, AMPA, L-NAME, D-NAME and carrageenan were purchased from Sigma Chemical Co. (St Louis, MO). Trans-ACPD was purchased from Tocris Neuramin (Essex, UK). Stock solutions of all drugs were made up fresh in preservative-free saline and diluted according to the concentration needed. Drugs were given i.t. in a volume of 1 µl followed by a flush with 10 µl saline. In all rats the effect of vehicle alone (saline) was examined.

Statistical analysis

Thermal withdrawal latencies and mechanical withdrawal thresholds are reported in seconds (sec) and grams (g), respectively or expressed as a percentage difference from time 0 (pre-drug) according to the formula: (trial - control)/control x

100 or as a difference score from the left (treated) and right (sham) hind paw using the same formula. Data are presented as mean±SEM. Changes in thermal withdrawal latencies were analysed using a one-way analysis of variance (ANOVA) followed by a post-hoc Fisher's test. Changes in mechanical withdrawal thresholds were analysed using the Kruskall-Wallis k-sample test. In all cases $p < 0.05$ was considered significant.

RESULTS

Acute hyperalgesia

The i.t. administration of NMDA (1 pmol) produced a rapid and transient facilitation of the TF reflex (from 4.2±0.1 to 3.3±0.2 sec; -28.6±1.7%) without evidence of a change in mechanical withdrawal threshold (Figure 1). In contrast, i.t. administration of AMPA + trans-ACPD (total dose, 20 nmol) produced a rapid and transient, decrease in mechanical withdrawal threshold (from 117.6±5.7 to 11.9±0.5 g; -89.8±0.6%) without a change in thermal withdrawal latency (Figure 1).

The acute thermal hyperalgesia produced by 1 pmol NMDA was completely abolished by prior treatment (10 min prior) with L-NAME (1 nmol, i.t.) (Fig. 2); D-NAME was without effect (data not shown, but see Meller et al.[25]). NMDA-produced facilitation of the TF reflex was completely recovered when tested 40 min after L-NAME (Figure 2). In contrast, the decrease in mechanical withdrawal threshold produced by AMPA + trans-ACPD was unaffected by L-NAME (Figure 2). The doses of L-NAME or D-NAME used did not significantly alter baseline TF latency or mechanical withdrawal threshold (Figure 2).

Persistent hyperalgesia

Sciatic nerve ligation

Prior to loose ligation of the sciatic nerve with chromic gut ligatures (day 0), there was no significant difference in withdrawal latencies between the left and the right hind paw (Fig. 3). However, 3 days after loose ligation of the left sciatic nerve with chromic gut ligatures, all rats showed evidence of a significantly faster withdrawal latency of the left compared to the right hind paw (Figure 3A). That is, all rats demonstrated a thermal hyperalgesia.

The i.t. administration of L-NAME (20 nmol), but not D-NAME (20 nmol) or saline blocked the thermal hyperalgesia in rats with chromic gut ligatures for a period of up to 3 hours (Figure 3B), suggesting that the production of NO is critical for the maintenance of thermal hyperalgesia. In contrast, i.t. administration of L-NAME, D-NAME or saline did not significantly change thermal nociceptive withdrawal latencies on the contralateral side (Figure 3C), suggesting that the production of NO is not involved in the reflex response to noxious heat.

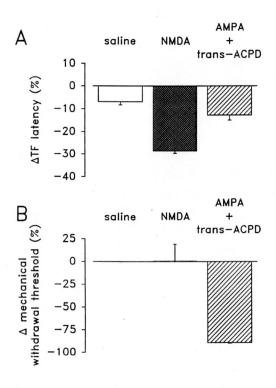

Figure 1. Excitatory amino acid produced thermal and mechanical hyperalgesia. Summary of the effects of i.t. administration of saline, NMDA (1 pmol) or AMPA + trans-ACPD (20 pmol) on changes in (A) tail-flick (TF) latency to heat and (B) mechanical withdrawal thresholds. Changes in TF latency or mechanical withdrawal thresholds are represented on the y-axis as a % change in latency or threshold calculated by the formula: (trial latency or threshold - control latency or threshold)/(control latency or threshold) x 100 and expressed as a percentage. All data points are expressed as mean±SEM.

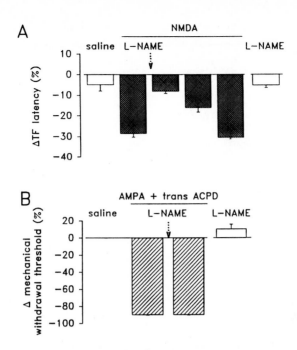

Figure 2. The role of NO in acute thermal and mechanical hyperalgesia. Summary of the effects of i.t. administration of L-NAME alone (1 nmol), and of L-NAME (1 nmol) on (A) the acute thermal hyperalgesia produced by i.t. administration of NMDA and (B) the acute mechanical hyperalgesia produced by i.t. administration of AMPA + trans-ACPD. In panel A, successive doses of NMDA were administered at 10 min intervals after i.t. administration of L-NAME. C. Effect of L-NAME alone, and of L-NAME. Changes in TF latency or mechanical thresholds are represented on the y-axis as a % change in latency or threshold calculated by the formula: (trial latency or threshold - control latency or threshold)/(control latency or threshold) x 100 and expressed as a percentage. All data points are expressed as mean±SEM.

Intraplantar carrageenan

Prior to intraplantar injection of carrageenan (time 0) there was no significant difference in thermal withdrawal latencies or mechanical withdrawal thresholds between the left and right hind paw (Figure 4). However, 3 hrs post-carrageenan, all rats showed evidence of a significantly faster thermal withdrawal latency and lower mechanical withdrawal threshold of the left hind paw compared to the right hind paw (Figure 4). That is, all rats demonstrated a marked thermal and mechanical hyperalgesia 3 hr post-carrageenan which was maintained for the 8 hrs that were examined post-carrageenan.

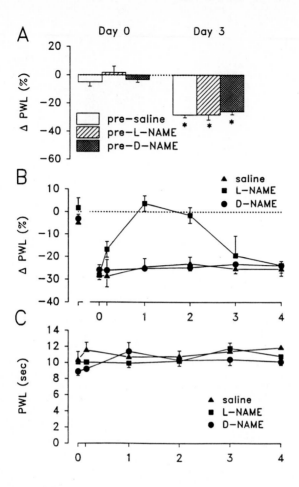

Figure 3. The role of NO in the persistent thermal hyperalgesia produced by loose ligation of the sciatic nerve with chromic gut sutures. A. Summary of the changes thermal withdrawal latencies (paw withdrawal latency; PWL) on day 0 (immediately prior to surgery) and on day 3 (day of maximal thermal hyperalgesia). B. Summary of the time course of the effect of i.t. administration of either saline, L-NAME (20 nmol) or D-NAME (20 nmol) on thermal hyperalgesia 3 days after loose ligation of the left sciatic nerve with chromic gut sutures. C. Summary of the time course of the effect of i.t. administration of either saline, L-NAME (20 nmol) or D-NAME (20 nmol) on withdrawal latencies of the right (contralateral) hind paw 3 days after loose ligation of the left sciatic nerve with chromic gut sutures. Thermal withdrawal latencies are represented on the y-axis as either withdrawal latency in seconds (sec) or as a percentage difference in withdrawal latencies between the left and the right hind paws according to the following formula: (left withdrawal latency - right withdrawal latency)/right withdrawal latency x 100. All data are presented as mean±SEM.

A

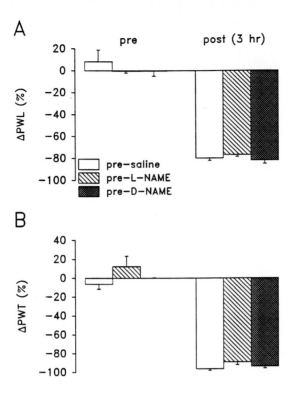

Figure 4. The effect of the intraplantar injection of carrageenan on changes in (A) thermal withdrawal latencies or (B) mechanical withdrawal thresholds at time 0 (immediately prior to injection; pre) and at 3 hr (time of maximal hyperalgesia; post). Changes in thermal withdrawal latencies (paw withdrawal latency; PWL) or mechanical withdrawal thresholds (paw withdrawal threshold; PWT) are represented on the y-axis as a percentage difference between the left and the right hind paws according to the following formula: (left - right)/right latency x 100. All data are presented as mean±SEM.

The i.t. administration of L-NAME (200 nmol), but not D-NAME (200 nmol) or saline, reversibly blocked the thermal hyperalgesia produced by intraplantar carrageenan for a period of 3 hours (Figure 5), suggesting that the production of NO is critical for the maintenance of thermal hyperalgesia. L-NAME, D-NAME or saline did not produce any significant change in thermal nociceptive withdrawal latencies in the non-injected paw, suggesting that production of NO is not involved in the reflex response to noxious heat. In contrast to an attenuation of the thermal hyperalgesia, L-NAME (or D-NAME or saline) did not affect the mechanical hyperalgesia produced by intraplantar carrageenan (Figure 5), suggesting that the production of NO is not involved in the maintenance of mechanical hyperalgesia produced in this model of persistent pain.

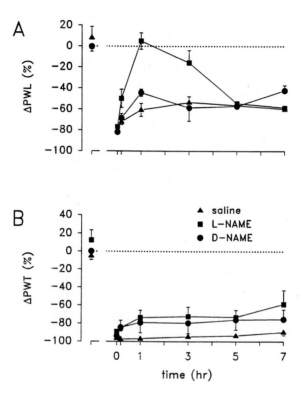

Figure 5. Summary of the time course of the effect of i.t. administration of either saline, L-NAME (200 nmol) or D-NAME (200 nmol) on (A) the thermal hyperalgesia or (B) the mechanical hyperalgesia produced by the intraplantar injection of 2 mg carrageenan. Changes in thermal withdrawal latencies (paw withdrawal latency; PWL) or mechanical withdrawal thresholds (paw withdrawal threshold; PWT) are represented on the y-axis as a percentage difference in between the left and the right hind paws according to the following formula: (left - right)/right x 100. All data are presented as mean±SEM.

DISCUSSION

Persistent pain is often associated with altered sensitivity to cutaneous stimuli which is manifest as hyperalgesia (increased sensitivity to noxious stimuli) and allodynia (non-noxious stimuli perceived as noxious).[36] As a consequence of tissue injury, inflammatory mediators are released at the site of injury, resulting in sensitization of nociceptors. The increased activity of afferent neurons leads to a neuronal 'plasticity' in the dorsal horn of the spinal cord, and these functional alterations contribute to the development of hyperalgesia and allodynia.[12,39,40] Although recent efforts to describe and define mechanisms underlying hyperalgesia indicate that NMDA receptors are intimately involved in mechanisms that result in long-term, use-dependent changes in neuronal excitability,[27] the role of other excitatory amino acid receptor subtypes and, in particular, the role of NO in hyperalgesia is still not well defined.

Thermal hyperalgesia

Excitatory amino acids

The NMDA receptor has been suggested to be involved in polysynaptic nociceptive transmission and plasticity in the spinal cord.[27] While the precise role that NMDA receptors play in spinal nociceptive processing is not clear, evidence suggests that nociceptive reflexes and responses of spinal dorsal horn neurons to noxious stimuli are largely unaffected by NMDA receptor antagonists, but facilitation of these responses to noxious stimuli are blocked by NMDA receptor antagonists.[5,6,9,10,16,20,38] For example, in a model of neuropathic pain in rats,[2] it has been demonstrated that i.t. administration of MK-801 (an NMDA receptor channel antagonist) reverses the thermal hyperalgesia,[22,42] suggesting that activation of the NMDA receptor in the lumbar dorsal horn is required for mechanisms of thermal hyperalgesia. In addition, Mao et al.[21] have shown that both AMPA and NMDA receptors are involved in the development of thermal hyperalgesia while only NMDA receptors are involved in the maintenance of thermal hyperalgesia.

The neuropathy model is not the only model of persistent pain that shows an involvement of NMDA receptors in thermal hyperalgesia. For example, the thermal hyperalgesia or hyperalgesic behavior associated with peripheral hind limb inflammation produced by complete Freund's adjuvant,[34] carrageenan[35,43] or formalin[7,8,31,32,41] have also been shown to be dependent on NMDA receptor activation, as has the prolonged facilitation of the flexor reflex produced by intraplantar injection of mustard oil.[38] Further, Coderre and Melzack[8] have shown that the enhanced response to intraplantar formalin is unaffected by CNQX (an AMPA receptor antagonist) or AP3 (a metabotropic glutamate receptor antagonist); only MK-801 blocked the nociceptive behavior. Consistent with a role for NMDA receptors in spinal hyperalgesia are reports that i.t. administration of NMDA, but not quisqualate or kainate, produces a marked hyperalgesia in thermal nociceptive tests in rats and mice.[1,6,17,18,19,20,25,33] Further, Coderre and Melzack[7] have shown that the increased response after intraplantar formalin is enhanced by NMDA, but not AMPA. Thus, there is a considerable amount of evidence to suggest a role for NMDA receptors (but not AMPA, KA or metabotropic glutamate receptors) in the mechanisms underlying thermal hyperalgesia.

Nitric oxide

As there is a significant amount of evidence to implicate NMDA in thermal hyperalgesia in the spinal cord, and as many of the effects of NMDA receptor activation are mediated through production of NO, we have previously proposed that NO plays a significant role in thermal hyperalgesia in the spinal cord.[25-27] In support of this hypothesis, several studies have recently demonstrated that NO does play a pivotal role in mechanisms of thermal hyperalgesia. For example, it has been shown that the i.t. administration of NMDA produces a rapid, transient, dose-dependent thermal hyperalgesia which is reversibly blocked by prior treatment with the selective NMDA receptor antagonist AP5,[18,25] suggesting that it is due to NMDA receptor activation. Importantly, the hyperalgesia was also reversibly blocked by prior i.t. administration of L-NAME[17,18,25] but not D-NAME.[17,25] In these studies, the doses of L-NAME or D-NAME used did not significantly alter baseline TF latency. Collectively, these results suggest that NMDA produces an acute thermal hyperalgesia through activation of NMDA receptors and subsequent production of NO. It also has been demonstrated that NMDA-produced thermal hyperalgesia is reversibly blocked by i.t. administration of hemoglobin,[17] suggesting that once NO is produced it must leave the neuron where it is produced and travel extracellularly to another neuron to activate soluble guanylate cyclase (GC-S) and subsequently increase production of cGMP.[25,26] If NO mediates the thermal hyperalgesia produced by NMDA, it might be expected that administration of L-arginine, which would increase the production of endogenous NO, might also produce an acute thermal hyperalgesia. In support, we have found that the i.t. administration of L-arginine, but not D-arginine, produced a rapid, transient, dose-dependent thermal hyperalgesia of similar magnitude and time-course to that produced by NMDA.[25] Collectively, these results suggest that the reflex withdrawal response to noxious heating of the tail is not mediated through activation of NMDA receptors and subsequent production of NO, but that NMDA-produced facilitation of thermal reflexes is NMDA- and NO-mediated.

More recently, we reported that NO mediated the thermal hyperalgesia produced in a model of persistent pain.[26] In those experiments, we found that the i.t. administration of L-NAME, but not the inactive enantiomer D-NAME, reversed the thermal hyperalgesia produced by chromic gut sutures for up to 3 hours. In sham rats, those same treatments produced no change in thermal nociceptive withdrawal latencies. From these data it appears that a sustained production of NO in the lumbar spinal cord is required for maintenance of thermal hyperalgesia produced in this model of neuropathic pain in the rat.

Given that the hyperalgesia and facilitation of nociception produced in other models of persistent pain, such as the inflammation produced by complete Freund's adjuvant,[34] carrageenan,[35,43] formalin[7,8,31,32,41] or mustard oil,[38] are all dependent on NMDA receptor activation, we suggested that NO may also mediate these responses.[25-27] In support, the present experiments demonstrate that thermal hyperalgesia produced by intraplantar injection of carrageenan is reversibly blocked by L-NAME, but not D-NAME or saline. Further, the experiments also show that L-NAME did not affect withdrawal latencies in the contralateral, non-inflamed hind paw. In addition, it has recently been reported that the facilitation found in electrophysiological[15] and behavioral experiments[20] following intraplantar injection of formalin are dependent on the production of NO; there is no available data on the role of NO in the hyperalgesia or behavioral response produced by mustard oil or capsaicin as yet.

Collectively, these data support our earlier hypothesis that thermal hyperalgesia, whether produced in models of acute or persistent pain, is mediated through production of NO and that NO does not play a role in the reflex response to thermal stimulation. It is of interest to note that 1 pmol L-NAME was able to completely block the acute thermal hyperalgesia produced by NMDA whereas 20 nmol L-NAME was required for the thermal hyperalgesia produced in the neuropathy model and 200 nmol was required for abolition of the thermal hyperalgesia produced in the carrageenan inflammation model. Further, the degree of maximum thermal hyperalgesia produced in these three models was -28.6±1.7, -28.2±3.6 and -61.0± 6.9%, respectively suggesting that a more intense stimulus may produce a greater degree of thermal hyperalgesia, increasing activity of NOS and requiring greater doses of L-NAME to attenuate the hyperalgesia.

It is likely that the neurotransmitters of primary afferents responsible for the reflex response to heat do not act on NMDA receptors or require the production of endogenous NO, but facilitation of the reflex response to heat produced by NMDA, and quite possibly by other neurotransmitters and neuromodulators, requires the production of endogenous NO.

Mechanical hyperalgesia

Excitatory amino acids

At present, very little is known about the excitatory amino acid receptor subtypes involved in mechanical hyperalgesia produced in acute or persistent models. However, Dougherty et al.[11] has recently demonstrated that the sensitization of spinothalamic tract neurons to mechanical stimulation after intra-articular injection of carrageenan was enhanced by non-NMDA receptor agonists such as quisqualate; NMDA was without effect. This electrophysiological data fits very well with our recent behavioral data in which we have shown that i.t. administration of NMDA does not produce any evidence of an acute mechanical hyperalgesia but that coactivation of AMPA and metabotropic glutamate receptors with either quisqualate or a 1:1 combination of AMPA and trans-ACPD results in a dose-dependent decrease in the mechanical threshold for reflexive withdrawal of the tail (i.e., an acute mechanical hyperalgesia).[29] In that study, we suggested that coactivation of AMPA and metabotropic receptors resulting in mechanical hyperalgesia was due to activity at both of these receptor subtypes that are not normally active (i.e., AMPA or trans-ACPD alone do not alter nociceptive thermal or mechanical withdrawal reflexes). It was further suggested that these same mechanisms may apply to the mechanical hyperalgesia produced in models of persistent pain. Preliminary findings by us using intraplantar injection of zymosan[28] and the study by Dougherty et al.[11] support these conclusions and we suggest that the maintenance of mechanical hyperalgesia is likely mediated by coactivation of AMPA and metabotropic receptor subtypes and not by production of NO. These data are further supported by several recent electrophysiological studies of spinal cord neurons that have shown cooperativity between the metabotropic glutamate receptor and ionotropic AMPA receptors.[3,4]

Nitric oxide

Recently, there have been several reports that have indicated that activation of excitatory amino acid receptor subtypes other than NMDA receptors are able to produce NO.[14,23,37] However, the present data suggest that the acute mechanical hyperalgesia produced by coactivation of ionotropic AMPA and metabotropic glutamate receptor subtypes is not mediated by the production of NO. In addition, in the present study, we have found that the carrageenan-produced mechanical hyperalgesia was unaffected by L-NAME, suggesting that NO is not involved in the maintenance of persistent mechanical hyperalgesia in this model. Further, our preliminary data suggests that the persistent mechanical hyperalgesia produced by intraplanatar injection of zymosan also is not mediated by production of NO.[82] Collectively, these data support the hypothesis that NO, whether produced in models of acute or persistent pain, is not involved in mechanisms underlying mechanical hyperalgesia.

In summary, under most physiological situations where there is low frequency input to the spinal cord, synaptic transmission is likely mediated by non-NMDA receptors. However, in situations of persistent pain, where high-frequency or sustained afferent input produces a prolonged depolarization, the Mg^{2+} block on spinal NMDA receptors is removed, allowing for NMDA receptor activation, an influx of Ca^{2+} and production of NO. These changes in Ca^{2+} and NO may lead to changes as a result of facilitation of synaptic transmission that would be manifest, for example, as thermal hyperalgesia. In contrast, an increase in afferent input also allows for the AMPA and metabotropic receptor subtypes involved in mechanical hyperalgesia to become active and lead to intracellular events that are not dependent on the production of NO, but do produce mechanical hyperalgesia.

Therefore, it is possible that drugs which are able to interfere with the production and subsequent actions of NO may serve as useful new and novel therapeutic analgesics, particularly in circumstances associated with thermal hyperalgesia. Further, it is likely that NO may only represent the first in a new and intriguing class of neurotransmitters that are involved in synaptic transmission and likely in nociceptive processing in the spinal cord. As our knowledge and understanding of these new systems emerge, the next few years should provide fruitful and interesting clarification of the mechanisms of persistent pain.

ACKNOWLEDGEMENTS: The authors wish to thank Drs. T.J. Maves and R.J. Traub, Ms. P.S. Pechman and Ms. C. Dykstra for their assistance and discussions and Mike Burcham for producing the graphics. Supported by DHSS grants DA 02879,· NS 29844 and an unrestricted pain research award from Bristol-Myers Squibb Co.

REFERENCES

1. AANONSEN, L.M. AND WILCOX, G.L. (1987) Nociceptive action of excitatory amino acids in the mouse: effects of spinally administered opioids, phencyclidine and sigma agonists. *J. Pharmacol. Exp. Ther.* **243**, 9-19.
2. BENNETT, G.J. AND XIE, Y.-K. (1988) A peripheral mononeuropathy in rat that produces disordrers of pain sensation like those seen in man. *Pain* **33**, 87-107.
3. BLEAKMAN, D., RUSIN, K.I., CHARD, P.S., GLAUM, S.R. AND MILLER,, R.J. (1992) Metabotropic glutamate receptors potentiate ionotropic glutamate responses in the rat dorsal horn, *Mol. Pharmacol.* **42**, 192-196.
4. CERNE, R. AND RANDIC, M. (1992) Modulation of AMPA and NMDA responses in rat spinal dorsal horn neurons by trans-1-aminocyclopentane-1,3-dicarboxyclic acid. *Neurosci. Lett.* **144**, 180-184.
5. CHAPMAN, V. AND DICKENSON, A.H. (1992) The combination of NMDA antagonism and morphine produces profound antinociception in the rat dorsal horn. *Brain Res.* **573**, 321-323.
6. CODERRE, T.J. AND MELZACK, R. (1991) Central neural mediators of secondary hyperalgesia following heat injury in rats: neuropeptides and excitatory amino acids. *Neurosci. Lett.* **131**, 71-74.
7. CODERRE, T.J. AND MELZAC, R. (1992) The contribution of excitatory amino acids to central sensitization and persistent nociception after formalin-induced tissue injury. *J. Neurosci.* **12**, 3665-3670.
8. CODERRE, T.J. AND MELZACK, R. (1992) The role of NMDA receptor-operated calcium channels in persistent nociception after formalin-induced tissue injury. *J. Neurosci.* **12**, 3671-3675.
9. DAVAR, G., HAMA, A., DEYKIN, A., VOS, B. AND MACIEWICZ, R. (1991) MK-801 blocks the development of thermal hyperalgesia in a rat model of experimental painful neuropathy. *Brain Res.* **553,** 327-330.

10. DICKENSON, A.H. AND AYDAR, E. (1991) Antagonism at the glycine site on the NMDA receptor reduces spinal nociception in the rat. *Neurosci. Lett.* **121**, 263-266.

11. DOUGHERTY, P.M., SLUKA, K.A., SORKIN, L.S., WESTLUND, K.N. AND WILLIS, W.D. (1992) Neural changes in acute arthritis in monkeys. I. Parallel enhancement of responses of spinothalamic tract neurons to mechanical stimulation and excitatory amino acids. *Brain Res. Rev.* **17**, 1-13.

12. DUBNER, R. AND RUDA, M.A. (1992) Activity-dependent neuronal plasticity following tissue injury and inflammation. *Trends in Neurosci* **15**, 96-103.

13. FORSTERMANN, U., SCHMIDT, H.H.W., POLLOCK, J.S., SHENG, H., MITCHELL, J.A., WARNER, T.D., NAKANE, M. AND MURAD, F. (1991) Isoforms of nitric oxide synathase. Characterization and purification from different cell types, *Biochem. Pharmacol.* **10**, 1849-1857.

14. GARTHWAITE, J., SOUTHAM, E. AND ANDERTON, M. (1989) A kainate receptor linked to nitric oxide synthesis from arginine. *J. Neurochem.* **53**, 1952-1954.

15. HALEY, J.E., DICKENSON, A.H. AND SCHACHTER, M. (1992) Electrophysiological evidence for a role of nitric oxide in prolonged chemical nociception in rat. *Neuropharmacol.* **31**, 251-258.

16. HALEY, J.E., SULLIVAN, A.F. AND DICKENSON, A.H. (1990) Evidence for spinal N-methyl-D-aspartate receptor involvement in prolonged chemical nociception in rat. *Brain Res.* **518**, 218-226.

17. KITTO, K.F., HALEY, J.E. AND WILCOX, G.L. (1992) Involvement of nitric oxide in spinally mediated hyperalgesia in the mouse. *Neurosci. Lett.* **148**, 1-5.

18. KOLHEKAR, R., MELLER, S.T. AND GEBHART, G.F. (1993) Characterization of the role of spinal NMDA receptors on thermal nociception in the rat. *Neuroscience* (in press).

19. MALMBERG, A.B. AND YAKSH, T.L. (1992) Hyperalgesia mediated by spinal glutamate or substance P receptor blocked by spinal cyclooxygenase inhibition. *Science* **257**, 1276-1279.

20. MALMBERG, A.B. AND YAKSH, T.L. (1993) Spinal nitric oxide synthesis inhibition blocks NMDA induced thermal hyperalgesia and produces antinociception in the formalin test in rats. *Pain* (in press).

21. MAO, J., PRICE, D.D., HAYES, R.L., LU, J. AND MAYER, D.J. (1992) Differential roles of NMDA and non-NMDA receptor activation in induction and maintenance of thermal hyperalgesia in rats with a painful mononeuropathy. *Brain Res.* **598**, 271-278.

22. MAO, J., PRICE, D.D., MAYER, D.J., LU, J. AND HAYES, R.L. (1992) Intrathecal MK 801 and local nerve anesthesia synergistically reduce nociceptive behaviors in rats with peripheral mononeuropathy. *Brain Res.* **576**, 254-262.

23. MARIN, P., QUIGNARD, J-.F., LAFON-CAZA, M. AND BOCKAERT, J. (1993) Non-classical glutamate receptors, blocked by both NMDA and non-NMDA antagonists, stimulate nitric oxide production in neurons. *Neuropharmacol.* **32**, 29-36.

24. MAVES, T.J., PECHMAN, P.S., GEBHART, G.F. AND MELLER, S.T. (1993) Possible chemical contribution from chromic gut sutures produce disorders of pain sensation like those seen in man. *Pain* (in press).

25. MELLER, S.T., DYKSTRA, C. AND GEBHART G.F. (1992) Production of endogenous nitric oxide and activation of soluble guanylate cyclase are required for N-methyl-D-aspartate-produced facilitation of the nociceptive tail-flick reflex. *Eur. J. Pharmacol.* **214**, 93-96.

26. MELLER, S.T., PECHMAN, P.S., GEBHART, G.F. AND MAVES, T.J. (1992) Nitric oxide mediates the thermal hyperalgesia produced in a model of neuropathic pain in the rat. *Neuroscience* **50**, 7-10.

27. MELLER, S.T. AND GEBHART, G.F. (1993) Nitric oxide (NO) and nociceptive processing in the spinal cord. *Pain* **52**, 127-136.

28. MELLER, S.T., DYKSTRA, C. AND GEBHART G.F. (1993) Characterization of the spinal mechanisms of thermal and mechanical hyperalgesia following intraplantar zymosan. *Soc. Neurosci. Abstr.* 19, (in press).

29. MELLER, S.T., DYKSTRA, C. AND GEBHART, G.F. (1993) Acute mechanical hyperalgesia in the rat is produced by coactivation of ionotropic AMPA and metabotropic glutamate receptors. *Neuroreport* (in press).

30. MELLER, S.T., DYKSTRA, C., PECHMAN, P.S., MAVES, T.J. AND GEBHART, G.F. (1993) Ethanol dose-dependently attenuates NMDA-mediated thermal hyperalgesia in the rat. *Neurosci. Lett.* (in press).

31. MURRAY, C.W., COWAN, A. AND LARSON, A.A. (1991) Neurokinin and NMDA anatogonists (but not a kainic acid antagonist) are antinociceptive in the mouse formalin model. *Pain* **44**, 179-185.

32. NASSTROM, J., KARLSONN, U. AND POST, C. (1992) Antinociceptive actions of different classes of excitatory amino acid receptor antagonists in mice. *Eur. J. Pharmacol.* **212**, 21-29.

33. RAIGORODSKY, G. AND URCA G. (1987) Intrathecal N-methyl-D-aspartate (NMDA) activates both nociceptive and antinociceptive systems. *Brain Res.* **422**, 158-162.

34. REN, K., HYLDEN, J.L.K., WILLIAMS, G.M., RUDA, M.A. AND DUBNER, R. (1992) The effects of a non-competitive NMDA receptor antagonist, MK-801, on behavioral hyperalgesia and dorsal horn neuronal activity in rats with unilateral inflammation. *Pain* **50**, 331-344.

35. REN, K., WILLIAMS, G.M., HYLDEN, J.L.K., RUDA, M.A. AND DUBNER, R. (1992) The intrathecal administration of excitatory amino acid receptor antagonists selectively attenuate carrageenan-induced behavioral hyperalgesia in rats. *Eur. J. Pharmacol.* **219**, 235-243.

36. WILLIS, W.D. (1992) Hyperalgesia and allodynia. Raven Press, New York.

37. WOOD, P.L., EMMETT, M.R., RAO, T.S., CLER, J., MICK, S. AND IYENGAR, S. (1990) Inhibition of nitric oxide synthase blocks N-methyl-D-aspartate-, quisqualate-, kainate-, harmaline-,and pentylenetetrazole-dependent increases in cerebellar cyclic GMP in vivo. *J. Neurochem.* **55**, 346-348.

38. WOOLF, C.J. AND THOMPSON, S.W.N. (1991) The induction and maintenance of central sensitization is dependent on N-methyl-D-aspartic acid receptor activation: implications for the treatment of post-injury pain hypersensitivity states. *Pain* **44**, 293-300.

39. WOOLF, C.J. (1992) Excitability changes in central neurons following peripheral damage: the role of central sensitization in the pathogenesis of pain. In: *Hyperalgesia and Allodynia.* ed. Willis, W.D. Raven Press, New York.

40. WOOLF, C.J. (1989) Recent advances in the pathophysiology of acute pain. *Br. J. Anaesth.* **63**, 139-146.

41. YAMAMOTO, T. AND YAKSH, T.L., (1992) Comparison of the antinociceptive effects of pre- and posttreatment with intrathecal morphine and MK801, an NMDA antagonist, on the formalin test in the rat. *Anesthesiology* **77**, 757-763.
42. YAMAMOTO, T. AND YAKSH, T.L. (1992) Spinal pharmacology of thermal hyperesthesia induced by incomplete ligation of sciatic nerve: Excitatory amino acids. *Pain* **49**, 121-128.
43. YAMAMOTO, T., SHIMOYAMA, N. AND MIZUGUCHI, T. (1993) The effects of morphine, MK-801, an NMDA antagonist, and CP-96,345, an NK1 antagonist, on the hyperesthesia evoked by carrageenan injection in the rat paw. *Anesthesiology* **78**, 124-133.

DYNAMIC CHANGES IN DORSAL HORN NEURONS

W. D. Willis, Jr.
Department of Anatomy and Neurosciences and Marine Biomedical Institute
University of Texas Medical Branch
Galveston, Texas 77555-0843
USA

INTRODUCTION

The responses of dorsal horn neurons to somatosensory stimulation can be altered under a variety of circumstances. For example, somatosensory responses of spinal cord dorsal horn neurons can be decreased by 1) habituation following repeated stimulation of the excitatory receptive field;[46] 2) stimulation of an inhibitory receptive field;[30] 3) activity in descending inhibitory pathways[81] and 4) pathological changes leading to loss of primary afferent fibers.[13] Conversely, somatosensory responses can be increased by such manipulations as 1) repeated stimulation of fine calibre primary afferent fibers ("wind-up");[47] 2) spatial summation of excitatory inputs from different parts of the receptive field;[49] 3) volleys in excitatory pathways descending from the brain;[80] and 4) sensitization of primary afferent fibers[37] or of dorsal horn neurons as a consequence of damage to peripheral tissue or peripheral nerves.[19,57]

The emphasis here will be on the sensitization process that causes increases after injury in the responses of dorsal horn neurons to mechanical stimuli. The particular dorsal horn neurons examined were primate spinothalamic tract (STT) cells, identified by antidromic activation from the contralateral ventral posterior lateral thalamic nucleus.[70] Changes in the responses of these output neurons of the dorsal horn may reflect changes in their own excitability, in the activity of primary afferent fibers or of excitatory or inhibitory dorsal horn interneurons in pathways that in turn modulate the activity of STT cells. In this sense, the study of the responses of STT cells is similar for the dorsal horn to investigations of motoneurons for the

NATO ASI Series, Vol. H 79
Cellular Mechanisms of Sensory Processing
Edited by Laszlo Urban
© Springer-Verlag Berlin Heidelberg 1994

ventral horn. Alterations in the responses of either STT cells or motoneurons may indicate changes in monosynaptic or polysynaptic transmission to these output neurons.[24] A major advantage in investigations of both types of neuron is that the basic functions of these cells are clear. STT cells transmit sensory information to the thalamus and motoneurons activate striated muscle. The sensations encoded by STT cells include pain, warm and cold, as well as some forms of tactile sense.[78] Some STT cells may also transmit proprioceptive information,[50] although there is no evidence that this is consciously perceived.[75] Our interest is primarily in the responses of STT cells that lead to pain sensation.

Most STT cells that we have investigated in monkeys respond to both innocuous and noxious mechanical stimulation of the skin.[26,56] This is true not only of STT cells encountered in the deep layers of the dorsal horn, but also of those found in the superficial layers. It is likely that our sample is biased towards the larger STT cells, since we have not observed the purely thermoreceptive STT cells that are known to occur in lamina I nor STT cells that have unmyelinated axons.[cf.16] Most STT cells, when we first record their activity, have only small to moderate responses to weak mechanical stimuli, such as brushing the skin or application of von Frey hairs with low bending forces. Much larger responses occur when the strength of the stimulus extends into the range that evokes pain in human subjects. It is our working hypothesis that the information provided to the thalamus by these cells relates only to pain sensation. In unanesthetized, behaving animals, we assume that these cells either do not respond to tactile stimuli or that the responses are so small that they would be regarded by higher levels of the pain system as noise. We further assume that the tactile functions of the STT are mediated by the small population of STT cells that respond best to innocuous stimuli.

If our assumption that most of the STT cells that we study signal pain and only pain is correct, then any enhancement of the somatosensory responses of these cells should cause an enhancement of pain sensation. Thus, an increase in responses to noxious stimuli would cause greater pain. Changes of this sort could contribute to the development of states of hyperalgesia. Furthermore, ordinarily non-painful (innocuous) mechanical stimuli might now evoke pain (provided that the increased signal exceeded the noise level). Such a change could help account for mechanical allodynia.

It has long been known that damage to the skin leads immediately to primary hyperalgesia in the area of damage, followed by a slower development of secondary hyperalgesia in the surrounding skin.[33,43] The area of secondary hyperalgesia expands during a period of 15 or more minutes, after which it regresses over 2 hours or more (see drawing of forearm in Figure 1 and line labelled A in the graph).[33]

Primary hyperalgesia is generally attributed to the sensitization of nociceptive primary afferent fibers.[6,28,42,48] The neural processes responsible for secondary hyperalgesia depend on the activation of primary afferent fibers, since the development of secondary hyperalgesia can be delayed by locally anesthetising the damaged skin (line B in graph of Figure 1). Secondary hyperalgesia is often associated with mechanical allodynia,[40,41] and there is considerable evidence that these abnormal sensations are due to changes in the central nervous system.[33,40,41,69; see 7,77]

We hypothesise that increases in the responses of STT cells to innocuous and noxious mechanical stimuli are an important component of the central mechanism underlying mechanical allodynia and hyperalgesia. Our experimental approach to this question has been to study changes in the responses of primate STT cells following intradermal injection of capsaicin.[20,65] When capsaicin is injected into the skin of humans, it produces immediate, severe pain, followed by the development of primary and secondary hyperalgesia.[40,41] We assume that the same happens in monkeys. Such injections of capsaicin in monkeys also produce a sensitization of STT cells, characterized by increased responses to innocuous and noxious mechanical stimuli.[20,65] We have induced a similar sensitization of STT cells in experiments in which we have released excitatory amino acids (EAAs) and substance P (SP) into the vicinity of STT cells, using microiontophoresis.[20,22] Furthermore, we have obtained evidence that the sensitization of STT cells following intradermal injections of capsaicin can be blocked by the introduction into the neighboring dorsal horn of selective antagonists of excitatory amino acid receptors,[21] NK1 peptide receptors,[79] or nitric oxide synthase.[61] These observations suggest that EAAs, SP and NO all play a role in the sensitization of the responses of STT cells to mechanical stimuli following injury. Thus, we hypothesise that these substances contribute to the central neural mechanism of secondary hyperalgesia and allodynia.

This evidence will now be described.

RESPONSES OF STT CELLS TO INTRADERMAL CAPSAICIN INJECTION

It is possible to record from an individual STT cell in the deep layers of the dorsal horn of the lumbar spinal cord in anesthetized monkeys for many hours. This permits extensive sensory testing, as well as pharmacological manipulations, such as those described later. The cells were identified by antidromic activation following stimulation in the contralateral VPL thalamic nucleus (criteria for antidromic activation included a constant latency action potential that followed high frequency stimulation and that collided with orthodromic action potentials during a critical interval).[70] Essentially all STT cells that we sample in our usual experiments can be activated by application of mechanical stimuli to a cutaneous receptive field on the ipsilateral hindlimb. Most of the cells also respond to noxious thermal stimuli, particularly to noxious heat pulses, but sometimes also to noxious cold pulses.[37,38,57]

Injection of capsaicin into the skin in human subjects causes pain, primary mechanical and thermal hyperalgesia and secondary mechanical hyperalgesia.[40,41,69]

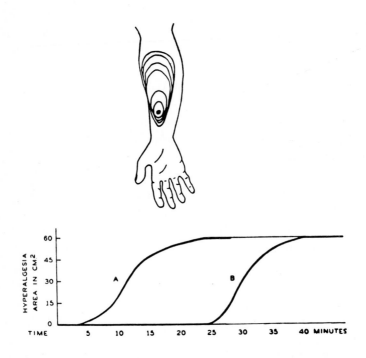

Figure 1. Development of secondary hyperalgesia following focal injury of the skin. The drawing of the arm shows the progressive spread of an area of secondary hyperalgesia in the skin surrounding a thermal injury at the site indicated by the dot. The line marked A in the graph shows the time course over which the area of secondary hyperalgesia developed to its maximum extent following the burn. The line marked B shows the time course of the development of secondary hyperalgesia when the area of skin to be damaged was first injected with the local anesthetic, procaine. (From Hardy, et al., 1952.)

Both forms of hyperalgesia are accompanied by mechanical allodynia. The secondary hyperalgesia and allodynia develop over a period of about 15 minutes, and they last hours.[41; cf. 33] Similar intradermal injections of capsaicin in monkeys evoke an intense discharge in STT cells that follows the time course of pain in humans.[65] As the heightened activity recedes, the neurons show increased responses and a lowered threshold to noxious heat stimuli applied over the injection site; responses to punctate noxious mechanical stimuli may also increase, although on average these are diminished, perhaps because of the inactivation of the terminals of nociceptors by the capsaicin. The increased responses to heat pulses and to punctate mechanical stimuli help account for the primary hyperalgesia that develops in the area of the injection site (there is also a small area of analgesia at the injection site) and are likely to be due to sensitization of nociceptors in the skin near the injection site.[4] The responses of the STT cells to innocuous and punctate noxious stimuli applied in an area of skin several cm from the injection site also increase, but there are no changes in the responses to thermal stimuli applied in this region.[65] These observations are consistent with the corresponding responses of human subjects to similar stimuli applied in the area of secondary hyperalgesia.[40,41] However, sensitization of primary afferent fibers in this region of the skin is not observed,[4,40] and so it is plausible to suggest that sensitization of dorsal horn neurons accounts for the sensory changes in humans[33,41,69] and is reflected in the altered responses of primate STT cells.

In recent years, we have employed a standard series of mechanical stimuli in order to characterize the STT cells on the basis of their responses to innocuous and noxious mechanical stimulation.[12,31] These stimuli include BRUSH (brushing the skin with a camel hair brush, a tactile stimulus), PRESS (application of pressure to the skin with an arterial clip, a compressive stimulus that is near pain threshold in humans), PINCH (application of another arterial clip that pinches the skin and is distinctly painful but that does not obviously harm the skin), and SQUEEZE (squeezing the skin with serrated forceps, a damaging stimulus). In experiments in which we wish to sensitise STT cells, we minimise the use of the SQUEEZE stimulus, since repeated applications of SQUEEZE can cause sensitization of these cells.[56] By contrast, the BRUSH, PRESS and PINCH stimuli can be repeated many times without any obvious change in the responses.

Figure 2 shows the effects of an intradermal injection of capsaicin on the responses of an STT cell to the BRUSH, PRESS and PINCH stimuli.[20] Following the recording of a period of background activity (Figure 2A), three series of mechanical stimuli were applied in succession to a series of 5 spots marked on the skin and spanning the receptive field. The 5 spots are indicated on the drawing of the hindlimb

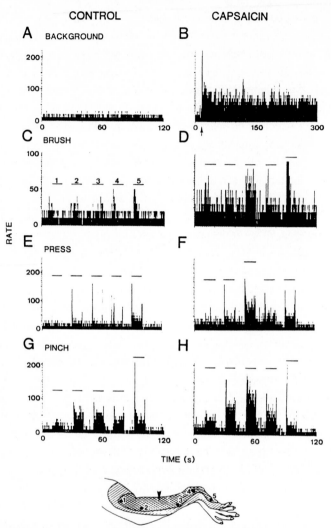

Figure 2. Enhancement of responses of a spinothalamic tract (STT) neuron to mechanical stimulation following intradermal injection of capsaicin. The peristimulus time histogram in A shows the background activity of the cell before capsaicin. The injection of capsaicin occurred at the time indicated by the arrow in B. Note the change in time scale. The horizontal lines in C-H indicates the times at which mechanical stimuli were applied to points 1-5 in the receptive field. C and D show the responses to BRUSH, E and F to PRESS and G and H to PINCH before and after capsaicin. The drawing shows the initial receptive field (doubly hatched area), the expanded receptive field after capsaicin (singly hatched area) and the site of the capsaicin injection (arrowhead).
(From Dougherty & Willis, 1992.)

at the bottom of the figure (the initial receptive field is doubly cross-hatched). The stimuli started with the weakest (BRUSH) and then progressed to higher intensities (PRESS and PINCH). The responses to these stimuli are shown in Figure 2C, E and G. After these and other control recordings were made, capsaicin was injected into the skin at the point indicated by the arrowhead in the drawing. The capsaicin evoked a substantial discharge that lasted more than 5 minutes (Figure 2B; time of injection is indicated by the arrow). Sensory testing began 15 minutes after the injection. At this time, the background activity was still elevated, and the responses to all of the mechanical stimuli were enhanced, at least at some spots within the receptive field (Figure 2D, F and H). In addition, it was observed that the receptive field had expanded (singly hatched area in the drawing).

Figure 3 shows the responses of the same STT cell to graded iontophoretic doses of several EAAs (glutamate, GLU; aspartate, ASP; N-methyl-D-aspartic acid, NMDA and quisqualic acid, QUIS). The control responses are in Figure 3A, C, E and G. After these were recorded, capsaicin was injected intradermally (see Figure 2). After the capsaicin injection, it was found that the responses to iontophoretic application of all of the EAAs tested were increased (Figure 3B, D, F and H).

In Figure 4 are shown the time courses of the changes in the responses of this cell (Figure 4A and B) and of another (Figure 4C and D) to both the mechanical stimuli and the EAAs. The responses increased over some 15 minutes after the capsaicin injection and then returned to near the control level in about 2 hours.

This type of experiment indicates that intradermal injections of capsaicin cause STT cells to become more responsive to mechanical stimuli applied to the skin and to chemical stimuli applied directly to the cells. These changes support the idea that the STT cells are sensitised by a neural mechanism activated by the capsaicin injection and the consequent barrage of nociceptive afferent discharges. Capsaicin is known to activate nociceptive afferent fibers, particular those supplied by C fibers,[27,44] and recordings consistent with this have been made from peripheral nerve fibers in both monkeys and humans following intradermal injection of capsaicin.[4,40] It is conceivable that the excitability of the STT cells is maintained by a continuous discharge of afferent fibers set in train by the capsaicin, but the evidence obtained to date is that capsaicin causes only a short-lasting discharge of afferent fibers, particularly of C fibers, near the injection site and does not affect afferent fibers supplying the area of secondary hyperalgesia.[4,40] It is interesting that the time course of the changes in the responses of the STT cells matches the time course of secondary hyperalgesia, including an increasing responsiveness during the first 15 minutes or so and a return to normal responsiveness over a period of a few hours. The increased sensitivity of the STT cells to EAAs suggests that afferent volleys that

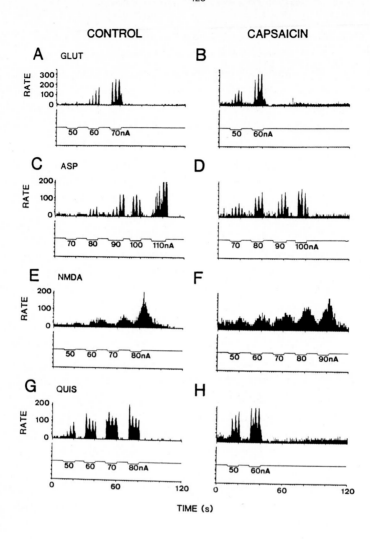

CONTROL   CAPSAICIN

A GLUT   B

C ASP   D

E NMDA   F

G QUIS   H

TIME (s)

Figure 3. Enhancement of responses of the same STT neuron whose responses are shown in Figure 2 to excitatory amino acids (EAAs) after intradermal injection of capsaicin. The iontophoretic currents used to release the EAAs and the duration of the currents are indicated. The responses to graded doses of glutamate (GLU) before and after capsaicin are shown in A and B, to aspartate (ASP) in C and D, to N-methyl-D-aspartate (NMDA) in E and F, and to quisqualate (QUIS) in G and H, respectively. (From Dougherty & Willis, 1992.)

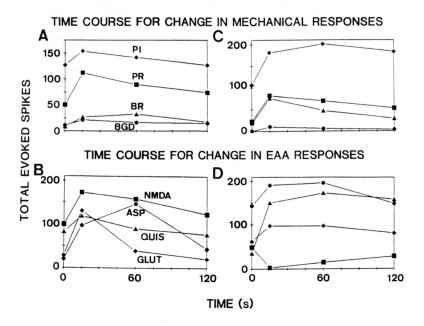

Figure 4. Time course of the changes in responses of 2 STT cells to mechanical stimuli applied to the receptive field and to iontophoretically released EAAs produced by intradermal injection of capsaicin. Background activity (BGD) and responses to BRUSH (BR), PRESS (PR) and PINCH (PI) are shown for one of the 2 STT cells in A and the responses to GLUT, ASP, NMDA and QUIS are shown in B. The comparable responses of the other STT cells are shown in C and D. (From Dougherty & Willis, 1992.)

release a constant amount of neurotransmitter (presumably EAAs) would be more effective in exciting the STT cells, thus accounting for the increased responses to mechanical stimuli.

THE ROLE OF EAAS AND SP IN CENTRAL SENSITIZATION

An intradermal injection of capsaicin is likely to evoke central activity by the synaptic actions of discharges conducted to the spinal cord dorsal horn largely in C fibers.[4,27,40,44,71] The neurotransmitters released by fine primary afferent fibers appear to include excitatory amino acids (EAAs), such as glutamate (GLU), and peptides, such as SP.[3,18,29,63,71,73] Release of these presumed neurotransmitters activates interneurons of the dorsal horn,[17,29,35,71] many of which can also release EAAs[60] or peptides.[36,68] Glutamate and SP have been shown to excite primate STT cells.[76] Some primary afferent fibers containing calcitonin gene-related peptide (CGRP), a substance that seems to be restricted in its distribution in the dorsal horn to primary afferent fibers,[14] have been found to synapse on STT cells.[10] STT cells are also contacted by numerous synaptic endings that contain GLU,[74] as shown in Figure 5, and by at least some synapses that contain SP.[9] Thus, STT cells are likely to be directly exposed to EAAs and peptides released into the dorsal horn by primary afferent fibers, as well as by interneurons or descending pathways.

Studies in which EAAs were released by microiontophoresis near STT cells have shown that these cells are highly responsive to EAAs acting both on N-methyl-D-aspartic acid (NMDA) and on non-NMDA receptors.[21,22] Particular EAAs that excite STT cells include the endogenous ligands, GLU and aspartate (ASP), as well as quisqualic acid (QUIS), α-amino-3-hydroxy-5-methyl-isoxazoleproprionic acid (AMPA), kainic acid (KAIN), and NMDA. SP can directly excite STT cells,[76] but more commonly SP appears to act as a neuromodulator that enhances the action of EAAs.[19,22]

The enhancement of the responses of an STT cell to NMDA by co-application of SP is shown in Figure 6. Graded currents were used to release graded doses of NMDA, and the same series of currents was applied 3 times at intervals of 5 minutes (Figure 6A-C). The release of SP alone had no obvious effect on the STT cell (Figure 6D). When NMDA and SP were co-released, the responses to the pulses of NMDA increased immediately (Figure 6E), and they were enhanced still more at 15 minutes after termination of the SP application (Figure 6F). Since there was no increment in the responses to NMDA upon repeated applications in this or other STT cells (Figure 6A-C, G), but rather a tendency for the responses to decrease, it can be concluded that SP had a modulatory effect that enhanced the responses to NMDA.

A particularly striking observation is that the co-application of an EAA and SP resulted in responses to EAAs that continued to increment for at least 15 minutes after termination of the SP. This behavior of STT cells is consistent with the time course of the onset of capsaicin sensitization and the development of secondary hyperalgesia after acute injury. Furthermore, some STT cells had a prolonged enhancement of their responses to later applications of the same EAA in the absence of additional SP.[19,22; cf. 62] This was observed in some STT cells when NMDA was co-applied with SP and in other STT cells when QUIS was co-applied with SP.

431

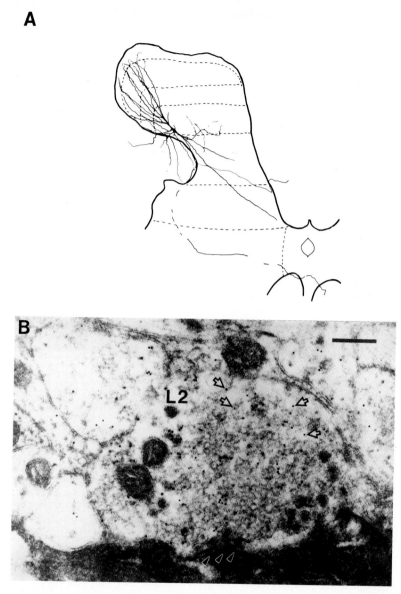

Figure 5. Glutamate immunoreactive synaptic ending on an STT cell labelled intracellularly with horseradish peroxidase (HRP). The STT cell was injected with HRP during an electrophysiological recording experiment. The reconstructed dendritic tree and the axons of the cell are shown in A. The electron micrograph in B shows a synaptic terminal on the labelled STT cell. The terminal is labelled immunocytochemically for glutamate using the immunogold technique. The black arrowheads at the bottom indicate an active zone. The open arrows point to gold particles. (From Westlund, et al., 1992.)

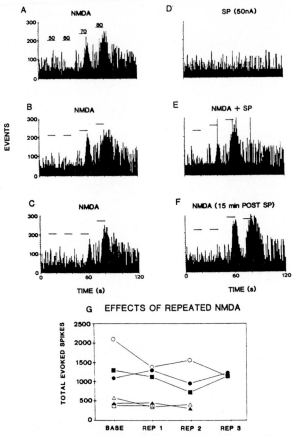

Figure 6. Responses of an STT cell to NMDA and substance P (SP). A graded series of iontophoretic currents were used to release NMDA. The responses to 3 series of current pulses are shown in A-C. When SP was released alone, D, there was no obvious effect at the dose employed. When NMDA was released during SP application, E, the responses to the NMDA increased. In F, the responses to another series of current pulses were increased still more 15 minutes after termination of the SP application. The graphs in G show that the responses of 6 different STT cells to repeated series of NMDA applications tended to decrease. (Dougherty & Willis, 1991.)

An example of this is shown in Figure 7 for an STT cell that was excited by graded iontophoretic doses of QUIS (Figure 7A). Co-application of the same series of QUIS pulses with SP resulted in larger responses for as long as 2 hours after termination of the SP application (Figure 7B-F).[22] Similarly, the responses of STT cells to NMDA were sometimes enhanced by co-application of SP, and these increased responses could be observed for several hours.[19] On the other hand, the responses of STT cells to AMPA did not increase for long periods after co-application with SP; instead, responses to AMPA generally returned to the control level within about 15 minutes.[22]

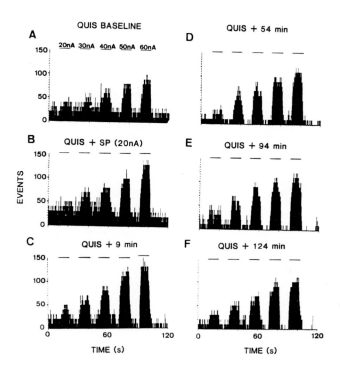

Figure 7. Responses of an STT cell to QUIS and SP. The current pulses used to release QUIS iontophoretically are indicated above the histogram in A above the responses of the neuron. In B, the responses to QUIS were increased during co-application of SP. C-F show that the responses to QUIS remained elevated for more than 2 hours after the termination of the SP application. (From Dougherty, et al., 1993.)

When the responses of an STT cell to an EAA, such as NMDA or QUIS, were enhanced following co-application of that EAA with SP, the responses of the same neurons to mechanical stimulation of the skin were generally also enhanced, as shown in Figure 8.[19,22] Thus, co-application of an EAA and SP can change the behavior of an STT cell in a manner similar to that seen after intradermal injection of capsaicin. We consider such STT cells to be sensitised.

SP was occasionally found to cause a reduction in the action of EAAs.[22] In some cases, the responses to activation of one type of EAA receptor were enhanced and those to activation of another type of EAA receptor were reduced (e.g., when responses to NMDA were enhanced, there was a reduction in QUIS or AMPA responses, and vice versa). This is illustrated in Figure 9. For cell A, SP caused an increase in the responses to NMDA but decreased the responses to QUIS, whereas for cell B, SP reduced the responses to NMDA while increasing those to AMPA. Alternatively, SP could cause a reduction of all EAA responses tested.[22]

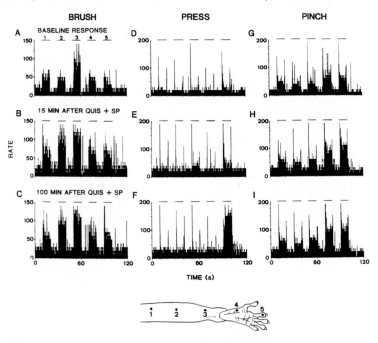

Figure 8. Increases in the responses of the same STT cell as in Fig. 7 to mechanical stimulation of the skin after iontophoretic application of QUIS and SP. A, D and G show the responses of the cell to BRUSH, PRESS and PINCH stimuli applied at 5 spots in the receptive field. B, E and H show the increases in the responses to mechanical stimuli tested 15 minutes after the co-application of QUIS and SP. C, F and I show partial recovery at 100 minutes after the drug applications. The drawing shows the spots stimulated in the receptive field. (From Dougherty, et al., 1993.)

From these observations, it appears that the changes seen in the responses of STT cells to EAAs and to mechanical stimulation of the skin following intradermal injection of capsaicin can be mimicked by iontophoretic co-application of EAAs and SP onto STT cells. However, this does not prove that these substances are in fact involved in the sensitization of STT cells that follows intradermal injection of capsaicin. Evidence that this is indeed the case was obtained using selective antagonists of EAA and SP receptors.[21,79] The way in which these experiments were conducted was to record from an STT cell using a multibarrelled electrode so that EAAs could be released by iontophoresis to test the responses of the cell to agonists of the NMDA or non-NMDA EAA receptors. After testing the responses of the STT cells both to EAAs and to mechanical stimulation of the skin, capsaicin was injected intradermally to sensitise the neuron. Repeated tests showed that the cell became more responsive to EAAs and to mechanical stimulation of the skin. After waiting several hours for the sensitization to regress, an antagonist to either non-NMDA receptors (CNQX), NMDA receptors (AP7) or NK1 SP receptors (CP96,345) was introduced into the dorsal horn adjacent to the STT cell through a microdialysis fiber.[21,79] In some experiments, an inactive isomer of the NK1 antagonist (CP96,344) was used instead of CP96,345 as a control for effects on calcium channels.[79] In experiments involving the release of the EAAs, we could time the arrival of an adequate concentration of antagonist at the location of the STT cell, as well as test for the selectiveness of the antagonism, by releasing the EAAs by iontophoresis.[21]

Figure 10 shows the responses of an STT cell to several EAAs before, during and after the administration of CNQX through the microdialysis fiber, and Figure 11 shows similar responses of another STT cell before, during and after administration of AP7.[21] It should be noted that these antagonists were rather selective, although CNQX in Figure 10G seems to have partially reduced the responses to NMDA. However, this observation is hard to interpret. The CNQX may have caused a hyperpolarization of the STT cell by blocking a depolarizing action of EAAs on non-NMDA receptors (note that the background activity was reduced by the CNQX). Hyperpolarization would permit a resumption of a magnesium block of the NMDA channels and thus reduce the responses to NMDA. Thus, the reduction of the NMDA responses need not indicate a lack of specificity of the antagonist.

The graphs in Figure 12 illustrate the effects of these antagonists on the responses of a sample of STT cells to graded mechanical stimuli (BRUSH , PRESS and PINCH) before and after intradermal injections of capsaicin.[21] In Figure 12A, it can be seen that CNQX prevented the initial response to capsaicin. It also prevented any increase in background discharge (Figure 12B). CNQX blocked the responses of

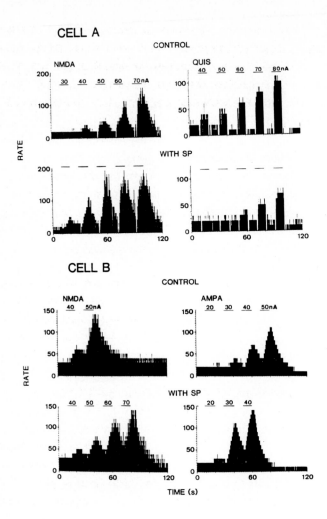

Figure 9. Reciprocal actions of SP on the responses of two STT cells to activation of NMDA and non-NMDA receptors. The first row of histograms show the control responses of cell A to graded iontophoretic doses of NMDA and of QUIS. The second row shows the effects of co-application of SP on these responses. The third row of histograms show the control responses of cell B to NMDA and AMPA. The fourth row shows the changes in the responses produced by co-application of SP. (From Dougherty, et al., 1993.)

STT cells to all of the mechanical stimuli, and capsaicin failed to enhance these in the presence of CNQX (Figure 12C-E). On the other hand, AP7 only reduced the responses to capsaicin (Figure 12A), and it did not significantly change the responses to the mechanical stimuli except that to PINCH (Figure 12C). However, AP7 prevented any change in background discharges or responses to mechanical stimuli after the second capsaicin injection (Figure 12B, C). The NK1 antagonist, CP96,345, had effects similar to those of AP7, but CP96,344 was without effect (not illustrated). [79]

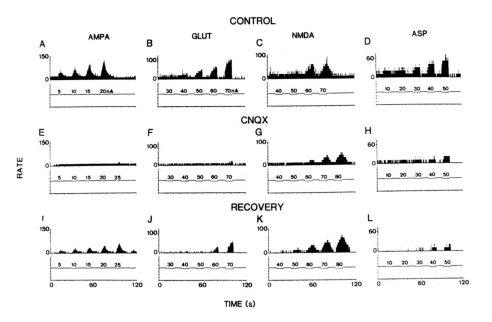

Figure 10. Selective antagonism of the responses of an STT cell to EAA agonists released with iontophoretic current pulses by CNQX administered through a microdialysis fiber. The control responses to graded doses of AMPA, GLUT, NMDA and ASP are shown in A-D. The non-NMDA receptor antagonist, CNQX, was then introduced into the dorsal horn through a microdialysis fiber, and after an hour, the responses in E-H were recorded. Administration of CNQX was then terminated, and after 4 hours there was partial recovery of the responses, as shown in I-L. (From Dougherty, et al., 1992.)

POSSIBLE MECHANISMS OF SENSITIZATION

It has been shown that EAAs and SP depolarise dorsal horn neurons and that the depolarization produced by SP has a slow time course.[32,52,72] However, the depolarization caused by SP lasts only a few minutes, and so it is insufficient to account for the duration of sensitization of STT cells.[72] Furthermore, a depolarization should make a cell more responsive to any constant stimulus impinging on the cell. However, a given STT cell can be sensitised to application of one EAA but show reduced responses to another (e.g., see Figure 9). Furthermore, responses to innocuous mechanical stimuli may be increased at a time that responses to noxious mechanical stimuli are unchanged (see Figure 12C and E). These observations suggest that some mechanism other than depolarization is involved in the sensitization process.

One obvious possibility is that second messenger systems are activated and

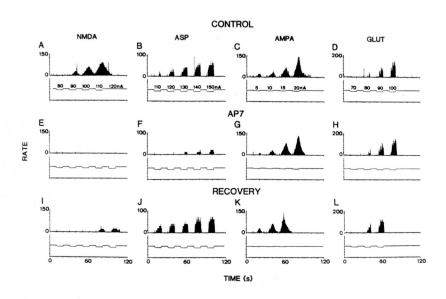

Figure 11. Selective antagonism of the responses of an STT cell to EAA agonists released iontophoretically by AP7 administered through a microdialysis fiber. Control responses to NMDA, ASP, AMPA and GLUT are shown in A-D. The NMDA receptor antagonist, AP7, was then introduced into the dorsal horn through a microdialysis fiber for 30 minutes, and the responses to the EAAs were again tested, as shown in E-H. Finally, the responses were retested 2 hours after termination of the AP7 infusion, and there was partial recovery of the responses, as shown in I-L. (From Dougherty, et al., 1992.)

that these cause sensitization of the responses of STT cells (or of interneurons in pathways that activate STT cells). It is well known that NMDA causes calcium influx through ion channels opened by NMDA receptors.[45] The increase in intracellular calcium ion concentration causes the activation of second messenger systems. For example, in some neurons, calcium influx activates nitric oxide synthase (NOS) by binding to calmodulin; NOS in turn, in the presence of NADPH and calcium, converts arginine to citrulline and nitric oxide (NO).[8,39] NO diffuses through the neuronal membrane and enters adjacent cells, where it activates guanylyl cyclase, which increases the concentration of cyclic GMP in the affected neurons.[23] We have recently obtained evidence for a role of NO in the sensitization of STT cells following intradermal injections of capsaicin.[61] Introduction of the NO synthase inhibitor, L-methyl-arginine methyl ester (L-NAME), but not its inactive isomer, D-NAME, into the dorsal horn through a microdialysis fiber prevents the sensitization of STT cells by intradermal injection of capsaicin.

The calcium influx produced by activation of NMDA receptors may also activate protein kinase C.[2,5,25] Protein kinase C, in turn, can increase NMDA currents by reducing the Mg^{++} block of the ion channels activated by NMDA.[11] We have recently found that direct activation of protein kinase C by administering a phorbol ester into the dorsal horn by microdialysis causes enhanced responses of STT cells to innocuous mechanical stimuli.[58] Administration of an inactive phorbol ester had no effect on the responses. Interestingly, the phosphorylation of NOS by protein kinase C (and also by CAMP-dependent protein kinase and calcium/calmodulin-dependent protein kinase II) can decrease NOS activity.[8] Thus, NO release may be regulated in opposite directions by the activation of NMDA receptors.

QUIS is thought to act both on AMPA receptors and on metabotropic EAA receptors.[15,51] AMPA has only relatively short-lasting actions on STT cells, even in the presence of SP, as noted above,[22] presumably because it acts only on inotropic receptors and these receptors are not upregulated by protein kinase C.[1;see 5] However, QUIS, in the presence of SP, can cause a prolonged increase in QUIS responses and in responses to mechanical stimulation of the skin. This may be due to activation of metabotropic EAA receptors. Consistent with this are recent observations that administration of trans-ACPD, an agonist of metabotropic EAA receptors, can cause an increase in the responses of STT cells to innocuous mechanical stimuli.[59] The actions of metabotropic glutamate receptors include a G-protein mediated increase in the intracellular levels of inositol triphosphate and diacylglycerol, as well as activation of protein kinase C.[64,66,67] Protein kinase C, in turn, activates metabotropic glutamate receptors and increases NMDA currents.[1]

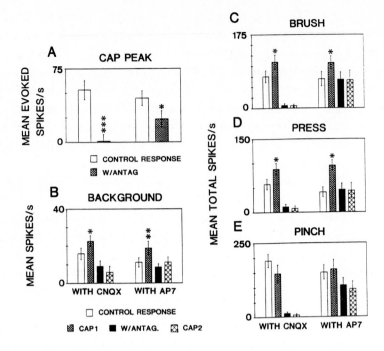

Figure 12. Effects of CNQX and AP7 on the responses of groups of STT cells to intradermal injection of capsaicin and to mechanical stimulation of the skin. The sets of bars at the left of each graph show the effects of CNQX, and those at the right show the effects of AP7. The open and filled bars represent control responses, and the hatched bars show responses after either the first or the second injection of capsaicin. In A, the response to capsaicin is shown to be reduced significantly by both EAA antagonists. In B, the first capsaicin injection produced a significant increase in the background activity measured 15 minutes after the injection. However, both EAA antagonists prevented the second capsaicin injection from having any effect on the background activity measured 15 minutes after the second injection. In C and D, the responses to BRUSH and PRESS were increased following the first injection of capsaicin. The responses were sensitised. However, both EAA antagonists prevented sensitization of the responses following the second injection of capsaicin. In E, the first capsaicin injection failed to change the responses to PINCH. The EAA antagonists reduced the pinch responses, but the responses were still unaffected by the second injection of capsaicin. (From Dougherty, et al., 1992.)

The role of SP in enhancing the responses to EAAs may also be due to the activation of a second messenger system complementary to those activated by the EAAs. SP is known to increase calcium influx into dorsal horn neurons.[53] In addition, SP causes the release of calcium from intracellular stores, and it activates the inositol phosphate system, at least in the brain (but perhaps not in the spinal cord).[34,55]

Although it is unclear at this time exactly how the activation of second messengers influences the responses of STT cells to EAAs or to mechanical stimuli, several possibilities are suggested by the findings in other systems mentioned above. For example, phosphorylation of NMDA ion channels by protein kinase C can result in increases in NMDA currents and hence in synaptic efficacy.[11] Another possible mechanism would be changes in the amount of transmitter released from presynaptic terminals. This is thought to occur in the hippocampus during long-term potentiation and has been attributed to the retrograde action of NO released from the postsynaptic cell and acting on presynaptic endings.[54]

CONCLUSIONS

Injury to the skin in humans causes pain, primary and secondary hyperalgesia. These sensory changes can be induced experimentally by injecting capsaicin into the skin. Changes in the responses of primate STT cells are also seen following intradermal capsacin injections. These changes include an initial high frequency discharge, enhanced responses to mechanical and heat stimuli applied at the site of the injection, and transiently increased responses to innocuous and noxious mechanical stimuli, but not to heat stimuli, in the area surrounding the injection site. We hypothesise that these changes in STT cells (and presumably in other nociceptive ascending tract cells) account for the development of primary hyperalgesia in the area of injury and of mechanical allodynia and secondary hyperalgesia in an undamaged region of skin surrounding an area of injury. We suggest that the immediate cause of these changes is the release of EAAs and peptides in the dorsal horn by nociceptive afferent fibers, as well as by interneurons (and possibly descending pathways). It seems likely that these neurotransmitters and modulators activate second messenger systems that, in turn, selectively alter the excitability of STT cells in response to particular stimuli. If our hypothesis is correct, the changes in the responses of STT cells lead to the observed changes in human perception. These findings offer the opportunity for pharmacological interventions that may be effective in reducing the hyperalgesia that is commonly associated with injury due to disease or surgery.

REFERENCES

1. ANIKSZTEJN, L., OTANI, S. AND BEN-ARI, Y. (1992) Quisqualate metabotropic receptors modulate NMDA currents and facilitate induction of long-term potentiation through protein kinase C. *Europ. J. Neurosci.* **4**, 500-505.
2. BABA, A., ETOH, S. AND IAWATA, H. (1991) Inhibition of NMDA-induced protein kinase C translocation by a Zn^{2+} chelator: implication of intracellular Zn^{2+}. *Brain Res.* **557**, 103-108.
3. BATTAGLIA, G. AND RUSTIONI, A. (1988) Coexistence of glutamate and substance P in dorsal root ganglion neurons of the rat and monkey. *J. Comp. Neurol.* **277**, 302-312.
4. BAUMANN, T.K., SIMONE, D.A., SHAIN, C.N. AND LAMOTTE, R.H. (1991) Neurogenic hyperalgesia: the search for the primary cutaneous afferent fibers that contribute to capsaicin-induced pain and hyperalgesia. *J. Neurophysiol.* **66**, 212-227.
5. BEN-ARI, Y., ANIKSZTEJN, L. AND BREGESTOVSKI, P. (1992) Protein kinase C modulation of NMDA currents: an important link for LTP induction. *TINS* **15**, 333-339.
6. BESSOU, P. AND PERL, E.R. (1969) Response of cutaneous sensory units with unmyelinated fibers to noxious stimuli. *J. Neurophysiol.* **32**, 1025-1043.
7. BONICA, J.J. *The management of pain.* (1990) 2nd ed. Lea & Febiger, Philadelphia.
8. BREDT, D.S. AND SNYDER, S.H. (1992) Nitric oxide, a novel neuronal messenger. *Neuron* **8**, 3-11.
9. CARLTON, S.M., LAMOTTE, C.C., HONDA, C.N., SURMEIER, D.J., DELANEROLLE, N.C. AND WILLIS, W.D. (1985) Ultrastructural analysis of substance P and other synaptic profiles innervating an identified primate spinothalamic tract neuron. *Neurosci. Abstr.* **11**, 578.
10. CARLTON, S.M., WESTLUND, K.N., ZHANG, D., SORKIN, L.S. AND WILLIS, W.D. (1990) Calcitonin gene-related peptide containing primary afferent fibers synapse on primate spinothalamic tract cells. *Neurosci. Lett.* **109**, 76-81.
11. CHEN, L. AND HUANG, L.Y.M. (1991) Sustained potentiation of NMDA receptor-mediated glutamate responses through activation of protein kinase C by a µ opioid. *Neuron* **7**, 319-326.
12. CHUNG, J.M., KENSHALO, D.R., JR., GERHART, K.D. AND WILLIS, W.D. (1979) Excitation of primate spinothalamic neurons by cutaneous C-fiber volleys. *J. Neurophysiol.* **42**, 1354-1369.
13. CHUNG, J.M., PAIK, K.S., KIM, J.S., NAM, S.C., KIM, K.J., OH, U.T., HASEGAWA, T., CHUNG, K. AND WILLIS, W.D. (1993) Chronic effects of topical application of capsaicin to the sciatic nerve on responses of primate spinothalamic neurons. *Pain* (in press).
14. CHUNG, K., LEE, W.T. AND CARLTON, S.M. (1988) The effects of dorsal rhizotomy and spinal cord isolation on calcitonin gene-related peptide-labeled terminals in the rat lumbar dorsal horn. *Neurosci. Lett.* **90**, 27-32.
15. COLLINGRIDGE, G.L. AND LESTER, R.A.J. (1989) Excitatory amino acid

receptors in the vertebrate central nervous system. *Pharmacol. Rev.* **40**, 143-210.

16. CRAIG, A.D. AND KNIFFKI, K.D. (1985) Spinothalamic lumbosacral lamina I cells responsive to skin and muscle stimulation in the cat. *J. Physiol.* **365**, 197-221.

17. CURTIS, D.R., PHILLIS, J.W. AND WATKINS, J.C. (1960) The chemical excitation of spinal neurones by certain acidic amino acids. *J. Physiol.* **150**, 656-682.

18. DE BIASI, S. AND RUSTIONI, A. (1988) Glutamate and substance P coexist in primary afferent terminals in superficial laminae of spinal cord. *Proc. Natl. Acad. Sci. USA* **85**, 7820-7824.

19. DOUGHERTY, P.M. AND WILLIS, W.D. (1991) Enhancement of spinothalamic neuron responses to chemical and mechanical stimuli following combined micro-iontophoretic application of N-methyl-D-aspartic acid and substance P. *Pain* **47**, 85-93.

20. DOUGHERTY, P.M. AND WILLIS, W.D. (1992) Enhanced responses of spinothalamic tract neurons to excitatory amino acids accompany capsaicin-induced sensitization in the monkey. *J. Neuroscience* **12**, 883-894.

21. DOUGHERTY, P.M., PALECEK, J., PALECKOVÁ, V., SORKIN, L.S. AND WILLIS, W.D. (1992) The role of NMDA and non-NMDA excitatory amino acid receptors in the excitation of primate spinothalamic tract cells by mechanical, chemical, thermal and electrical stimuli. *J. Neuroscience* **12**, 3025-3041.

22. DOUGHERTY, P.M., PALECEK, J., ZORN, S. AND WILLIS, W.D. (1993) Combined application of excitatory amino acids and substance P produces long-lasting changes in responses of primate spinothalamic tract neurons. *Brain Res. Rev.*, Accepted.

23. EAST, S.J. AND GARTHWAITE, J. (1990) Nanomolar N^G-nitroarginine inhibits NMDA-induced cyclic GMP formation in rat cerebellum. *Eur. J. Pharmacol.* **184**, 311-313.

24. ECCLES, J.C. (1964) *The physiology of synapses.* Springer-Verlag, New York.

25. ETOH, S., BABA, A. AND IWATA, H. (1991) NMDA induces protein kinase C translocation in hippocampal slices of immature rat brain. *Neurosci. Lett.* **126**, 119-122.

26. FERRINGTON, D.G., SORKIN, L.S. AND WILLIS, W.D. (1987) Responses of spinothalamic tract cells in the superficial dorsal horn of the primate lumbar spinal cord. *J. Physiol.* **388**, 681-703.

27. FITZGERALD, M. (1983) Capsaicin and sensory neurones--a review. *Pain* **15**, 109-130.

28. FITZGERALD, M. AND LYNN, B. (1977) The sensitization of high threshold mechanoreceptors with myelinated axons by repeated heating. *J. Physiol.* **265**, 549-563.

29. GERBER, G., CERNE, R. AND RANDIC, M. (1991) Participation of excitatory amino acid receptors in the slow excitatory synaptic transmission in rat spinal dorsal horn. *Brain Res.* **561**, 236-251.

30. GERHART, K.D., YEZIERSKI, R.P., GIESLER, G.J. AND WILLIS, W.D. (1981) Inhibitory receptive fields of primate spinothalamic tract cells. *J. Neurophysiol.* **46**, 309-1325.

31. GIESLER, G.J., YEZIERSKI, R.P., GERHART, K.D. AND WILLIS, W.D. (1981) Spinothalamic tract neurons that project to medial and/or lateral thalamic nuclei: evidence for a physiologically novel population of spinal cord neurons. *J. Neurophysiol.* **46**, 1285-1308.

32. GU, Y.P. AND HUANG, L.Y.M. (1989) Effects of excitatory amino acids on neurons isolated from spinal trigeminal nuclei. *Neurosci. Abstr.* **15**, 947.

33. HARDY, J.D., WOLFF, H.G. AND GOODELL, H. (1952) *Pain sensations and reactions.* Williams & Wilkins, New York (reprinted by Hafner, New York, 1967).

34. HELKE, C.J., KRAUSE, J.E., MANTYH, P.W., COUTURE, R. AND BANNON, M.J. (1990) Diversity in mammalian tachykinin peptidergic neurons: multiple peptides, receptors, and regulatory mechanisms. *FASEB J.* **4**, 606-1615.

35. HENRY, J.L. (1976) Effects of substance P on functionally identified units in cat spinal cord. *Brain Res. Bull.* **114**, 439-451.

36. HUNT, S.P., KELLY, J.S., EMSON, P.C., KIMMEL, J.R., MILLER, R.J. AND WU, J.Y. (1981) An immunohistochemical study of neuronal populations containing neuropeptides or γ-aminobutyrate within the superficial layers of the rat dorsal horn. *Neuroscience* **6**, 1883-1898.

37. KENSHALO, D.R., JR., LEONARD, R.B., CHUNG, J.M. AND WILLIS, W.D. (1979) Responses of primate spinothalamic neurons to graded and to repeated noxious heat stimuli. *J. Neurophysiol.* **42**, 1370-1389.

38. KENSHALO, D.R., JR., LEONARD, R.B., CHUNG, J.M. AND WILLIS, W.D. (1982) Facilitation of the responses of primate spinothalamic cells to cold and to tactile stimuli by noxious heating of the skin. *Pain* **12**, 41-152.

39. KNOWLES, R.G., PALACIOS, M., PALMER, R.M.J. AND MONCADA, S. (1989) Formation of nitric oxide from L-arginine in the central nervous system: A transduction mechanism for stimulation of the soluble guanylate cyclase. *Proc. Natl. Acad. Sci. USA* **86**, 5159-5162.

40. LAMOTTE, R.H., LUNDBERG, L.E.R. AND TOREBJÖRK, H.E. (1992) Pain, hyperalgesia and activity in nociceptive C units in humans after intradermal injection of capsaicin. *J. Physiol.* **448**, 749-764.

41. LAMOTTE, R.H., SHAIN, C.N., SIMONE, D.A. AND TSAI, E.F.P. (1991) Neurogenic hyperalgesia: psychophysical studies of underlying mechanisms. *J. Neurophysiol.* **66,** 190-211.

42. LAMOTTE, R.H., THALHAMMER, J.G. AND ROBINSON, C.J. (1983) Peripheral neural correlates of magnitude of cutaneous pain and hyperalgesia: a comparison of neural events in monkey with sensory judgments in human. *J. Neurophysiol.* **50**, 1-26.

43. LEWIS, T. (1942) *Pain.* Macmillan, New York.

44. LYNN, B. (1990) Capsaicin: actions on nociceptive C-fibres and therapeutic potential. *Pain* **41**, 61-69.

45. MACDERMOTT, A.B., MAYER, M.L., WESTBROOK, G.L., SMITH, S.J. AND BARKER, J.L. (1986) NMDA-receptor activation increases cytoplasmic calcium concentration in cultured spinal cord neurones. *Nature* **321**, 519-522.

46. MAUNZ, R.A., PITTS, N.G. AND PETERSON, B.W. (1978) Cat spinoreticular neurons: locations, responses and changes in responses during repetitive stimulation. *Brain Res.* **148**, 365-379.

47. MENDELL, L.M. (1966) Physiological properties of unmyelinated fiber projection to the spinal cord. *Exp. Neurol.* **16**, 316-332.

48. MEYER, R.A. AND CAMPBELL, J.N. (1981) Myelinated nociceptive afferents account for the hyperalgesia that follows a burn to the hand. *Science* **213**, 1527-1529.

49. MILNE, R.J., FOREMAN, R.D., GIESLER, G.J. AND WILLIS, W.D. (1981) Convergence of cutaneous and pelvic visceral nociceptive inputs onto primate spinothalamic neurons. *Pain* **11**, 163-183.

50. MILNE, R.J., FOREMAN, R.D. AND WILLIS, W.D. (1982) Responses of primate spinothalamic neurons located in the sacral intermediomedial gray (Stilling's nucleus) to proprioceptive input from the tail. *Brain Res.* **234**, 227-236.

51. MONAGHAN, D.T., BRIDGES, R.J. AND COTMAN, C.W. (1989) The excitatory amino acid receptors: their classes, pharmacology, and distinct properties in the function of the central nervous system. *Annu. Rev. Pharmacol. Toxicol.* **29**, 365-402.

52. MURASE, K., RYU, P.D. AND RANDIC, M. (1989) Excitatory and inhibitory amino acids and peptide-induced responses in acutely isolated rat spinal dorsal horn neurons. *Neurosci. Lett.* **103**, 56-63.

53. MURASE, K., RYU, P.D. AND RANDIC, M. (1989) Tachykinins modulate multiple ionic conductances in voltage-clamped rat spinal dorsal horn neurons. *J. Neurophysiol.* **61**, 854-865.

54. O'DELL, T.J., HAWKINS, R.D., KANDEL, E.R. AND ARANCIO, O. (1991) Tests of the roles of two diffusible substances in long-term potentiation: evidence for nitric oxide as a possible early retrograde messenger. *Proc. Natl. Acad. USA* **88**, 11285-11289.

55. OSBORNE, N.N. AND GHAZI, H. (1989) The effect of substance P and other tachykinins on inositol phospholipid hydrolysis in rabbit retina, superior colliculus and retinal cultures. *Vision Res.* **29**, 757-764.

56. OWENS, C.M., ZHANG, D. AND WILLIS, W.D. (1992) Changes in the response states of primate spinothalamic tract cells caused by mechanical damage of the skin or activation of descending controls. *J. Neurophysiol.* **67**, 1509-1527.

57. PALECEK, J., DOUGHERTY, P.M., KIM, S.H., PALECKOVÁ, V., LEKAN, H., CHUNG, J.M., CARLTON, S.M. AND WILLIS, W.D. (1992) Responses of spinothalamic tract neurons to mechanical and thermal stimuli in an experimental model of peripheral neuropathy in primates. *J. Neurophysiol.* **68**, 1951-1966.

58. PALECEK, J., PALECKOVÁ, V., DOUGHERTY, P.M. AND WILLIS, W.D. (1993) The effect of phorbol esters on the responses of primate spinothalamic neurons to mechanical and thermal stimuli. Submitted.

59. PALECEK, J., PALECKOVÁ, V., DOUGHERTY, P.M. AND WILLIS, W.D. (1993) The effect of trans-ACPD, a metabotropic excitatory amino acid agonist, on the responses of primate spinothalamic tract neurons. Submitted.

60. PALECKOVÁ, V., PALECEK, J., MCADOO, D.J. AND WILLIS, W.D. (1992) The non-NMDA antagonist CNQX prevents release of amino acids into the rat spinal cord dorsal horn evoked by sciatic nerve stimulation. *Neurosci. Lett.* **148**, 19-22.

61. PALECEK, J., PALECKOVÁ, V. AND WILLIS, W.D. (1993) An inhibitor of nitric

oxide synthase blocks sensitization of spinothalamic neurons after intradermal injection of capsaicin in primates. Submitted.

62. RANDIC, M., HECIMOVIC, H. AND RYU, P.D. (1990) Substance P modulates glutamate-induced currents in acutely isolated rat dorsal horn neurones. *Neurosci. Lett.* **117**, 74-80.

63. RANDIC, M., RYU, P.D. AND URBÁN, L. (1986) Effects of polyclonal and monoclonal antibodies to substance P on slow excitatory transmission in rat spinal dorsal horn. *Brain Res.* **383**, 15-27.

64. SCHOEPP, D.D. AND JOHNSON, B.G. (1988) Excitatory amino acid agonist-antagonist interactions at 2-amino-4-phosphobutyric acid-sensitive quisqualate receptors coupled to phosphoinositide hydrolysis in slices of rat hippocampus. *J. Neurochem.* **50**, 1605-1613.

65. SIMONE, D.A., SORKIN, L.S., OH, U., CHUNG, J.M., OWENS, C., LAMOTTE, R.H. AND WILLIS, W.D. (1991) Neurogenic hyperalgesia: central neural correlates in responses of spinothalamic tract neurons. *J. Neurophysiol.* **66**, 228-246.

66. SLADECZEK, F., RÉCASENS, M. AND BOCKAERT, J. (1988) A new mechanism for glutamate receptor action: phosphoinositide hydrolysis. *TINS* **11**, 545-549.

67. SUGIYAMA, H., ITO, I. AND HIRONO, C. (1987) A new type of glutamate receptor linked to inositol phospholipid metabolism. *Nature* **325**, 531-533.

68. TESSLER, A., HIMES, B.T., ARTYMYSHYN, R., MURRAY, M. AND GOLDBERGER, M.E. (1981) Spinal neurons mediate return of substance P following deafferentation of cat spinal cord. *Brain Res.* **230**, 263-281.

69. TOREBJÖRK, H.E., LUNDBERG, L.E.R. AND LAMOTTE, R.H. (1992) Central changes in processing of mechanoreceptive input in capsaicin-induced secondary hyperalgesia in humans. *J. Physiol.* **448**, 765-780.

70. TREVINO, D.L., COULTER, J.D. AND WILLIS, W.D. (1973) Location of cells of origin of spinothalamic tract in lumbar enlargement of the monkey. *J. Neurophysiol.* **36**, 750-761.

71. URBÁN, L. AND DRAY, A. (1992) Synaptic activation of dorsal horn neurons by selective C-fibre excitation with capsaicin in the mouse spinal cord *in vitro*. *Neuroscience* **47**, 693-702.

72. URBÁN, L. AND RANDIC, M. (1984) Slow excitatory transmission in rat dorsal horn: possible mediation by peptides. *Brain Res.* **290**, 336-341.

73. URBÁN, L., WILLETTS, J., RANDIC, M. AND PAPKA, R.E. (1985) The acute and chronic effects of capsaicin on slow excitatory transmission in rat dorsal horn. *Brain Res.* **330**, 390-396.

74. WESTLUND, K.N., CARLTON, S.M., ZHANG, D. AND WILLIS, W.D. (1992) Glutamate-immunoreactive terminals synapse on primate spinothalamic tract cells. *J. Comp. Neurol.* **322**, 519-527.

75. WHITE, J.C. AND SWEET, W.H. (1969) *Pain and the neurosurgeon*. Thomas. Springfield. 76. Willcockson, W.S., Chung, J.M., Hori, Y., Lee, K.H. and Willis, W.D. (1984) Effect of iontophoretically released peptides on primate spinothalamic tract cells. *J. Neuroscience* **4**, 741-750.

77. WILLIS, W.D. (Ed.) (1992) *Hyperalgesia and allodynia*. Raven Press, New York.

78. WILLIS, W.D. and Coggeshall, R.E. (1991) *Sensory mechanisms of the spinal cord*. 2nd ed., Plenum Press, New York.

79. WILLIS, W.D., PALECEK, J., PALECKOVÁ, V., RAGLAND, J. AND

DOUGHERTY, P.M. (1992) Neurokinin receptor antagonists modify the responses of primate STT neurons to cutaneous stimuli. *Neurosci. Abstr.* **18**, 1023.

80. YEZIERSKI, R.P., GERHART, K.D., SCHROCK, B.J. AND WILLIS, W.D. (1983) A further examination of effects of cortical stimulation on primate spinothalamic tract cells. *J. Neurophysiol.* **49**, 424-441.

81. ZHANG, D., OWENS, C.M. AND WILLIS, W.D. (1991) Two forms of inhibition of spinothalamic tract neurons produced by stimulation of the periaqueductal gray and the cerebral cortex. *J. Neurophysiol.* **65**, 1567-1579.

POSTSYNAPTIC CHANGES DURING SUSTAINED PRIMARY AFFERENT FIBER STIMULATION AS REVEALED BY C-FOS IMMUNOHISTOCHEMISTRY IN THE RAT SPINAL CORD

Catherine Abbadie, Prisca Honoré and Jean-Marie Besson
Physiopharmacologie du Système nerveux
INSERM U 161, 2 rue d'Alésia, 75014 Paris
France

INTRODUCTION

It was initially reported by Hunt et al.[36] that physiological stimulation of rat primary sensory neurons causes the expression of c-*fos*-like protein immunoreactivity in nuclei of postsynaptic neurons of the dorsal horn of the spinal cord. In these experiments it was demonstrated that noxious heat or chemical stimuli resulted in a rapid appearance of Fos-like immunoreactivity (Fos-LI) in the superficial laminae of the dorsal horn, while activation of low threshold cutaneous afferents resulted in fewer labeled cells with a different laminar distribution. The work of Hunt et al.[36] has been at the origin of numerous studies related to pain research. After several years of investigations, there is accumulating evidence that various nociceptive peripheral stimuli result in c-*fos* expression at the spinal cord level. These stimuli include noxious heat,[10,11,35,36,48,56,57,58,59,61] noxious chemical stimulation,[31,36,42,52,59] noxious mechanical stimulation,[2,10,11,12,,42] acute inflammation,[25,37,46,48,49] intense electrical transcutaneous stimulation[13,35,44] and visceral stimulation.[7,8,9,32,45,54] These data are in good agreement with numerous electrophysiological investigations showing that a very high proportion of neurons located either in the superficial laminae or in the neck of the dorsal horn are driven by noxious stimuli (see Refs in 4). It is reasonable to assume therefore that those dorsal horn cells driven by noxious stimulation may be those which preferentially express c-*fos*. This assertion is strongly supported by the fact that stimulation of the sciatic nerve at Aδ/C intensity, but not at Aα/β, induced c-*fos* expression in lumbar spinal cord neurons.[35] Moreover, morphine, at doses which strongly depress the

NATO ASI Series, Vol. H 79
Cellular Mechanisms of Sensory Processing
Edited by Laszlo Urban
© Springer-Verlag Berlin Heidelberg 1994

responses of dorsal horn neurons to thin Aδ and C fiber stimulation without affecting responses due to the activation of Aα and Aβ fibers[43] also dose-dependently blocked Fos-LI; this effect is prevented by the combined administration of naloxone and morphine.[3,32,52,56]

In our present study we have investigated the distribution and intensity of Fos-LI in spinal cord neurons during chronic arthritis, and after noxious cold stimulation.

Adjuvant-induced arthritis (AIA) in the rat which resembles human rheumatoid polyarthritis has been largely used as a chronic pain model (see refs in 5). The time course of the disease has been extensively studied.[15,20,21,23] We report here quantitative analysis of Fos-LI in lumbar spinal cord neurons during the development of AIA in the absence of any intentional stimulation. Fos-LI evoked by calibrated mechanical stimulation was also evaluated in both arthritic and normal rats. The effects of various analgesics (morphine, aspirin and acetaminophen) on Fos-LI were then evaluated. Some of these results have been published previously.[1,2,3]

Several earlier studies have demonstrated an increase in Fos-LI after noxious heat stimulation. Although no systematic or quantitative study was performed to consider the appropriate duration and the intensity of noxious stimulation, it appears that the heat stimulation should be at least above 46°C (i.e. noxious) to induce c-*fos* expression.[58] A dense labelling was observed for even a brief (5s) noxious stimulation at 52°C.[58] It has been shown that the number of Fos-LI neurons in the superficial dorsal horn increased with the duration of the stimulation.[58] To our knowledge, no experiment have considered the effects of a cold stimulation on Fos-LI. This may be important as follows:

(1) Some cells located in lamina I are excited by innocuous skin cooling.[17,39] In addition to their dynamic discharges, cold receptors show a background discharge at normal skin temperatures and a static one which during cooling signals the temperature levels (see Refs in 60). It was thus interesting to know if a non-noxious cold stimulation leads to labeling in the marginal zone of the dorsal horn.

(2) The available information on specific cold nociceptors is extremely poor. This is well illustrated when considering the classification of sensory receptors published by Perl[50] and Willis and Coggeshall.[60] In fact only a small number of electrophysiological studies have been devoted to this problem;[14,29,30,3941,53] the data are extremely difficult to interpret since only a few units were recorded, some of them being also activated by thermal and mechanical nociceptive stimuli, while a few of them were classified as cutaneous high threshold cold receptors. In addition, it is extremely difficult to compare these data since the modality of cold stimulation varied greatly between studies, and only a small number of neurons were studied with very

low temperatures. Thus the Fos-LI technique we used in the present study could be useful to gauge postsynaptic activation during innocuous or noxious stimulation yielding indirect information on peripheral processes.

Materials and methods have been previously described.[1,2,3]

C-*FOS* EXPRESSION IN THE LUMBAR SPINAL CORD OF ARTRITIC RATS

Experiments were performed on male Sprague-Dawley rats. Polyarthritis was induced by intradermal injection into the base of the tail of Freund's adjuvant (killed *Mycobacterium butyricum* suspended in mineral oil).[51] This disease predominantly affects hindpaw joints. The dramatic clinical signs appear from the 10th day post-inoculation, peak three weeks later, and last over several weeks. Among the observed changes, the most marked are decreases in locomotion, increases in scratching behavior and increases in sensitivity to paw pressure or flexion and extension of inflamed joints, loss of weight and hyperventilation (see Refs. in 5).

The expression of the immediate-early gene c-*fos* was studied initially during the development of chronic arthritis and secondly following calibrated mechanical noxious pressure applied to the ankle at a time when the behavioral effects were maximal.

Fos-LI during the development of adjuvant-induced arthritis

A detailed parallel clinical and behavioral study of AIA in the rat described four stages in the time course of the disease.[15] Thus, our study took these stages into consideration. For this purpose, we considered Fos-LI at various times of AIA (one, two, three, 11 and 22 weeks after the inoculation).

We found that Fos-LI was absent in mid-thoracic and cervical segments, and predominated in lumbar segments. The time course of Fos-LI in the lumbar segment during the development of AIA is illustrated in Figure 1A. Considering the mean total number of Fos-LI cells in the whole spinal segment from L2 to L6, there was a significant difference between the 6 groups (control, one week, two, three, 11 and 22 after AIA injection) of animals. Fos-LI was nearly absent in control and at one week,

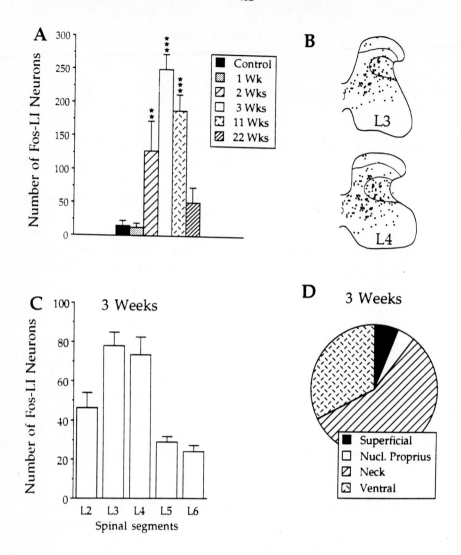

Figure 1. Fos-like immunoreactivity (Fos-LI) during the development of Adjuvant-induced polyarthritis. **A**: Number of Fos-LI neurons in the lumbar (L2-L6) segment (15 sections). Significance is expressed using PLSD Fisher's test, taking the control group as reference (**p<0.01, ***p<0.001). **B**: Camera lucida drawings showing Fos-LI distribution in L3 and L4 segments (3 sections superimposed) 3 weeks after Freund adjuvant injection. **C**: Rostrocaudal quantification of Fos-LI in lumbar enlargement (3 sections per segment). **D**: Laminar distribution of Fos-LI in L3-L4 segment.

moderate at 2 weeks, maximal at 3 weeks, slightly decreased at 11 weeks, and then did not differ from control values at 22 weeks. Considering the animals at 3 weeks as reference, which corresponds to the peak of this distribution and when hyperalgesia is maximal, all groups except 11 weeks presented a significantly lower number of Fos positive cells ($p<0.01$ for 2 weeks, and $p<0.001$ for 22 weeks, 1 week and for the control).

On analysing the rostrocaudal distribution of Fos-LI in the lumbar spinal cord, we observed no significant difference between the 5 lumbar segments for control, 1 week, 2 weeks and 22 weeks, but a significant difference was noticed at 3 weeks ($p<0.0001$) and 11 weeks ($p<0.005$). At 3 weeks, maximal labeling was present in L3-L4 (60.5 %: number of Fos-LI cells in L3-L4 / total number of Fos-LI cells in the L2-L6 enlargement; Figures 1B and C). The segmental pattern of labeling followed the somatotopic organization of the afferent fibers that innervate the hindpaw.[40,47,54] The maximal labeling observed in the lumbar enlargement corresponded to the clinical signs of arthritis i.e. hindpaws predominantly affected.

The laminar distribution is illustrated in Figures 1B and D. In AIA animals, Fos-LI was maximal in the neck of the dorsal horn (laminae V and VI), rather high in the ventral horn, and very low in the superficial laminae (laminae I and II) and the nucleus proprius (laminae III and IV). At 3 weeks, the regional distribution in L3-L4 was ≈5 % in the superficial laminae, ≈5 % in the nucleus proprius, ≈55 % in the neck and ≈35 % in the ventral horn.

These data demonstrate that c-*fos* is expressed without any stimulation in polyarthritic animals. From the behavioral point of view, the absence of significant labeling one week after the induction of the disease is in good agreement with the fact that during the preclinical stage, the clinical signs and the behavioral modifications do not appear. In contrast, the increase in the number of Fos-LI neurons at two weeks and particularly at three weeks corresponds to the acute stage of the disease defined as a lack of mobility and exploring behavior, a dramatic increase in hindpaw and forepaw joint diameters, radiological abnormalities and a maximal hyperalgesia. The maximal label observed at three weeks, corresponds to the peak of the behavioral modifications. These observations indirectly suggest that Fos-LI can be used as a marker of abnormal neuronal activity during chronic pain, at least for AIA. However, we still observed a sustained labelling 11 weeks after the induction of the disease during which time the animals were recovering[15] and behavioral scores were returning to control values. Nevertheless, it must be pointed out that at this time post-inoculation, mean joint diameters and radiological scores were still increased. We did not observe any Fos-LI at 22 weeks. Thus, compared to previous studies which have shown an acute, short lived immediate early gene (IEG) expression,[13,36,52] AIA induces a sustained activation (several weeks) of this immediate early gene.

The basal Fos labelling we observed during AIA coincides with electrophysiological data obtained in the dorsal horn of polyarthritic rats.[16,45] Neurons in this area are normally silent or display low activity in healthy un-anesthetized spinalized animals while 4 weeks after Freund's Adjuvant injection, they display a high level of spontaneous activity.[45]

In un-stimulated AIA animals, Fos-LI was mainly present in the neck of the lumbar dorsal horn, and to a lesser extent in the ventral horn. Surprisingly, the number of labelled cells was low in the superficial laminae ($\approx$5%). Thus the labeling we obtained three weeks after Freund's adjuvant injection into the base of the tail strongly contrasts with previous investigations performed during acute inflammation. Indeed in these latter experiments, dense Fos-LI was observed in laminae I and II after complete Freund's adjuvant injection[46] or carrageenan injection.[25,49] This labeling was observed a few hours (1 to 24 hours) after the injection. In our experiments maximal labeling appears at 3-4 weeks. Our data indicate that c-*fos* induced by chronic inflammation is expressed to a greater extent in deeper laminae than in superficial ones. It is likely that the neurons we labelled during the development of AIA were probably wide dynamic range neurons. Our data tend to suggest that neurons located in deeper laminae are more sensitive to the changes occurring during chronic pain conditions.

Effects of a chronic treatment with aspirin or acetaminophen on Fos-LI in the non-stimulated arthritic rat

Aspirin and acetaminophen are commonly and widely used in patients suffering chronic pain. The effects of these two compounds on the Fos-LI present in chronic arthritic animals was investigated (aspirin: 150 mg/kg i.v.; lysine acetylsalicylate injectable preparation; Synthélabo France; proacetaminophen: 300 mg/kg i.v.; propacetamol hydrochloride injectable preparation; 1g propacetamol liberates 0.5g paracetamol; UPSA France). Chronic treatment with these NSAIDs was begun three weeks after the inoculation. Acute treatment with these compounds had no effect on Fos-LI. A chronic (14 days) oral treatment with aspirin (300 mg/kg/day), or acetaminophen (500 mg/kg/day) which started three weeks after the inoculation of Freund's adjuvant did not significantly reduce the number of Fos-LI neurons in the treated groups as compared to the control (Figure 2B).

When the chronic NSAID treatment, was begun one week after the AIA inoculation, the number of Fos-LI in the treated groups was significantly (p<0.001) decreased as compared to the control group (Figure 2A). The number of Fos-LI cells counted in the whole grey matter was reduced by 52% (as compared to control value) in the aspirin treated group and by 41% (as compared to control value) in the acetaminophen treated group. In this earlier treatment, we showed a clear correlation between the clinical signs and Fos-LI. Indeed both drugs clearly prevented most of the clinical symptoms of the disease when considering mobility, exploration, paw diameters and weight, and also the expression of c-*fos* in spinal cord neurons.

In contrast, when the chronic drug treatment was started three weeks after AIA induction, there was no correlation between the modifications of the clinical signs of the disease and Fos-LI. Indeed although both aspirin and acetaminophen reduced the signs of arthritis, the number of Fos-LI neurons was not significantly different between the control and the two treated groups.

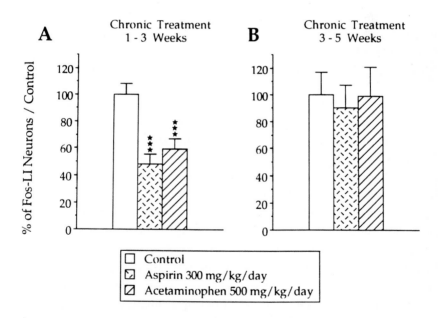

Figure 2. Fos-like immunoreactivity (Fos-LI) following a two week oral chronic treatment with aspirin or acetaminophen. The number of Fos-LI neurons in the lumbar segment of adjuvant-induced arthritis rats significantly decreases if the chronic treatment started one week after Freund adjuvant (FA) injection (A), but not if the treatment started three weeks after FA injection (B). Significance is expressed using PLSD Fisher's test, taking the control group as reference (***p<0.001).

These observations suggest that the use of Fos-LI technique for pharmacological investigations should be used with caution and question the suitability of the Fos-LI technique to gauge the effects of NSAIDs and acetaminophen. At present, despite *in vitro* studies showing that the half-life of the Fos protein is approximately two hours, we do not know the *in vivo* characteristics of the basal labelling during the disease. The knowledge of the Fos protein half-life *in vivo* would be required to fully evaluate the effects of pharmacological compounds. Nevertheless it would be of special interest to gauge the effects of a large variety of NSAIDs during the development of arthritis using the same experimental approach as that reported here.

Comparison of Fos-LI induced by mechanical stimulation in adjuvant-induced arthritis and in normal rats

These experiments were performed three weeks after the inoculation at the time when clinical symptoms peak and mechanical hyperalgesia was at its maximum. In this study, stimuli were applied under 100 mg/kg i.p. ketamine anesthesia, 10 min after the anesthetic injection. Mechanical stimulation consisted of intermittent pressure to the ankle joint over a 10 min period (20 pressures every 2 min delivered through calibrated forceps (4.0 N/cm^2). This pressure was considered noxious as judged by its ability to evoke vocalization and a brief limb withdrawal.

Figure 3. compares Fos-LI evoked by mechanical stimulation in normal and AIA rats. In both groups, mechanical stimulation induced c-*fos* expression in the ipsilateral lumbar spinal cord. The total number of Fos-LI nuclei dramatically increased for both stimulated arthritic and stimulated normal rats as compared to non-stimulated rats ($p < 0.001$). More interestingly, the total number of Fos-LI neurons in the lumbar segment was significantly higher ($p < 0.001$) in stimulated arthritic as compared to stimulated normal rats. The number of Fos-LI neurons differed according to the lumbar segment, as shown in Figure 3C. In both stimulated normal and arthritic rats, maximal labeling was present in L3-L4 (55-65 % of number of the total number of Fos-LI cells in the L2-L6 enlargement was present in L3-L4). As observed for the total number of Fos-LI neurons in the lumbar spinal enlargement, the number of Fos-LI per lumbar segment was significantly higher for every lumbar spinal segment in stimulated arthritic rats as compared to stimulated normal group.

The laminar distribution of Fos-LI induced by the ankle stimulation is illustrated in Figure 3D. In stimulated normal and stimulated arthritic rats Fos-LI was intense in the superficial laminae and in the neck of the dorsal horn, and also in the ventral horn in arthritic rats. These data are in good agreement with numerous electrophysiological investigations showing that a very high proportion of neurons located either in the superficial laminae or in the neck of the dorsal horn are driven by noxious stimuli (see Refs in 4). It is likely therefore that dorsal horn neurons receiving noxious input preferably express *c-fos*. Data obtained from the chronic arthritic group (appearance of "basal" Fos labeling in dorsal horn neurons in the absence of any intentional stimulation) may relate to the well known clinical observations in human rheumatoid disease i.e. the flashes of pain which can spontaneously appear. Similarly the increased number of Fos-LI neurons in stimulated arthritic rats as compared to stimulated normal animals is in good agreement with the hyperalgesia described in such a chronic pain model and to pain reactions evoked in humans by weak

stimulation of the inflamed joint. The origine of these modifications could be due either to peripheral mechanisms i.e. activation and/or sensitization of thin peripheral fibers induced by various chemical agents released at the periphery (see Refs: Dray and Wood,[26] Handwerker,[33] Reeh, this volume) during arthritis and to central components related to central nervous system plasticity described during inflammatory processes.[27]

Effects of analgesics on the Fos-LI induced by mechanical stimulation in the arthritic rat

An acute administration of a single dose of aspirin (150 mg/kg i.v.) or proacetaminophen (300 mg/kg i.v., 1g proacetaminophen liberates 0.5g acetaminophen) produced no change in the number of Fos-LI neurons induced by the ankle stimulation (Figure 4A). We then studied the effect of a 10 day chronic treatment with acetaminophen (250 or 500 mg/kg/day orally), this treatment had also no effect on the number of Fos-LI neurons (Figure 4B).

Several reasons could be put forward to explain the lack of effect of aspirin and acetaminophen on the Fos-LI induced by mechanical stimulation. (1) The technique we used is only able to undertake a restricted quantitative approach by counting Fos-LI neurons without taking into account the intensity of the labeling for each neuron;

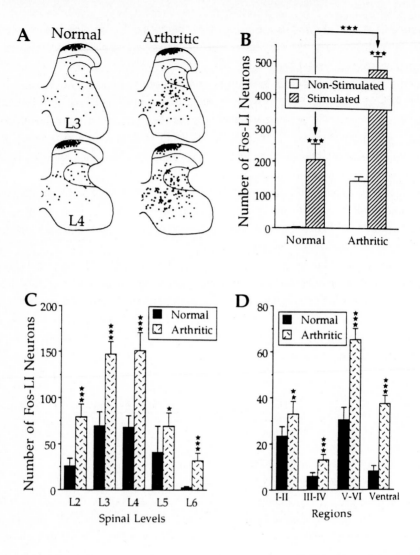

Figure 3. Comparison of Fos-like immunoreactivity (Fos-LI) after calibrated mechanical ankle-joint stimulation of normal and AIA rats. A: Camera lucida drawings showing Fos-LI distribution in L3 and L4 segments (3 sections superimposed). B: Number of Fos-LI neurons in the lumbar enlargement (L2-L6; 15 sections). C: Rostrocaudal distribution in lumbar segments (3 sections per segment). D: Laminar distribution of Fos-LI neurons in L3-L4 segment. Significance is expressed using PLSD Fisher's test (*p<0.05, **p<0.01, ***p<0.001).

in this respect, the effect of the phasic stimulation we used in this experiment (repeated pressure) could be less sensitive to NSAIDs than sustained pain encountered in clinical situations. (2) Both aspirin and acetaminophen are

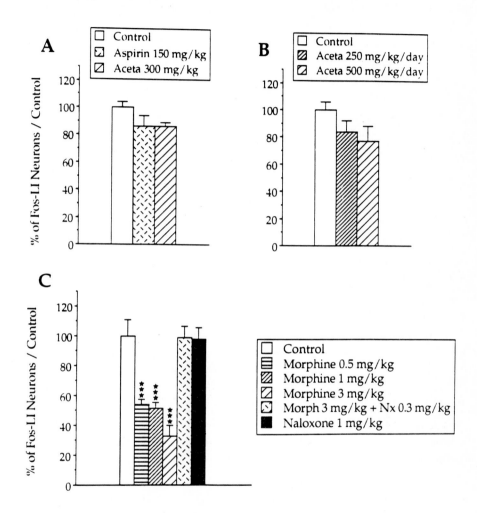

Figure 4. Effects of analgesic compounds on Fos-like immunoreactivity (Fos-LI) in lumbar segments of AIA rats after mechanical stimulation of the ankle joint. A: Acute pretreatment with i.v. aspirin or acetaminophen has no effect on the number of Fos-LI neurons. B: A 10 day oral chronic treatment with acetaminophen has no effect on the number of Fos-LI neurons. C: Pretreatment with i.v. morphine significantly decreases the number of Fos-LI neurons; whereas naloxone and morphine combined or naloxone alone did not change the number of Fos-LI neurons. Significance is expressed using PLSD Fisher's test, taking the control group as reference (***p<0.001).

classified as minor analgesics, the activity of which could not be detected in the present experimental conditions. This lack of sensitivity is further emphasised by the fact that under the same experimental conditions, we found a clear effect of morphine. Acute pretreatment with morphine (0.5-3 mg/kg i.v.) significantly ($p < 0.001$) reduced the number of Fos-LI neurons in stimulated arthritic animals (Figure 4C). In the superficial laminae, pretreatment with a single morphine injection of either 0.5 or 1 mg/kg reduced by more than 50% the number of Fos-LI neurons and at 3 mg/kg completely abolished the labeling evoked by the stimulation. In the neck of the dorsal horn, the decrease produced by morphine was less striking if the whole number of Fos labelled cells was counted ($\approx$40% with 0.5 mg/kg, $\approx$45% with 1 mg/kg and $\approx$55% with 3 mg/kg; percentage decrease vs control value). However if the number of Fos-LI neurons counted in the side contralateral to the stimulation, corresponding to the basal Fos-LI, is subtracted from the ipsilateral side, the decrease caused by morphine is more marked ($\approx$60% with 0.5 mg/kg, $\approx$75% with 1 mg/kg and $\approx$88% with 3 mg/kg). Morphine effects were antagonised by naloxone, but the effect of naloxone was not significant.

Our data are in good agreement with previous studies reporting that opioid agonists (s.c., i.v. or i.c.v.) suppress Fos labeling induced by various types of peripheral stimuli[31,32,52,56]. These effects were marked with doses of 0.5 and 1 mg/kg i.v. and the evoked labeling was almost abolished by 3 mg/kg. For this latter dose, the amount of Fos-LI in the superficial laminae and in the neck of the dorsal horn were 4% and 12% of the control values respectively; there was no significant difference in the effects of morphine in these 2 regions. This finding contrasts with previous studies, in which maximal inhibition of c-*fos* expression was greater in the deeper laminae than in the superficial ones[31,52,56] but was reminiscent of a recent study in which the decrease in Fos-LI was similar for all laminae.[31] Our experiments show that the measure of Fos-LI is a sensitive method for detecting the effects of morphine irrespective of the nature of afferent stimulation. This is relevant to the fact that most nociceptive dorsal horn neurons receive noxious inputs from C polymodal nociceptors (see Refs in 4). We would also like to emphasise the sensitivity of the technique since with the lowest dose of morphine we used (0.5 mg/kg), in our experimental conditions (the applied pressure intensity was 4N/cm^2), the evoked labeling was about 50% of the control values in the superficial laminae and in the neck of the dorsal horn. However, it is difficult to compare our data with previous studies since the effects of morphine depend on various parameters: anesthesia, intensity, duration and nature of the stimulation.

C-*FOS* EXPRESSION IN RAT LUMBAR SPINAL CORD INDUCED BY INTENSE COLD STIMULATION

Experiments were performed under urethane (1500 mg/kg i.p.) anesthesia. One hindpaw of the rat was dipped up to the ankle in a water and alcohol solution:
- for the study of the effect of temperature: for three min at 15°C, 10°C, 5°C, 0°C, -10°C, -15°C, -17.5°C and -20°C;
- for the study of the effect of duration of the stimulation: 1, 3 and 5 min at -20°C.

Fos-LI was absent in the lumbar spinal cord when the hindpaw of the anesthetised rat was maintained in a cold bath at 15, 10°C or 5°C for 3 min. Surprisingly, for colder stimulation (0°C and -10°C) there was very sparse Fos-LI (2-5 neurons per section in the lamina I of L3-L4 segment; Fig. 5). More numerous Fos-LI neurons appeared when the intensity of the stimulation was -15°C, and then a dramatic increase was observed for further decreases in temperature (-17.5°C and -20°C; Fig. 5). Considering the group stimulated at -17.5°C, 3 out of 6 rats exhibited moderate Fos-LI whereas the other 3 exhibited a great number of Fos-LI nuclei.
In fact these two groups differed ($p<0.05$), and the one which had fewer Fos-LI did not significantly differ from the group stimulated at -15°C, and the one which had intense Fos-LI did not differ from the group stimulated at -20°C. These observations of Fos labeling are in good agreement with clinical observations of the effects of the stimulation. Two hours following stimulation at -17.5°C the foot and ankle was apparently normal, these animals displayed weak Fos-LI. In those animals which did exhibit significant Fos-LI at this temperature there was a clear increase in the volume of the paw and associated erythema. In contrast, at -20°C, the large increase in Fos-LI was always associated with paw inflammation.

For the stimulation at -20°C, the rostrocaudal and laminar distributions of Fos-LI neurons are illustrated in Fig. 6. Fos-LI nuclei were largely present in the lumbar enlargement (L2-L6). In adjacent segments (rostral to L2 and caudal to L6), Fos-LI nuclei were sparse (about four per one section). The number of Fos-LI was the greatest in L3 and L4 segments and to a lesser extent in L5. The analysis of the laminar distribution revealed that Fos-LI was maximal in the superficial dorsal horn (65 %), weaker in the deep dorsal horn (18 %) and in the ventral horn (14 %); it was almost absent in the nucleus proprius (3 %).

When the temperature of the stimulation was at - 20°C, the number of Fos-LI neurons increased with the duration of the stimulation i.e. from 1 to 3 and to 5 min (Figure 5B). This increase predominantly affected the superficial laminae of L3-L4 segments (Fig. 6). There is a clear relationship between the number of Fos-LI neurons and the duration of the stimulation since in L4 segment the mean number (± SEM) of Fos-LI neurons was 20.3±3 per section (n=4) for 1 min, 114.6 ± 7.2 (n=9) for 3 min and 168.3 ± 7.5 (n=5) for 5 min.

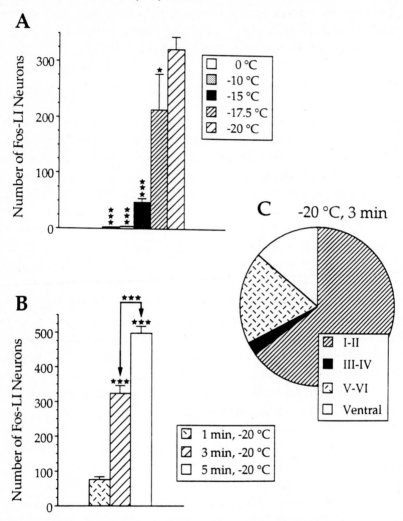

Figure 5. Fos-like immunoreactivity (Fos-LI) in lumbar segments (L2-L6; 1 section per segment), induced by noxious cold stimulation of the hindpaw. A: Note that 0°C or -10°C (3 min) does not induce c-fos expression, and that the number of Fos-LI nuclei increases with the intensity of the stimulation. B: The number of Fos-LI nuclei increases with the duration of the stimulation. C: Fos-LI is greater in the superficial laminae of the dorsal horn after cold stimulation. Significance is expressed using PLSD Fisher's test, taking the "-20°C group" as reference in A, and the "1min group" in B (*p<0.05, **p<0.01, ***p<0.001).

Pretreatment with morphine significantly decreased the Fos-LI induced by the cold stimulation (-20°C, 3 min). This effect was reversed by co-application of naloxone. The decrease in the number of Fos-LI nuclei was more marked with 10 mg/kg s.c. ($p<0.001$; decrease of 53% as compared to control values, in the whole grey matter) than with 5 ($p<0.05$; decrease of 32%), however there was no significant difference between these two doses. The effects of morphine were more marked in the deeper laminae of the dorsal horn than in the superficial ones.

In our experimental conditions, under urethane anesthesia, the cold stimulation requires very low temperature values in order to induce c-*fos* expression in lumbar spinal cord. At temperatures from 0°C to -10°C, there was only a small number of labelled nuclei located in lamina I. The threshold seems to be at -15°C. For colder temperatures (-17.5 and -20°C), there was a great increase in the mean number of Fos-LI neurons, and this increase was consistent with decrease in temperature. Since few studies have used very cold stimuli, it is difficult to interpret our data. Considering psycho-physiological studies in humans, cold pain thresholds vary considerably from one subject to another, and from the stimulation conditions e.g. the location and area of stimulation. Extreme values of pain thresholds are 18.3°C and -4.8°C (see Refs in 19). The temperature used in the present experiment have been shown to be clearly nociceptive in humans. Indeed, dipping the hand of ten subjects in a water and alcohol solution, pain thresholds were felt after 13.5±1.9 seconds at 0°C and after 6.0±0.8 at -10°C. Thus, even if it is difficult to extrapolate our data in humans, it is obvious that a three minutes stimulation at -15°C, the intensity which approximately corresponds to the threshold for consistent Fos-LI, is clearly in the noxious range. This is supported by the fact that in animals, nociceptive reactions to cold stimulation have been induced at 5°C[24]. Thus, there is a clear difference between nociceptive reaction threshold in freely moving animals and threshold for c-*fos* expression in dorsal horn neurons. Several lines of evidence indicate that the use of anesthesia is not responsible for these differences. Indeed the numerous investigations which have studied the electrophysiological characteristics of peripheral nociceptors to various modalities of stimulation either under various anesthesia regimes or in spinalized non-anesthetised animals did not reveal any major differences in their properties (see Refs in 60). The unexpected very low temperature threshold which induced c-*fos* expression is certainly not the result of a general depressive effect of urethane on synaptic transmission between primary afferent fibers and dorsal horn neurons. Indeed, under the same anesthesia condition, we observed numerous Fos-LI neurons in the dorsal horn following either mechanical or heat noxious stimulation.[2] With this latter stimulation, the temperature threshold inducing Fos-LI (46°C)[58] corresponds to the threshold of nociceptive reactions in freely moving animals. Under the same anesthesia and stimulating the same area, at 52°C, only a few seconds (15 sec) are necessary to induce more numerous Fos-LI neurons (number of Fos-LI neurons per one section in L4: 74±6), than a longer duration of stimulation, one minute at -20°C (number of Fos-LI neurons per section in L4: 30±3). Even if it is difficult to compare noxious cold stimulation to noxious heat stimulation, it seems that the latter stimulation is more effective in inducing c-*fos* expression. If one speculates, this could be due to different patterns of activity of primary afferent fiber and/or from different neurotransmitter release (peptides, excitatory amino acids) at the superficial dorsal horn level. Another explanation could be that nociceptors responding to noxious cold are very few in number.

It is also difficult to compare our results with electrophysiological studies on primary afferent fibers because few studies have used very cold stimuli. According to Chery-Croze,[19] a very cold stimulation (-40°C) probably activates cold mechano-thermal receptors,[6,14,29,30,38] polymodal nociceptors,[14,29] thermal nociceptors,[29] and perhaps a particular type of cold receptor.[28] According to Georgopoulos,[29] mechano-thermal receptors responding only to cold and heat have thresholds between 31°C and 0°C; he found the same for thermal nociceptors. For Chéry-Croze,[18] the threshold temperature for five polymodal nociceptors lay between 20-15°C. Although the experimental conditions in the above mentioned studies[6,14,28,29,30,38] differ markedly, our data clearly indicate that there was no Fos labelling at temperatures within the physiological range of afferent fibers sensitive to noxious cold stimuli.

As already mentioned, several speculative hypotheses could be proposed to explain these results, but it appears that under our experimental conditions, the Fos-LI technique is not sensitive enough to detect noxious cold stimulation. Despite this lack of sensitivity, for temperatures below -15°C, the number of Fos-LI neurons increases with the decrease in temperature. In addition, at -20°C, there is a clear relationship between the number of Fos-LI neurons and the duration of the stimulation. These data suggest that the labeling does not reflect the acute activation of cold nociceptors and/or polymodal nociceptors following the application of the stimulus, but is probably due to their delayed activation following secondary phenomena related to vasoconstriction. In this respect, Daum et al.[23] in comparable experimental situations described that at -5°C and -15°C, freezing of the hindpaw did not take place, but did occur below -15°C, when there is a loss of vascular integrity. This latter study is in good agreement with our rough clinical observations in which anesthetised animals which display no or weak Fos-LI, did not show any evident modification of the stimulated paw while for the groups which displayed intense Fos-

LI, there was a clear increase in the volume of the paw associated with a large erythema. This finding is confirmed when considering the group of rats stimulated at -17.5°C (see results).

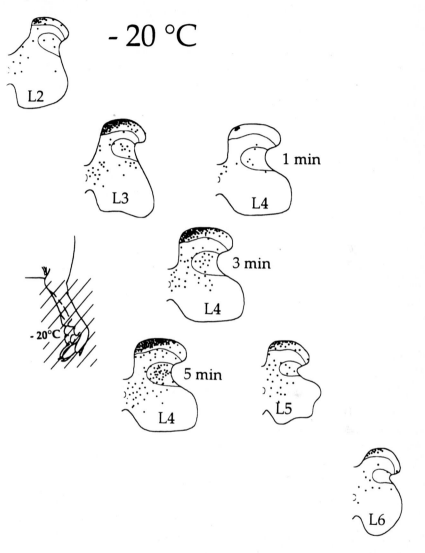

Figure 6. Fos-like immunoreactivity (Fos-LI) induced by noxious cold stimulation of the hindpaw. Note that after cold stimulation (-20°C, 3 min) Fos-LI is intense in the superficial laminae of L3 and L4 segments and that the number of Fos-LI increases with the duration of the stimulation.

As already mentioned, stimulation at temperatures between 25 and 15°C did not induce c-*fos* expression. Since at these temperatures there is an activation of cold receptors which display phasic and static discharges,[60] our data clearly suggest that activation of nociceptors is essential to induce c-*fos* expression. This is in good agreement with numerous previous investigations using various modalities of peripheral stimulation. This is confirmed by the fact that after 10 mg/kg s.c. morphine, the number of Fos-LI neurons was decreased by 50%.

CONCLUDING REMARKS

In the first part of these studies, we have demonstrated that c-*fos* expression induced by chronic inflammation was markedly expressed in the deeper laminae of the dorsal horn and in the ventral horn of the L3 and L4 segments of the spinal cord. The number of Fos-LI neurons correlated with behavioral studies i.e. three weeks after AIA inoculation, which was the peak of Fos-LI distribution corresponding to the maximal hyperalgesia. In addition, the increased number of Fos-LI neurons in stimulated arthritic rats compared to stimulated normal animals is reminiscent of hyperalgesia to mechanical stimulation observed during this chronic disease. The fact that Fos-LI was blocked by a chronic treatment with acetaminophen or aspirin during the development of arthritis, but not when the same treatments started at the maximal stage of the disease, suggest that in pharmacological investigations, the Fos-LI technique needs to be employed with caution under defined conditions.

In the second part of these studies, we unexpectedly found that only damaging cold stimulation was effective in inducing consistent c-*fos* expression. As previously demonstrated with noxious heat stimulation, the labeling induced by intensive cold stimulation was mainly localised in the superficial dorsal horn. C-*fos* expression following heat, but not cold, stimulation, is consistent with previous electrophysiological, behavioral and psycho-physiological studies relevant to nociception and pain in various species. Fos-LI induced by extremely cold stimulation, which seems to reproduce frostbite, may reflect activation of nociceptors due to vasoconstriction.

ACKNOWLEDGEMENTS: This study was supported by INSERM funds and by an unrestricted grant from Bristol-Myers Squibb.

REFERENCES

1. ABBADIE, C. AND BESSON, J.-M. (1992) C-*fos* expression in rat lumbar spinal cord during the development of adjuvant-induced arthritis. *Neuroscience* **48**, 985-993.
2. ABBADIE, C. AND BESSON, J.-M. (1993) C-*fos* expression in rat lumbar spinal cord following peripheral stimulation in adjuvant-induced arthritis and in normal rats. *Brain Res.* **607**, 195-204.
3. ABBADIE, C. AND BESSON, J.-M. (1993) Effects of morphine and naloxone on basal and evoked Fos-like immunoreactivity in lumbar spinal cord neurons of arthritic rats. *Pain* **52**, 29-39.
4. BESSON, J.-M. AND CHAOUCH, A. (1987) Peripheral and spinal mechanisms of nociception. *Physiol. Rev.* **67**, 67-186.
5. BESSON, J.-M. AND GUILBAUD, G. (1988) *The Arthritic Rat as a Model of Clinical Pain?* Elsevier Science Publishers B. V., Amsterdam.
6. BESSOU, P. AND PERL, E.R. (1969) Response of cutaneous sensory units with unmyelinated fibers to noxious stimuli. *J. Neurophysiol.* **32**, 1025-1043.
7. BIRDER, L.A. AND DEGROAT, W.C. (1992) Increased c-*fos* expression in spinal neurons after irritation of the lower urinary tract in the rat. *J. Neurosci.* **12(12)**, 1878-4889.
8. BIRDER, L.A. AND DEGROAT, W.C. (1992) The effect of glutamate antagonists on c-*fos* expression induced in spinal neurons by irritation of the lower urinary tract. *Brain Res.* **580**, 115-120.
9. BIRDER, L. A., J. R. ROPPOLO, M. J. IADAROLA, AND W. C. DEGROAT. (1991) Electrical stimulation of visceral afferent pathways in the pelvic nerve increases c-*fos* in the rat lumbosacral spinal cord. *Neurosci. Lett.* **129**, 193-196.
10. BULLITT, E. (1989) Induction of c-*fos*-like protein within the lumbar spinal cord and thalamus of the rat following peripheral stimulation. *Brain Res.* **493**, 391-397.
11. BULLITT, E. (1990) Expression of c-*fos*-like protein as a marker for neuronal activity following noxious stimulation in the rat. *J. Comp. Neurol.* **296**, 517-530.
12. BULLITT, E. (1991) Somatotopy of spinal nociceptive processing. *J. Comp. Neurol.* **312**, 279-290.
13. BULLITT, E., LEE, C.L., LIGHT, A.R. AND WILLCOCKSON, H. (1992) The effect of stimulus duration on noxious-stimulus induced c-*fos* expression in the rodent spinal cord. *Brain Res.* **580**, 172-179.
14. BURGESS, P.R. AND PERL, E.R. (1973) Cutaneous mechanoreceptors and nociceptors. In: *Handbook of Sensory Physiology.* ed. A. Iggo. Springer, New-York.
15. CALVINO, B., CREPON-BERNARD, M.-O. AND LE BARS, D.(1987) Parallel clinical and behavioral studies of adjuvant-induced arthritis in the rat: possible relationship with "chronic pain". *Behav. Brain Res.* **24**, 11-29.

16. CALVINO, B., VILLANUEVA, L. AND LE BARS, D.(1987) Dorsal horn (convergent) neurones in the intact anaesthetized arthritic rat. I. Segmental excitatory influences. *Pain* **28**, 81-98.

17. CHRISTENSEN, B.N. AND PERL, E.R. (1970) Spinal neurons specifically excited by noxious or thermal stimuli: marginal zone of the dorsal horn. *J. Neurophysiol.* **33**, 293-307.

18. CHÉRY-CROZE, S. (1981) La douleur thermique cutanée: caractéristiques psychophysiques et mécanismes nerveux périphériques, *Doctorat d'Etat es Sciences*, Lyon.

19. CHÉRY-CROZE, S. (1983) Painful sensation induced by a thermal cutaneous stimulus. *Pain* **17**, 109-137.

20. COLPAERT, F.C., BERVOETS, K.J.W. AND VAN DEN HOOGEN, R.H.W.M. (1987) Pharmacological analysis of hyperventilation in arthritic rats. *Pain* **30**, 243-258.

21. COLPAERT, F.C., DE WITTE, P.A., MAROLI, N., AWOUTERS, F., NIEMEGEERS, C.J.E. AND JANSSEN, P.A. (1980) Self-administration of the analgesic suprofen in arthritic rats: evidence of mycobacterium butyricum-induced arthritis as an experimental model of chronic pain. *Life Sci.* **27**, 921-928.

22. DAUM, P.S., BOWERS, W.D. TEJADA, J. MOREHOUSE, D. AND HAMLET, M.P. (1991) Cooling to heat of fusion (HOF), followed by rapid rewarming, does not reduce the integrity of microvascular corrosion casts. *Cryobiology* **28**, 294-301.

23. DE CASTRO COSTA, M., DE SUTTER, P., GYBELS, J. AND VAN HEES, J. (1981) Adjuvant-induced arthritis in rats: a possible animal model of chronic pain. *Pain* **10**, 173-185.

24. DESMEULES, J.A., V. KAYSER, J. WEIL-FUGAZZA, A. BERTRAND AND G. GUILBAUD (1993) Major role of the sympathetic nervous sytem in the development of pain-related behaviour in rats with sciatic nerve constriction used as a model of neuropathic pain. *Pain, Suppl.*

25. DRAISCI, G. AND IADAROLA, M.J. (1989) Temporal analysis of increases in c-*fos*, preprodynorphin and preproenkephalin mRNAs in rat spinal cord. *Mol. Brain Res.* **6**, 31-37.

26. DRAY, A. AND WOOD, J.N. (1991) Nonopioid molecular signaling mechanisms involved in nociception and antinociception. In: *Towards a New Pharmacotherapy of Pain.* eds. A.I. Basbaum and J.-M. Besson. John Wiley and Sons, Chichester.

27. DUBNER, R. (1991) Neuronal plasticity and pain following peripheral tissue inflammation or nerve injury. *Proceeding of the VIth World Congress on Pain.* eds. M.R. Bond, J.E. Charlton, and C.J. Woolf. Elsevier Science Publichers BV, Amsterdam.

28. DUCLAUX, R., SCHÄFER, K. AND HENSEL, H. (1980) Response of cold receptors to low skin temperatures in the nose of the cat. *J. Neurophysiol.* **43**, 1571-1578.

29. GEORGOPOULOS, A.P. (1976) Functional properties of primary afferent units probably related to pain mechanisms of primate glabrous skin. *J. Neurophysiol.* **39**, 71-84.

30. GEORGOPOULOS, A. P. (1977) Stimulus response relations in high threshold mechanothermal fibers inervating primate glabrous skin. *Brain Res.* **128**, 547-552.

31. GOGAS, K.R., PRESLEY, R.W., LEVINE, J.D. AND BASBAUM, A.I. (1991). The antinociceptive action of supraspinal opioids results from an increase in descending inhibitory control: correlation of nociceptive behavior and c-*fos* expression. *Neuroscience* **42**, 617-628.

32. HAMMOND, D.L., PRESLEY, R.W., GOGAS, K.R. AND BASBAUM, A.I. (1992) Morphine or U-50,488 suppresses Fos protein-like immunoreactivity in the spinal cord and nucleus tractus solitarii evoked by a noxious visceral stimulus in the rat. *J. Comp. Neurol.* **315**, 244-253.

33. HANDWERKER, H.O. (1991) What peripheral mechanisms contribute to nociceptive transmission and hyperalgesia? In: *Towards a New Pharmacotherapy of Pain.* eds. A.I. BASBAUM AND J.-M. BESSON, John Wiley and Sons, Chichester.

34. HARDY, J.D., WOLF, H.G., AND GOODEL, H. (1952) *Pain Sensations and Reactions*, Williams and Wilkins Company, Baltimore.

35. HERDEGEN, T., KOVARY, K., LEAH, J. AND BRAVO, R.(1991) Specific temporal and spatial distribution of JUN, FOS and KROX-24 proteins in spinal neurons following noxious transsynaptic stimulation. *J. Comp. Neurol.* **313**, 178-191.

36. HUNT, S.P., PINI, A. AND EVAN, G. (1987) Induction of c-*fos*-like protein in spinal cord neurons following sensory stimulation. *Nature* **328**, 632-634.

37. HYLDEN, J.L.K., NOGUCHI, K. AND RUDA, M.A. (1992) Neonatal capsaicin treatment attenuates spinal Fos activation and dynorphin gene expression following peripheral tissue inflammation and hyperalgesia. *J. Neurosci.* **12(5)**, 1716-1725.

38. IGGO, A. (1959) Cutaneous and cold receptors with slowly conducting (C) afferent fibers. *Q. J. Exp. Physiol.* **44**, 362-370.

39. KUMAZAWA, T. AND PERL, E.R. (1977) Primate cutaneous receptors with unmyelinated (C) fibers abd their projection to the substansia gelatinosa. *J. Physiol. (Paris)* **73**, 287-304.

40. LAMOTTE, C.,S. KAPADIA, E. AND SHAPIRO, C.M. (1991) Central projections of the sciatic, saphenous, median, and ulnar nerves of the rat demonstrated by transganglionic transport of choleragenoid-HRP (B-HRP) and wheat germ agglutinin-HRP (WGA-HRP). *J. Comp. Neurol.* **311**, 546-562.

41. LAMOTTE, R.H. AND THALAMMER, J.G. (1982) Response properties of high threshold cutaneous cold receptors in the primate. *Brain Res.* **244**, 279-287.

42. LEAH, J.D., SANDKUHLER, J., MURASHOV, A. AND ZIMMERMANN, M. (1992) Potentiated expression of Fos protein in the rat spinal cord following bilateral noxious cutaneous stimulation. *Neuroscience* **48**, 525-532.

43. LE BARS, D., GUILBAUD, G., JURNA, I. AND BESSON, J.-M. (1976) Differential effects of morphine on responses of dorsal horn lamina V type cells elicited by A and C fibre stimulation in the spinal cat. *Brain Res.* **115**, 518-524.

44. LEE, J.-H. AND BEITZ, A.J. (1992) Electroacupuncture modifies the expression of c-*fos* in the spinal cord induced by noxious stimulation. *Brain Res.* **577**, 80-91.

45. MENÉTREY, D. AND BESSON, J.-M. (1982) Electrophysiological characteristics of dorsal horn cells in rats with cutaneous inflammation resulting from chronic arthritis. *Pain* **13**, 343-364.
46. MENÉTREY, D., GANNON, A., LEVINE, J.D. AND BASBAUM, A.I. (1989) Expression of c-*fos* protein in interneurons and projection neurons of the rat spinal cord in response to noxious somatic, articular and visceral stimulation. *J. Comp. Neurol.* **285**, 177-195.
47. MOLANDER, C. AND GRANT, G. (1986) Laminar distribution and somatotopic organization of primary afferent fibers from hindlimb nerves in the dorsal horn. A study by transganglionic transport of horseradish peroxidase in the rat. *Neuroscience* **19**, 297-312.
48. NARANJO, J.R., MELLSTRÖM, B., ACHAVAL, M. AND SASSONE-CORSI, P. (1991) Molecular pathways of pain: Fos/Jun-mediated activation of a noncanonical AP-1 site in the prodynorphin gene. *Neuron* **6**, 607-617.
49. NOGUCHI, K., KOWALSKI, K., TRAUB, R., SOLODKIN, A. IADAROLA, M.J. AND RUDA, M.A. (1991) Dynorphin expression and Fos-like immunoreactivity following inflammation induced hyperalgesia are colocalized in spinal cord neurons. *Molec. Brain Res.* **10**, 227-233.
50. PERL, E.R. (1984) Characterization of nociceptors and their activation of neurons in the superficial dorsal horn: first step for the sensation of pain. In: *Advances in Pain Research and Therapy.* eds. L. Kruger and J.C. Liebeskind. Raven Press, New-York.
51. PEARSON, C.M. AND WOOD, F.D. (1959) Studies of polyarthritis and other lesions induced in rats by injection of mycobacterial adjuvant. I. General clinical and pathologic caracteristics and some modifying factors. *Arthritis Rheum.* **2**, 440-459.
52. PRESLEY, R.W., MENÉTREY, D., LEVINE, J.D. AND BASBAUM, A.I. (1990) Systemic morphine suppresses noxious stimulus-evoked Fos protein-like immunoreactivity in the rat spinal cord. *J. Neurosci.* **10**, 323-335.
53. SAUMET, J.-L., S. CHÉRY-CROZE, AND R. DUCLAUX. (1985) Response of cat skin mechanothermal nociceptors to cold stimulation. *Brain Res. Bull.* **15**: 529-532.
54. SWEET, J.E. AND C.J. WOOLF (1985) The somatotopic organization of primary afferent terminals in the superficial laminae of the dorsal horn of the rat spinal cord. *J. Comp. Neurol.* **231**, 66-77.
55. TRAUB, R.J., PECHMAN, P.M., IADAROLA, J. AND GEBHART, G.F. (1992) Fos-like proteins in the lumbosacral spinal cord following noxious and non-noxious colorectal distension in the rat. *Pain* **49**, 393-403.
56. TÖLLE, T.R., CASTRO-LOPES, J.M., COIMBRA, A. AND ZIEGLGÄNSBERGER, W. (1990) Opiates modify induction of c-*fos* proto-oncogene in the spinal cord of the rat following noxious stimulation. *Neurosci. Lett.* **111**, 46-51.
57. TÖLLE, T.R., CASTRO-LOPES, J.M. AND ZIEGLGÄNSBERGER, W. (1991) C-*fos* induction in the spinal cord following noxious stimulation: prevention by opiates but not by NMDA antagonists. In: *Proceedings of the VIth World Congress on Pain.* eds. M.R. Bond, J.E. Charlton, and C.J. Woolf. Elsevier, Amsterdam.
58. WILLIAMS, S., PINI, A., EVAN, G. AND HUNT, S.P. (1989) Molecular events in the spinal cord following sensory stimulation. In: *Processing of Sensory*

Information in the Superficial Dorsal Horn of the Spinal Cord. eds. F.
Cervero, J. Bennett, and M. Headley. Plenum Publishing Corporation.

59. WILLIAMS, S., EVAN, G.I. AND HUNT, S.P. (1990) Changing patterns of c-*fos*
induction in spinal neurons following thermal cutaneous stimulation in the
rat. *Neuroscience* **36**, 73-81.

60. WILLIS, W.D. AND COGGESHALL, R.E. (1991) *Sensory Mechanisms of the
Spinal Cord*, Plenum Press, New-York.

61. WISDEN, W., ERRINGTON, M.L., WILLIAMS, S., DUNNETT, S.B., WATERS, C.,
HITCHCOCK, S., EVAN, G., BLISS, T.V.P. AND HUNT, S.P. (1990)
Differential expression of immediate early genes in the hippocampus and
spinal cord. *Neuron* **4**, 603-614.

STRUCTURAL PLASTICITY OF PRIMARY AFFERENT TERMINALS IN THE ADULT DORSAL HORN - REGENERATIVE SPROUTING INDUCED BY PERIPHERAL NERVE INJURY

Clifford J. Woolf
Department of Anatomy and Developmental Biology
University College London
London WC1E 6B
Unite Kingdom

THE PATHOPHYSIOLOGY OF PERIPHERAL NEUROPATHIC PAIN

This chapter will review evidence that a structural reorganization of the central terminals of axotomized primary afferents contributes to the pathogenesis of peripheral neuropathic pain. Peripheral neuropathic or neurogenic pain is that pain resulting from a lesion to or disorder of the peripheral nervous system and includes a number of diverse conditions, the commonest of which are; trigeminal neuralgia, postherpetic neuralgia, painful diabetic neuropathy, the reflex sympathetic dystrophies, mononeuropathies and peripheral nerve injury. Patients typically present with a characteristic set of sensory disorders; a constant burning pain, a partial loss of sensitivity, tactile or cold allodynia (the production of pain in response to low intensitiy stimuli) and hyperpathia (abnormal painful sensations) with repeated stimulation.

The treatment for peripheral neuropathic pain is generally inadequate.[6,7] Non-surgical treatment including sympatholytics, anticonvulsants, antidepressants, calcium channel blockers, steroids, topical aspirin or capsaicin, and transcutaneous nerve stimulation, have benefit but often only for a limited period.[7] Surgical intervention in the periphery is in many cases ineffective or may worsen the situation.[37,68,69] New insights into the pathogenesis of peripheral neuropathic pain are required if the management of this condition is to improve.

Two general mechanisms appear to operate to produce neuropathic pain;

NATO ASI Series, Vol. H 79
Cellular Mechanisms of Sensory Processing
Edited by Laszlo Urban
© Springer-Verlag Berlin Heidelberg 1994

abnormal peripheral input and abnormal central sensory processing. Abnormal central sensory processing includes functional and structural alterations in the CNS. Before discussing the structural changes in detail, a brief review of the other mechanisms will be presented.

INVOLVEMENT OF ABNORMAL PERIPHERAL INPUT

Acute Input

Damage to a peripheral nerve initiates an acute injury discharge in the axotomized afferent fibers.[66] This discharge lasts for tens of seconds and is due to a sudden depolarization of the peripheral membrane consequent on ionic shifts. Because the discharge will involve many, if not all of the axotomized afferents, an enormous and highly abnormal input will enter the CNS. Apart from producing intense and excruciating pain, such input appears to produce long-lasting changes in the dorsal horn. The evidence for this is that animal models of neuropathic pain are prevented if a local anaesthetic is administered topically prior to damage to a nerve.[24,45]

Brief afferent inputs have the capacity to produce relatively long lasting changes in excitability[67,70] as a result of the summation of C-fiber mediated slow synaptic potentials in the spinal cord.[60] The summation operates via glutamate acting on the N-methyl-D-aspartate and (NMDA) receptors[60] although neuropeptides may also be involved. Activation of the NMDA receptor results in calcium entry into the cell which can directly activate protein kinases and nitric oxide synthase, although substance P and other neuropeptides can also activate kinases through other second messenger systems. The activated protein kinases produce a number of changes in the neuron, including phosphorylating ion channels, such as the NMDA receptor ion channel.[12] Blocking the NMDA receptor with specific antagonists eliminates the summation of slow potentials,[60] the excitability increase produced by afferent input[73] and neuropathic pain.[18,46] The excitability increases produced by brief electrical stimulation of a peripheral nerve, however[67] only lasts for an hour or so. How could such changes contribute to persistent neuropathic pain. One possibility is that the NMDA receptor mediated change in second messengers may have consequences other than just the short-lived phosphorylation of receptors or ion channels. Nerve injury results, for example in the persistent increase in the expression of the immediate-early proto-oncogene c-fos,[13,47] which may control the expression of a variety of late effector genes. This could result in a maintained increase in excitability way beyond the initiating input, in a manner analogous to the synaptic plasticity in the hippocampus that is thought to determine memory and learning. Alternatively NMDA receptor activation might lead to an excitotoxic effect on dorsal horn neurons leading to cell death.[2] If a selective death of inhibitory interneurons occurred, this would result in a permanent disinhibition, or excitability increase. Indirect evidence from this idea has been produced[57] but whether actual degeneration of specific subpopulations of neurons occurs has not been established yet.

Chronic Input

A few days after the acute injury discharge, an ectopic afferent input begins to be generated, first in myelinated and later in unmyelinated injured axons, at the proximal stump (neuroma) along the axon and also from cell bodies in the dorsal root ganglion.[19,36,65] Ectopic activity appears to be the consequence of the development of abnormal pacemaker properties, due to the accumulation of sodium channels in the injured neuron.[8] While the pacemaker may become autonomous, running as a rhythmic oscillator, a feature of injured neurons is the development of abnormal sensitivity to mechanical, thermal and chemical stimuli.[8,19] Sensitivity to circulating and locally released catecholamines in axotomized and unaxotomized fibers following nerve injury[65] is of particular importance because of its possible role in the aetiology of sympathetic maintained pains. Cross-excitation may occur between sensory fibers, so that abnormal activity in one fiber might initiate firing in other fibers due to abnormal proximity of the fibers, loss of Schwann cells, accumulation of potassium or the formation of junctions between adjacent membranes.[19] It also might develop between postganglionic sympathetic neurons and primary sensory neurons so that normal sympathetic reflex output might generate an input in sensory fibers.

The simplest explanation for how ectopic afferent input produces neuropathic pain would be that such activity in nociceptive A delta and C-fibers would initiate sensory signals in the neural pathways in the central nervous system that ultimately lead to the sensation of pain. In other words the CNS remains normal, it's just the ongoing input in 'pain' fibers that produces the chronic pain. That this is not the case for the tactile hyperalgesia or mechanical allodynia associated with neurogenic pain has now been definitely established.[9,38] Such pain is initiated by activity in low threshold mechanoreceptor primary afferents. Blockade of conduction in large myelinated fibers eliminates the touch evoked allodynia, while leaving C-fiber mediated thermal and pain sensitivity intact. How does this occur? - The answer lies in abnormal central processing.

ABNORMAL CENTRAL PROCESSING

Two general categories of abnormal central processing can occur; an increase in excitability (**central sensitization**, a form of functional plasticity) and a re-wiring of synaptic connections (**structural reorganization**). Both may occur together.

Central sensitization

This is the phenomenon whereby the response of dorsal horn neurons to normal afferent input is augmented or facilitated. The hypersensitivity state can be produced by brief bursts of activity in C afferents[71] as a result of an NMDA, tachykinin or nitric oxide mediated action on spinal neurons.[73,76] Experimentally a 20 second stimulation of cutaneous C-fibers produce an excitability increase that lasts up to 10 minutes while muscle afferents produce an effect that lasts up to an hour.[67,74] Recently this phenomenon has been demonstrated directly in human subjects.[61] Central sensitization results from the modification of the receptive field properties of dorsal horn neurons including a reduction in threshold, an increase in responsiveness, recruitment of novel inputs and an increase in size of the receptive field.[17,52,72]

Any ongoing input in C-fibers would produce an ongoing but afferent-dependent state of central sensitization. The maintenance of an altered central processing by an abnormal peripheral input has been demonstrated both for experimental allodynia in human subjects[31] and in a small group of patients with painful neuropathy.[23] In this respect some component of the pain of peripheral neuropathy in certain patients may be similar to the pain resulting from acute tissue injury which also depends on induction of central sensitization.[71] The difference being that the inducing stimulus in the case of acute tissue injury is transient, as opposed to the persistent ectopic C input associated with nerve injury.

The pain of reflex sympathetic dystrophy can also be explained by this model. Reflex activity in postganglionic sympathetic neurons may begin to drive C-afferents, which have developed an adrenergic sensitivity as a result of axotomy[10]. This C-afferent input would then produce central sensitization. Once central sensitization is present, either as a result of ectopic pacemaker activity in C-fibers or secondary to sympathetic drive, it will result in abnormal responses to all other inputs including A beta afferents.

Structural Reorganization

Peripheral nerve injury results in a complex series of changes in the cell bodies of the axotomized neurons in the dorsal root ganglion. The changes include alterations in morphology (the chromatylytic reaction), reductions in the levels of transmitters and chemical changes that provide the molecular machinery for regeneration to occur. The latter includes decreases in the levels of cytoskeletal proteins and the upregulation of growth-associated proteins that are normally expressed only during development.[53]

Although regeneration of the injured axon in the periphery has been extensively investigated and thought to contribute to post nerve-injury sensory disorders by either a failure of regeneration or an innappropriate peripheral innervation, recently it has become clear that structural changes also occur in the central terminals of primary sensory neurons in the dorsal horn after damage to a peripheral nerve. Evidence for this has emerged from studies on the growth associated protein GAP-43.

GAP-43

GAP-43 is a membrane bound protein,[3,16,53] expressed at high levels in neurons during development (Figure 2) and incorporated into axonal growth cones.[4,22,26,28,29,55] After neural injury in the adult, GAP-43 is re-expressed in those neurons where there is successful regeneration[5,54,59,62,74] (Figure 2). Sustained re-expression is not seen in neurons that do not retain the capacity to regenerate[20,59]. Modification of the level of the protein in cells *in vitro*, show that it is directly involved in process formation.[27,48,77,78]

Both intrinsic spinal and primary sensory neurons express high levels of GAP-43 mRNA during the first postnatal week in rats (Figure 1). By 3 weeks the levels have decreased to the low levels present in the adult.[14] Injury to the peripheral axon of adult primary sensory neurons results in the re-expression of GAP-43 mRNA (Figure 2) or protein (Figure 3) in dorsal root ganglion (DRG) cells.[5,14,25,54,56,62,63] Initially the GAP-43 is found only in small DRG cells but within a week, both large and small cells express the protein[56] (Figures 3 & 4).

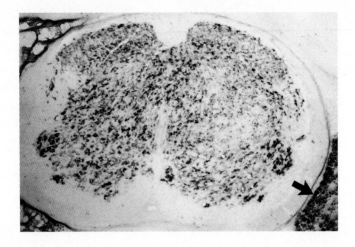

Figure 1. In-situ hybridization for GAP-43 mRNA in a transverse section through a neonatal rat lumbar spinal cord (P0). Note staining in all the dorsal and ventral horn neurons and in the dorsal root ganglion (arrow) but not in the white matter. (Modified from Chong et al., Eur. J. Neurosci. 4:883 1992)

Peripheral nerve injury produces an axotomy of motor as well as primary sensory neurons and there is an increase in GAP-43 mRNA in the axotomized motor neurons in the spinal cord[14] (Fig. 5). There is no change, however, in dorsal horn GAP-43 mRNA levels, indicating that no transynaptic signal has induced an upregulation in the intrinsic dorsal horn neurons.

The increased protein produced in DRG cells as a result of a peripheral nerve section is transported to the injured axon in the periphery,[5,54] where it is believed to contribute directly to the successful reinnervation of target tissues by enabling neurite formation, elongation and guidance. The protein is, however, also distributed along the central axons of the DRG cells, even though they are uninjured and remain in contact with their CNS targets. This can be detected by GAP-43 immunohistochemistry.[30,44,74] Figure 6 shows the appearance of GAP-43 label in the superficial laminae of the lumbar dorsal horn after a sciatic nerve section. That this GAP-43 is of primary afferent origin can be demonstrated by its disappearance if the L3, L4 and L5 dorsal roots are sectioned following the sciatic nerve injury.[15] An ultrastructural analysis shows that the GAP-43 is contained largely within unmyelinated fiber bundles with a small number of labelled synaptic terminals (Figure 7).

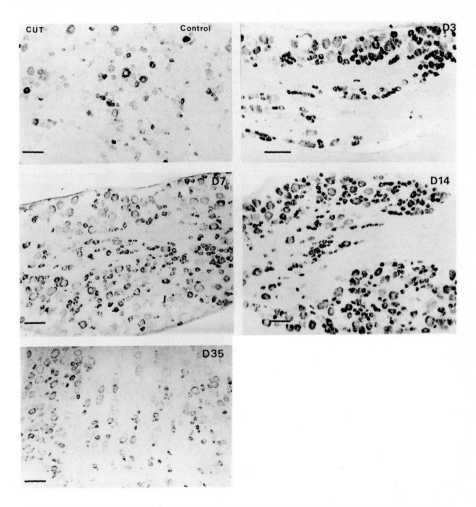

Figure 2. Re-expression of GAP-43 mRNA in sections cut through the adult L4 dorsal root ganglion at different times after sciatic nerve transection, day 3 (D3) to 35 (D35). Scale bar 100μm. Reproduced with permission from Chong et al., (Eur. J. Neurosci. 4: 883-895, 1992.)

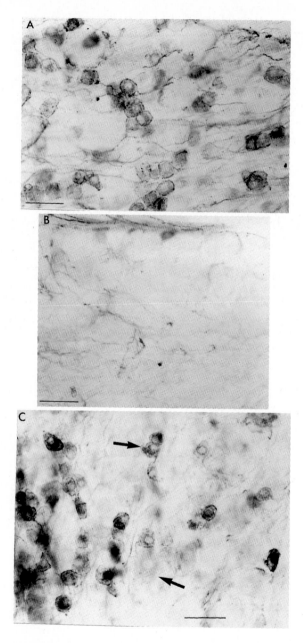

Figure 3. Photomicrographs of 50um thick longitudinal sections through the L5 dorsal root ganglion showing GAP-43 immunoreactivity in DRG cells and axonal profiles ipsilateral (A and C) and contralateral (B) to a sciatic nerve section. A and B are from an animal where the sciatic nerve was sectioned 4 days earlier and C from an animal where the section was performed 14 days before. The arrows show immunostained profiles <30µm and >50um. Scale bars: 75µm. (Modified from Sommervaille et al., Neuroscience 45: 213-220 1991.)

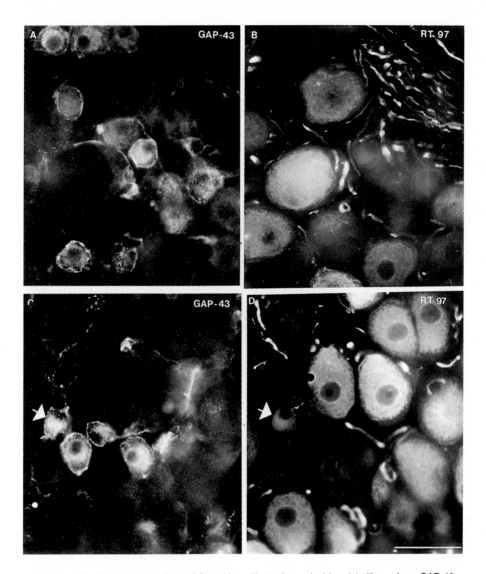

Figure 4. Fluorescent photomicrographs illustrating double labelling for GAP-43 immunoreactivity (A and C) with a FITC label and for RT 97 (B and D) with a Texas Red label in the same L5 dorsal root ganglion sections 4 days (A and B) and 14 days (C and D) following sciatic nerve section. No double labelled cell profiles are present in A and B, all the GAP-43 immunoreactive cells are small (A) and all the RT 97 positive cells are large. In C and D the arrow indicates a GAP-43 positive cell that is also RT 97 positive. Scale 50μm. (Reproduced with permission from Sommervaille et al., Neuroscience 45:213-220 1991)

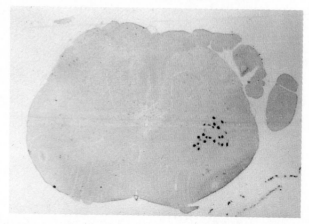

Figure 5. Re-expression of GAP-43 mRNA in a transverse section of an adult rat lumbar spinal cord 14 days after a sciatic nerve crush on one side. Note that increased staining is confined to axotomized sciatic motorneuron pool. (modified from Chong et al., Eur. J. Neurosci. 4: 883-895, 1992)

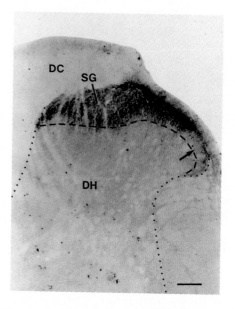

Figure 6. Transverse sections of the dorsal half of the spinal cord showing GAP-43 staining in the ipsilateral superficial laminae of the dorsal horn (DH) including the substantia gelatinosa (SG) 14 days after a sciatic nerve crush.The dotted line outlines the grey/white boundary. The interrupted line indicates the lamina 2/3 boundary Bar=50µm. DC, dorsal column. Note the mediolateral distribution is identical to that of the sciatic nerve terminals at this level with no staining in the lateral third of the dorsal horn in lamina 2 (arrow). Modified from Woolf et al., Neuroscience 34: 465-478, 1990)

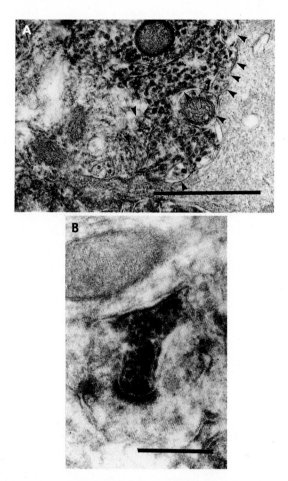

Figure 7. A. Electron micrographs of GAP-43 immunolabelled bundles of unmyelinated axons in laminae I and II of the lumbar dorsal horn 14 days following an ipsilateral sciatic nerve section. The arrow heads indicate some of the individual axons. B. An electron micrograph of an immunolabelled presynaptic terminal ending on a dendrite in the superficial dorsal horn. Note that the synaptic thickening is of the asymmetric variety and that synaptic vesicles are present. Scale bars 500 nm. Modified from Coggeshall et al., Neuroscience Lett. 131:37-41 1991.

When serial electron microscopic sections of GAP-43 labelled material are made then it becomes apparent that at least some of the large fiber bundles are likely to be filopodia emerging from a growth cone-like structure[15] (Fig. 8). The GAP-43 label in the dorsal horn after a nerve injury might be a marker, therefore, of substantial structural change in the terminal arbors of the axotomised primary sensory neurons.

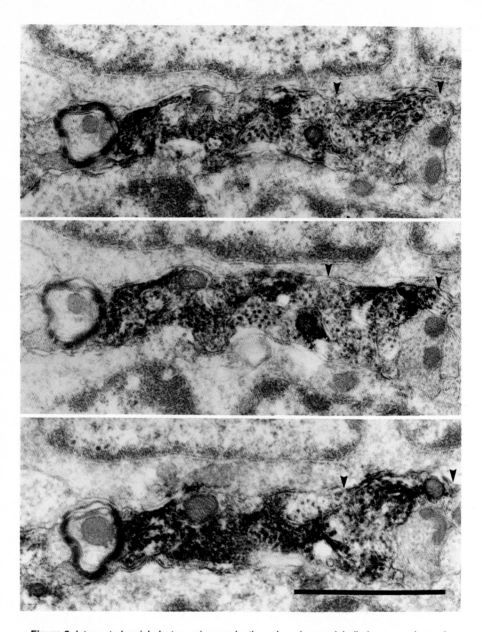

Figure 8. Interrupted serial electron micrographs through an immunolabelled presumed growth cone in lamina I of a rat whose sciatic nerve was transected 2 weeks previously. Section B is 4000 A (5 thin sections) from section A and section C is a further 4000 A along the labelled element. Note in A the labelled structure comprises a bundle of many (21) contiguous labelled processes resembling small unmyelinated axons. In B the number of separable processes is fewer and in C essentially a single large element is stained with a few subdivisions. Scale bar 500 nm. (Reproduced with permission from Coggeshall et al., Neurosci. Lett. 131:37-41 1991)

STRUCTURAL CHANGES IN THE DORSAL HORN

Two general kinds of structural change are possible in primary afferent central terminals in the dorsal horn after a peripheral nerve injury; degeneration/atrophy and regeneration/sprouting. Until our recently, only degenerative changes had been described.[1] These are thought to arise either from the death of dorsal root ganglion cells consequent on the nerve injury or a transganglionic atrophy of terminals due a lack of trophic support from the periphery. The net effect in any case is the same the withdrawal of primary afferent synapses in the dorsal horn. Such a loss has been found for C-fiber terminals in the superficial dorsal horn.[11] Sprouting of afferent terminals has been studied largely in relation to the effect of denervation on the terminal projection areas of neighbouring intact afferents. The first report of such sprouting was made by Liu and Chambers in 1958 using a spared root preparation, but this finding has been disputed. Sprouting of uninjured neurons has been found after denervation produced in the neonate.[21,49] In order to get substantial sprouting outside of the highly somatotopically organised existing nerve terminal field in the adult[58] the primary sensory neurons have to be primed for growth. This can be achieved by a peripheral nerve crush lesion,[33,35] precisely the lesion that produces an upregulation of GAP-43. Peripheral nerve lesions also produce sprouting within

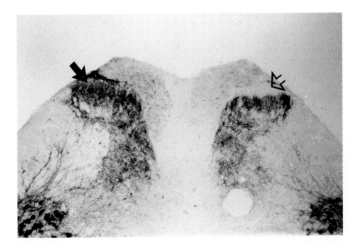

Figure 9. A photomicrograph of a transverse section through the dorsal horn at the L4 segment showing the central terminal label present when B-HRP was injected into a sciatic nerve cut 2 weeks previously and into the contralateral intact nerve. On the cut side B-HRP label is present in lamina II (solid arrow) but not on the control side (open arrow). (Scale bar 200µm).

CONTROL

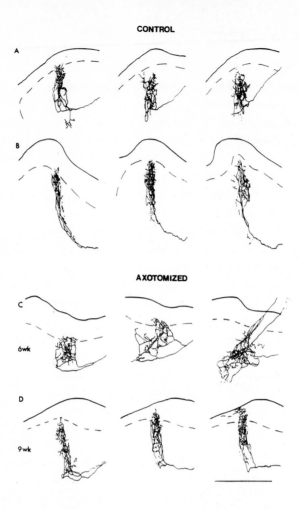

AXOTOMIZED

Figure 10. Camera lucida reconstructions from transverse sections of the spinal cord of the complex terminal arbors of four single sural A beta afferent fibers. Each row shows three adjacent arbors from a single afferent, two controls (A & B) and two from axotomized sural nerves (C &D). The solid line above each drawing represents the dorsal most surface of the dorsal horn, the dotted line the lamina II/III border. Each arbor has a collateral axon arising from a stem axon running longitudinally in the dorsal columns (not shown). This collateral axon, for hair follicle afferent fibers, terminates in a 'flame-shaped' branching pattern (A & B), with mediolaterally restricted branches extending dorsally from lamina IV to the lamina II/III border and only a few sparse terminals in some cases reaching inner lamina II. C. Illustrates arbors which possess a branching pattern not seen in control animals, a wide mediolateral spread, dorsal extension up to II_o and a disruption of the flame-shaped pattern. D. Shows arbors from an axotomized afferent which while retaining the flame-shape, extend in some cases right up to the marginal zone (lamina I). Scale bars 250 μm. (Reproduced with permission from Woolf et al., Nature 355:75-78 1992)

the nerve central terminal field. This can be detected by looking at the laminar termination patterns of different HRP labelled conjugates. HRP conjugated to the lectin wheat germ agglutinin predominantly labels C-fibers producing terminal label in lamina II.[58] HRP conjugated to the B-fragment of cholera toxin (B-HRP) only labels myelinated Aß and Aδ afferents producing a pattern of terminal label where all laminae in the dorsal horn are labelled except lamina II (Figure 9)[42]. Following nerve injury B-HRP central terminal begins within 7 days post section to spread into lamina II[75] (Figure 9), indicating the growth of the central terminals of the peripherally axotomized neurons into a novel territory. This finding is of interest firstly in showing that the neurobiological response to a nerve lesion in the adult includes a remodelling of central terminal projections in the spinal cord and secondly that such a remodelling includes low threshold afferent terminals invading an area where nociceptive afferents normally terminate. This structural reorganization may play a major role in the development of sensory disorders after nerve injury, particularly of touch-induced allodynia, where low intensity stimuli begin to elicit severe pain. That the anatomical changes seen by bulk labelling do represent a genuine growth of Aß afferents, can be seen by filling single axotomized fibers with HRP and studying their terminal patterns.[50,75] Figure 10 indicates the results from such an approach and shows the hair follicle like afferents sprout into lamina II.

The combination of central terminals with the molecular machinery for growth (e.g. GAP-43) and vacant synapses resulting from degeneration/atrophy together provide the mechanism and opportunity for growth to occur.

CONCLUSION

At the time of peripheral injury, an abnormal injury discharge may be sufficient to produce long term changes in the excitability of the spinal cord and/or an excitoxic death of dorsal horn neurons. The maintenance of sensory disorders may result both from an ongoing ectopic input generated in the injured axons, which might persistently induce a state of central sensitization, and from the structural reorganization of synaptic connections in the dorsal horn. Structural changes may explain why the sensory disorders associated with nerve injury are persistent and resistant to most forms of treatment. The presence of such structural alterations also indicates that regenerative changes in the adult nervous system might not always be beneficial and that chronic neuropathic pain might be the manifestation of a maladaptive form of neuroplasticity.

REFERENCES

1. ALDSKOGIUS, H., ARVIDSSON, J. AND GRANT, G. (1985) The reaction of primary sensory neurons to peripheral nerve injury with particular emphasis on transganglionic changes. *Brain Res.* **373**: 15-21.
2. BENNETT, G.J. (1991) Evidence from animal models on the pathogenesis of painful peripheral neuropathy: relevance for pharmacotherapy. In: *Towards a new pharmacotherapy of pain* (eds. Basbaum A.I. and Besson J.M.), pp. 365-379, John Wiley & Sons, Chichester.
3. BENOWITZ, L.I. AND ROUTTENBERG, A. (1987) A membrane phosphoprotein associated with neural development, axonal regeneration, phospholipid metabolism and synaptic plasticity. *Trends Neurosci.* **10**:527-531.
4 BIFFO, S., VERHAAGEN, J., SHRAMA, L.H., SCHOTMAN, P., DANHO, W. AND MARGOLIS, F.L. (1990) B-50/GAP-43 expression correlates with process outgrowth in the embryonic mouse nervous system. *Eur. J. Neurosci.* **2**: 487-499.
5. BISBY, M.A. (1988) Dependence of GAP-43 (B50,F1) transport on axonal regeneration in rat dorsal root ganglion neurons. *Brain Res.* **458**: 157-161.
6. BOWSHER, D. (1991) Neurogenic pain syndromes and their management. *Brit. Med. Bull.* **47**: 644-666
7. BULLITT, E. (1992) The treatment of hyperalgesia following nerve injury. In: *Hyperalgesia and allodynia*, (ed) Willis WD Jr, pp. 345-361, Raven Press, New York.
8. BURCHIEL, K.B. (1984) Effects of electrical and mechanical stimulation on two foci of spontaneous activity which develop in primary afferent neurons after peripheral axotomy. *Pain* **18**: 249-265
9. CAMBELL, J.N., RAJA, S.N., MEYER, R.A. AND MCKINNON, S.E. (1988) Myelinated afferents signal the hyperalgesia associated with nerve injury. *Pain* **32**: 89-94
10. CAMBELL, J.N., MEYER, R.A., DAVIS, K.D. AND RAJA, S.N. (1992) Sympathetically maintained pain. A unifying hypothesis. In: *Hyperalgesia and allodynia*, (ed) Willis WD Jr, pp 141-149, Raven Press, New York,.
11. CASTRO-LOPES, J.M., COIMBRA, A., GRANT, G. AND ARVIDSSON, J. (1990) Ultrastructural changes of the central scalloped (C_1) primary afferent endings of synaptic glomeruli in the substantia gelatinosa Rolandi of the rat after peripheral neurotomy. *J. Neurocytol.* **19**: 329-337
12. CHEN L., HUANG L-Y. M. (1992) Protein kinase C reduces MG_{2+} block of NMDA-receptor channels as a mechanism of modulation. *Nature* **356**: 521-523
13. CHI, S-J., LEVINE, J.D. AND BASBAUM, A.I. (1989) Time course of peripheral neuroma-induced expression of Fos protein immunoreactivity in spinal cord of rats and effects of local anesthetics. *Neurosci. Abst.* **15**: 155
14. CHONG, M.S., FITZGERALD, M., WINTER, J., HU-TSA, M., EMSON, P.C., WIESE, U. AND WOOLF, C.J. (1992) GAP-43 mRNA in rat spinal cord and dorsal root ganglia neurons: Developmental changes and re-expression following peripneral nerve injury. *Eur. J. Neurosci.* **4**:883-895.
15. COGGESHALL, R.E., REYNOLDS, M.L. AND WOOLF, C.J. (1991) Distribution

of the growth association protein GAP-43 in the central processes of axotomized primary afferents in the adult rat spinal cord; presence of growth cone-like structures. *Neuroscience Lett.* **131**: 37-41.

16. COGGINS, P.J. AND ZWIERS, H. (1991) Biochemistry and functional neurochemistry of a neuron-specific phosphoprotein. *J. Neurochem.* **56**:1095-1106.

17. COOK, A.J., WOOLF, C.J., WALL, P.D. AND MCMAHON, S.B. (1987) Dynamic receptive field plasticity in rat spinal cord dorsal horn following C-primary afferent input. *Nature* **325**: 151-153

18. DAVAR, G., HAMA, A., DEYKIN, A., VOS, B. AND MACIEWICZ, R. (1991) MK-801 blocks the development of thermal hyperalgesia in a rat model of experimental painful neuropathy. *Brain Res.* **553**: 327-330

19. DEVOR, M. (1991) Neuropathic pain and injured nerve: peripheral mechanisms. *Brit. Med. Bull.* **47**: 619-630

20. DOSTER, K.S., LOZANO, A.M., AGUAYO, A.J. AND WILLARD, M.A. (1991) Expression of growth-associated protein GAP-43 in adult rat retinal ganglion cells following axon injury. *Neuron* **6**: 635-647.

21. FITZGERALD, M., WOOLF, C.J. AND SHORTLAND, P. (1990) Collateral sprouting of the central terminals of cutaneous primary afferent neurons in the rat spinal cord: Pattern, morphology, and influence of targets. *J. Comp. Neurol.* **300**: 370-385.

22. FITZGERALD, M., REYNOLDS, M.L. AND BENOWITZ, L.I. (1991) GAP-43 expression in the developing rat lumbar spinal cord. *Neurosci.* **41**: 187-199.

23. GRACELY, R.H., LYNCH, S.A. AND BENNETT, G.J. (1992) Painful neuropathy: Altered central processing, maintained dynamically by peripheral input. *Pain* **51**: 175-194.

24. GONZÁLEZ-DARDER, J.M., BARBERÁ, J. AND ABELLÁN, M.J. (1986) Effects of prior anaesthesia on autotomy following sciatic transection in rats. *Pain* **24**: 87-91

25. HOFFMAN, P.N. (1989) Expression of GAP-43, a rapidly transported growth-associated protein and class II beta tubulin, a slowly transported cytoskeletal protein, are coordinated in regenerating neurons. *J. Neurosci.* **9**: 893-897.

26. JACOBSON, R.D., VIRAG, I. AND SKENE, J.H.P. (1986) A protein associated with axonal growth, GAP-43, is widely distributed and developmentally regulated in rat CNS. *J. Neurosci.* **6**: 1843-1855.

27. JAP, TJOEN, SAN, E.R.A., SCHMIDT-MICHELS, M., OESTREICHER, A.B., GISPEN, W.H. AND SCHOTMAN, P. (1992) Inhibition of nerve growth factor-induced B-50/GAP-43 expression by antisense oligomers interferes with neurite outgrowth of PC 12 cells. *Biochem. Biophys. Res. Comm.* **187**: 839-846.

28. KALIL, K. AND SKENE, J.H.P. (1986) Elevated synthesis of an axonally transported protein correlates with axonal outgrowth in normal and injured pyramidal tracts. *J. Neurosci.* **6**: 2563-2570.

29. KARNS, L.R., NG S-C., FREEMAN, J.A. AND FISHMAN, M.C. (1987) Cloning of complementary DNA for GAP-43, a neuronal growth-related protein. *Science* **236**: 597-560.

30. KNIYHAR-CSILLIK, E., CSILLIK, B. AND OESTRICHER, A.B. (1992) Light and

electron microscopic localization of B-50 (GAP-43) in the rat spinal cord during transganglionic degenerative atrophy and regeneration. *J. Neurosci. Res.* **32**: 93-109.

31. KOLTZENBURG, M., LUNDBERG, L.E.R. AND TOREBJÖRK, H.E. (1992) Dynamic and static components of mechanical hyperalgesia in human hairy skin. *Pain* **51**: 207-220.

32. LAMOTTE, C.C., KAPADIA, S.E. AND KOCOL, C.E. (1989) Deafferentation-induced expansion of sciatic terminal field labelling in the adult rat dorsal horn following pronase injection of the sciatic nerve. *J. Comp. Neurol.* **288**: 311-325.

32. LIU, C.N. AND CHAMBERS, W.W. (1958) Intraspinal sprouting of dorsal root axons. *Arch. Neurol. Psychiat.* **79**: 46-61.

33. MCMAHON, S.B. AND KETT-WHITE, (1991) Sprouting of peripheral regenerating primary sensory neurones in the adult central nervous system. *J. Comp. Neurol.* **304**: 307-315.

34. MELLER, S.T. AND GEBHARDT, G.F. (1993) Nitric oxide (NO) and nociceptive processing in the spinal cord. *Pain* **52**: 127-136.

35. MOLANDER, C., KINNMAN, E. AND ALDSKOGIUS, H. (1988) Expansion of spinal cord primary sensory afferent projection following combined sciatic nerve resection and saphenous nerve crush: A horseradish proxidase study in the adult rat. *J. Comp. Neurol.* **276**: 436-441.

36. NORDIN, M., NYSTROM, B., WALLIN, U. AND HAGBARTH, K-E. (1984) Ectopic sensory discharges and paraesthesias in patients with disorders of peripheral nerves, dorsal roots and dorsal columns. *Pain* **20**: 231-245.

37. NOORDENBOS, W. AND WALL, P.D. (1981) Implications of the failure of nerve resection and graft to cure chronic pain produced by nerve lesions. *J. Neurol. Neurosurg. Psychiat.* **44**: 1068-1073.

38. PRICE, D.D., BENNETT, G.J. AND RAFFII, M. (1989) Psychological observations on patients with neuropathic pain relieved by a sympathetic block. *Pain* **36**: 273-288

39. RICH, K.M., LUSZCZYNSKI, J.R., OSBORNE, P.A., JOHNSON, J.R.E.M. (1987) Nerve growth factor protects adult sensory neurons from cell death and atrophy caused by nerve injury. *J. Neurocytol.* **16**: 261-268.

40. RICHARDSON, P.M. AND ISSA, V.M.K. (1984) Peripheral nerve injury enhances central regeneration of primary sensory neurones. *Nature* **309**: 791-793.

41. RICHARDSON, P.M. AND VERGE, V.M.K. (1987) Axonal regeneration in dorsal spinal roots is accelerated by peripheral axonal transection. *Brain Res.* **411**: 406-408.

42. ROBERTSON, B. AND GRANT, G. (1985) A comparison between wheat germ agglutinin- and choleragenoid-horseradish peroxidase as anterogradely transported markers in central branches of primary sensory neurones in the rat with some observations in the cat. *Neuroscience* **14**: 895-905.

43. SATO, J. AND PERL, E.R. (1991) Adrenergic excitation of cutaneous pain receptors induced by peripheral nerve injury. *Science* **251**: 1608-1610.

44. SCHREYER, D.J. AND SKENE, J.H.P. (1991) Fate of GAP-43 in ascending spinal axons of DRG neurons after peripheral nerve injury: delayed accumulation and correlation with regenerative potential. *J. Neurosci.* **11(12)**: 3738-3751.

45. SELTZER, Z., BEILIN, B.Z., GINZBURG, R., PARAN, Y. AND SHIMKO, T.

(1991) The role of injury discharge in the induction of neuropathic pain behaviour in rats. *Pain* **46**: 327-336

46. SELTZER, Z., COHN, S., GINZBURG, R. AND BELLIN, B.Z. (1991) Modulation of neuropathic pain behaviour in rats by spinal disinhibition and NMDA receptor blockade of injury discharge. *Pain* **45**: 69-75.

47. SHARP, F.R., GRIFFITH, J., GONZALEZ, M.F. AND SAGAR, S.M. (1989) Trigeminal nerve section induces Fos-like immunoreactivity (FLI) in brainstem and decreases FLI in sensory cortex. *Mol. Brain. Res.* **6**: 217-220.

48. SHEA, T.B., PERRONE-BIZZOZERO, N.I., BEERMANN, M.L., BENOWITZ, L.I. (1991) Phospholipid-mediated delivery of anti-GAP-43 antibodies into neuroblastoma cells prevents neuritogenesis. *J. Neurosci.* **11**: 1685-1690.

49. SHORTLAND, P., MOLANDER, C., WOOLF, C.J. AND FITZGERALD, M. (1990) Neonatal capsiacin treatment induces invasion of the substantia gelatinosa by the terminal arborization of hair follicle afferents in the rat dorsal horn. *J. Comp. Neurol.* **296**: 23-31.

50. SHORTLAND, P. AND WOOLF, C.J. (1993) Chronic peripheral nerve section results in a rearrangement of the central terminals of axotomized A beta primary afferent neurons in the rat spinal cord. *J. Comp. Neurol.* **330**: 65-82.

51. SIEGAL, J.D., KLIOT, M., SMITH, G.M. AND SILVER J. (1990) A comparison of the regenerating potential of dorsal root fibers into grey or white matter of the adult rat spinal cord. *Exp. Neurol.* **109**: 90-97.

52. SIMONE, D.A., SORKIN, L.S., OH, U.T., CHUNG, J.M., OWENS, C., LAMOTTE, R.H. AND WILLIS, W.D. (1991) Neurogenic hyperalgesia: Central neural correlates in responses of spinothalamic tract neurons. *J. Neurophysiol.* **66**: 228-246.

53. SKENE, H.J.P. (1989) Axonal growth associated proteins. *Ann. Rev. Neurosci.* **12**: 127-156.

54. SKENE, J.H.P. AND WILLARD, M. (1981) Axonally transported proteins associated with axon growth in rabbit cental and peripheral nervous system. *J. Cell. Biol.* **89**: 96-103.

55. SKENE, J.H.P., JACOBSON, R.D., SNIPES, G.J., MCGURIE, C.B., NORDEN, J.J. AND FREEMAN, J.A. (1986) A protein induced during nerve growth (GAP-43) is a major component of growth cone membranes. *Science* **233**: 783-786.

56. SOMMERVAILLE, T., REYNOLDS, M.L. AND WOOLF, C.J. (1991) Time-dependent differences in the increase in GAP-43 expression in dorsal root ganglion cells after peripheral axotomy. *Neurosci.* **45**: 213-220.

57. SUGIMOTO, T., BENNETT, G.J. AND KAJANDER, K.C. (1990) Transsynaptic degeneration in the superficial dorsal horn after sciatic nerve injury: effects of a chronic constriction injury, transection and strychnine. *Pain* **42**: 205-213.

58. SWETT, J.E. AND WOOLF, C.J. (1985) Somatotopic organization of primary afferent terminals in the superficial dorsal horn of the rat spinal cord. *J. Comp. Neurol.* **231**: 66-71.

59. TETZLAFF,, W., ZWIERS, H., LEDERIS, K., CASSAR, L., RICHARDSON, P. AND BISBY M.A. (1989) Axonal transport and localization of B-50/GAP-43-like immunoreactivity in regenerating sciatic and facial nerves of the

rat. *J. Neurosci.* **9**: 1303-1313.

60. THOMPSON, S.W.N., KING, A.E. AND WOOLF, C.J. (1990) Activity-dependent changes in rat ventral horn neurons *in vitro*; summation of prolonged afferent evoked postsynaptic depolarizations produce a D-2-amino-5-phosphonovaleric acid sensitive windup. *Eur. J. Neurosci.* **2**: 638-649.

61. TOREBJÖRK, H.E., LUNDBERG, L.E.R. AND LAMOTTE, R.H. (1992) Central changes in processing of mechanoreceptor input in capsaicin-induced sensory hyperalgesia in humans. *J. Physiol.* **448**: 765-780.

62. VAN DER ZEE, C.E.E.M., NIELANDER, H.B., VOS, J.P., DA SILVA, S.L., VERHAAGEN, J., OESTREICHER, A.B., SCHRAMA, L.H., SCHOTMAN, P. AND GISPEN, W.H. (1989) Expression of growth-associated protein B-50 (GAP43) in dorsal root ganglia and sciatic nerve during regenerative sprouting. *J. Neurosci.* **9**: 3505-3512.

63. VERGE, V.M., TETZLAFF, W., BISBY M.A. AND RICHARDSON, P.M. (1990) Influence of nerve growth factor on neurofilament gene expression in mature primary sensory neurons. *J. Neurosci.* **10**: 2018-2025.

64. VERGE, V.M., TETZLAFF, W., RICHARDSON, P.M. AND BISBY, M.A. (1990) Correlation between GAP43 and Nerve growth factor receptors in rat sensory neurons. *J. Neurosci.* **10**: 926-934.

65. WALL, P.D. AND GUTNICK, M. (1974) Ongoing activity in peripheral nerves: the physiology and pharmacology of impulses originating from a neuroma. *Exp. Neurol.* **43**: 580-593.

66. WALL, P.D., WAXMAN S. AND BASBAUM, A.I. (1974) Ongoing activity in peripheral nerve: injury discharge. *Exp. Neurol.* **45**: 576-589.

67. WALL, P.D. AND WOOLF, C.J. (1984) Muscle but not cutaneous C-afferent input produces prolonged increases in the excitability of the flexion reflex in the rat. *J. Physiol. (Lond).* **356**: 443-458.

68. WHITE, J.C. AND SWEET, W.H. (1969) *Pain and the neurosurgeon. A forty-year experience.* C.C. Thomas, Springfield, ILL.

69. WIRTH, F.R. AND RUTHERFORD, R.B. (1970) A civilian expeience with causalgia. *Arch. Surg.* **100**: 633-638.

70. WOOLF, C.J. (1983) Evidence for a central component of post-injury pain hypersensitivity. *Nature* **306**: 686-688.

71. WOOLF, C.J. (1991) Generation of acute pain: Central mechanisms. *Brit. Med. Bull.* **47**: 523-533.

72. WOOLF, C.J. AND KING, A.E. (1990) Dynamic alterations in the cutaneous mechanoreceptive fields of dorsal horn neurons in the rat spinal cord. *J. Neurosci.* **10**: 2717-2726.

73. WOOLF, C.J. AND THOMPSON, S.W.N. (1991) The induction and maintenance of central sensitization is dependent on N-methyl-D-aspartic acid receptor activation; implications for the treatment of post-injury pain hypersensitivity states. *Pain* **44**: 293-299.

74. WOOLF, C.J. AND WALL, P.D. (1986) The relative effectiveness of C primary afferent fibres of different origins in evoking a prolonged facilitation of the flexor reflex in the rat. *J. Neurosci.* **6**: 1433-1443.

74. WOOLF, C.J., REYNOLDS, M.L., MOLANDER, C., O'BRIEN, C., LINDSAY, R.M. AND BENOWITZ, L.I. (1990) GAP-43, a growth associated protein, appears in dorsal root ganglion cells and in the dorsal horn of the rat spinal cord following peripheral nerve injury. *Neuroscience* **34**: 465-478.

75. WOOLF, C.J., SHORTLAND, P. AND COGGESHALL, R.E. (1992) Peripheral nerv einjury triggers central sprouting of myelinated afferents. *Nature* **355**: 75-78.

76. XU, X-J., MAGGI, C.A. AND WIESENFELD-HALLIN, Z. (1991) On the role of NK-2 tachykinin receptors in the mediation of spinal reflex excitability in the rat. *Neuroscience* **44**: 483-490.

77. YANKER, B.A., BENOWITZ, L.I., VILLA-KOMAROFF, L. AND NEVE, R.L. (1990) Transfection of PC12 cells with the human GAP-43 gene: effects on neurite outgrowth and regeneration. *Molec. Brain. Res.* **7**: 39-44.

78. ZUBER, M.X., GOODMAN, D.W., KARNS, L.R. AND FISHMAN, M.C. (1989) The neuronal growth-associated protein GAP-43 induces filopodia in non-neuronal cells. *Science* **244**: 1193-1195.

LIST OF INVITED SPEAKERS

Dr Belmonte, Carlos
Univ. of Alicante
Campus de San Juan
Ap. Correos 374
E-03080 Alicante
Spain

Dr Besson, Jean-Marie
INSERM
Port Royal
75014 Paris
France

Dr Bregestovski Piotr
INSERM, U
161-2 Rue d'Alesia
75014 Paris
France

Dr Dolphin, Annette, C.
Dept. of Pharmacology
Royal Free Hosp. Sch. of Medicine
Rowland Hill St.
London NW3 2PF
Great Britain

Dr Dray, Andy
Sandoz Inst. for Medical Research
5 Gower Pl.
London WC1E 6BN
Great Britain

Dr French, Andrew, S.
Dept. Physiology
Faculty of Medicine
Univ. of Alberta
Edmonton, T6G 2H7
Canada

Dr Henry, James, L.
Dept. of Physiology
McGill University
McIntyre Med. Sci. Bld.
3655 Drummond St.
Montreal, QC, H3G 1Y6
Canada

Dr Holzer, Peter
Dept. Exp. and Clin. Pharmacol.
Univ. of Graz
Universitatsplatz 4
A-8010 Graz
Austria

Dr Hunt, Stephen, P.
Molecular Neurobiology Unit
MRC Centre Hills Rd.
Cambridge CB2 2QH
Great Britain

Dr Iadarola, Michael, J.
Neurobiol. and Anesthesiol. Branch
NIDR, NIH
Bethesda, Maryland 20892
U.S.A.

Dr Jeftinija, Srdija
Dept. Vet. Anatomy
Iowa State Univ.
Ames, IA 50011
U.S.A.

Dr Mendell, Lorne, M.
Dept. of Neurobiol. and Behavior
SUNY at Stony Brook
College of Arts and Sciences
Stony Brook, N.Y. 11794-5230
U.S.A.

Dr Lev-Tov, Aharon
Dept. Anatomy
The Hebrew Univ. Med. Sch.
Jerusalem 91010
Israel

Nistri, Andrea
SISSA
Strada Costiera 11
34014 Trieste
Italy

Dr Lodge, David
Lilly Res CTR Ltd.
Erl Wood Manor
Windlesham
Surrey GU20 6PH
Great Britain

Dr Reeh, Peter, W.
Inst. of Physiol. and Biocybernetics
Univ. of Erlangen-Nurnberg
Universitatsstr. 17.
D-8520 Erlangen
Germany

Dr Maggi, Carlo, A.
Ind. Farmac. Riunite Menarini
Pharmacol. Dept. Research Labs.
Via Sette Santi
3 I-50131 Firenze
Italy

Dr Schaible, Hans-Georg
Dept. Physiology
Univ. Würzburg, Röntgenring 9
D-8700 Würzburg
Germany

Dr Meller, Stephen, T.
Dept. Pharmacology
University of Iowa
Iowa City, IA 52242
U.S.A.

Dr Schmidt, Robert, F.
Dept. Physiology
Univ. Würzburg
Röntgenring 9
D-8700 Würzburg
Germany

Dr Stoney, David, S. Jr.
Dept. of Physiol. and Endocrinol.
Med. Coll. of Georgia
Augusta, Ga 30912
U.S.A.

Dr Surprenant, Annmarie
Vollum Institute for Advanced
Biomedical Research
Oregon Health Sciences University
L-474, 3181 SW. Sam Jackson Rd.
Portland, Oregon 97201-3098
U.S.A.

Dr Urban, Laszlo
Dept. Pharmacology
Sandoz Inst. for Medical Research
5 Gower Pl.
London WC1E 6BN
Great Britain

Dr Weihe, Eberhard
Dept. of Anatomy
Johannes Gutenberg-Univ.
Saarstr. 19-21
D-6500 Mainz
Germany

Dr Wiesenfeld-Hallin Zsuzsanna
Dept. Clinical Neurophysiology
Huddinge Univ. Hospital Karolinska
Institute S-141 86 Huddinge
Sweden

Dr Willis, William D.
Dept. of Anat. and Neurosciences
Marine Biomed Inst.
Univ. of Texas, Medical
Branch at Galveston
200 University Boulevard
Galveston TX 77550-2772.
U.S.A.

Dr Woolf, Clifford, J.
Cerebral Function Group
Dept. of Anatomy
University College of London
Gower St.
London
WC1E 6BT
Great Britain

SUBJECT INDEX

1,S,3R-ACPD, 178

2-amino-5-phosphonovaleric acid (APV), 246

8 Br-Cyclic AMP, 386

Absolute re refractory period, 67
Acetaminophen, 454
Acetylcholine, 123
Adaptation, 24
    and Ca-ions, 27
Allodynia, 475
Aminocyclopentane-dicarboxylic acid (ACPD), 178
AMPA receptors, 165,173,405
    interaction with NMDA, 165
Arthritis
    and *fos* expression, 450
    carrageenan, 407
    Freund's adjuvant, 450
L-aspartate, 174,185
Axon reflex, 139
Axotomy, 10, 361
    and neuropeptides, 361
    and protooncogenes, 300

Bradykinin (BK), 94,120,279,387
    and EAA release, 189
    B2 receptors, 280
    mechanism of action, 280
BDNF, 283
Branch point filtering, 63
    and geometrical ratio, 76
    and safety factor, 76
    in DRG cells, 65

C fiber, 87,89,196
    and hyperexcitability, 380
    c-fos, and *c-jun* (see also protooncogenes), 297
C neuron, 70
CCK, 366
Calcium channel, 5,48,98
    voltage dependent, 47
Capsaicin, 96,134

    and EAA release, 187
    and extravasation, 278
    and ion channels, 100
    and protons, 278
    and STT cells, 423
Carbon dioxide, 92
Carrageenan, 407
CGRP, 95,142,340,347,381
Chemoreceptors, 87
Chemosensitivity, 78,119
    and neuroma, 109
    and pH, 105
    ionic basis, 98
Choline acetyltransferase (ChAT), 38
cIEG transcription factor, 323
CNQX, 176,196,202
Conduction velocity
    and temperature, 73
    computer simulation, 76
Cornea
    and polymodal receptors, 89
Current
    L type, 49,227
    P type, 49
    N type, 75,277
CP 96,345, 220,240
Cytokines, 284,353

Des-Arg^9-Leu^8-BK, 280
Diltiazem, 102
DNQX, 176
Dorsal horn neurons
    anatomical classification, 232
    and sensory fibers, 232
    functional classification, 234
    molecular plasticity, 350

Dorsal root ganglion (DRG) cells, 3
    and conduction velocity, 72
    and EAA release, 185
    and ionic currents, 4,48
    and types, 6,73
    effect of trophic factors
    in organotypic culture, 186

Enteric nervous system, 35

EPSP
    and AP4 receptors, 156
    monosynaptic, motoneurons, 152
    polysynaptic, motoneurons, 155
Excitatory amino acid (EAA) receptors
    and hyperexcitability, 209,379,399
    in inflammation, 195
    in mechanical hyperalgesia, 414
    in the hippocampus, 161
    in thermal hyperalgesia, 411
    in the spinal cord, 151,173
    metabotropic, 167,178
    non-NMDA, 176
    pharmacology, 174
    release, 185
Experimental inflammation
    knee joint, 197
Extravasation, 278

Flare, 139

GABA receptor, 55
    in primary afferents, 340
Galanin, 361
    and autotomy, 364
    and spinal inhibition, 364
GAP 43, 305
    and sprouting, 477
    in inflammation, 347
Gel mobility shift assay, 315
Glia
    and EAA release, 189
L-glutamate, 174,185
G protein, 41, 51, 276
GTP-gamma-S, 41,49
GYKI52466, 177

H neuron, 70
Habituation, 421
Heat sensitivity, 129
Hippocampus, 161
Histamine, 123
HPLC, 186
Hyperalgesia
    and receptor sensitization, 128
    effects of L-NAME, 405

Inflammation
    and neuropeptides, 346
    and silent fibers, 292
    neurogenic, 133
Inflammatory
    "soup", 96,120
    substances,94,119

Ketamine, 201
Knee joint
    and inflammation, 195

Least conduction interval (LCI), 67

Magnesium ions
    and NMDA receptors, 208,385
Mechanoreceptors, 87
    and ion channels, 21
    and sensitization, 129
Merkel cell
    action on nociceptors, 343
Motoneurons, 152
    and EAA receptors, 152

N neuron, 105
L-NAME, 245,405,439
    and acute hyperalgesia, 405
    and carrageenan, 407
    and chronic hyperalgesia, 405
NBQX, 176
Nerve ligarion, 405
    effects of L-NAME, 406
Neurokinin 1-3 receptors,218
    NK1 receptor upregulation, 346
Neurokinins (see also tachykinins)
    neurokinin A, 218,340,386
    neurokinin B, 218
    NK1 receptor upregulation, 346
Neuroma, 109
Neuropeptides
    and herpes virus, 348
    release, 138
Neurotrophins, 283
NGF
    and DRG, 9,274,283
    and expression of receptors, 283
    and hyperalgesia, 284,343
Nitric oxide (NO)126,353
    and axotomy, 352
    and hyperalgesia, 401
    and NMDA receptors, 401,439
    and SP, 244
NMDA receptors, 161
    and desensitization, 163
    and EPSP, 152
    and hyperexcitability, 379, 427
    and PKC, 162,385
    in neuropathy, 474
    modulation, 161
NMDA current
    time course, 162
Nociception
    and cellular phenotype, 337

in inflamed joint, 202
in normal joint, 199
Nociceptive neurons, 87
and polymodality, 87
Nociceptor, 88
and hypertonic saline, 96
and protons, 91
and sensitization, 119
in the cornea, 88
types, 89
Non-NMDA receptors
and EPSP, 152
NPY, 339
Opioid peptides
and immune cells, 344
in peripheral antinociception, 345
Opioid receptors
induction in inflammation, 344
role in peripheral fibers, 274

PC12 pheochromocytoma cells, 321
Peripheral nerve injury
and nitric oxide, 362
and neuropeptides, 361
and upregulation of CCK, 366,368
Polymodality
of sensory neurons, 103
Potassium conductance
and sensrymotor neurons, 40
and TRH in motoneurons, 262
PPT gene, 217
Primary afferent fibers, 63,88,
and chemical environment, 273
and opioid receptors, 274
as local effectors, 133, 340
heterogeneity, 135
plasticity of central terminals, 473
silent fibers, 289
Pro-dynorphin (see also opioid), 339
Pro-enkephalin (see also opioid), 339
Prostaglandins
PGE2, 95,120
Protein kinase C (PKC), 162
role in receptor interaction, 385
Protons, 91,105
and capsaicin, 278
Protooncogenes, 297,314,449
and nerve lesion, 300
and neurotrophins, 306
expression afterstimulation, 298
dynorphin gene expression, 322
induced by cold stimulation, 461
in sustained hyperactivity, 449
in vitro expression, 304

Quisqualate, 173

Receptive field, 206
and EAA receptor blockers, 206
Receptors
chemo-, 78,119
in sensorymotor neurons, 42
mechano-, 18
tachykinin, 217
RP 67,580, 220
Ruthenium red, 187

Safety factor, 76
Sensitization
central mechanisms, 438,476
of silent fibers, 292
of substantia gelatinosa, 232
Sensorymotor neurons, 35
and plasticity, 297
Serotonin (5-HT), 120
Silent primary afferents, 289
during inflammation, 291
in normal joint, 290
Somatostatin, 361
Spatio-temporal filtering, 81
Spinothalamic tract cells (STT), 421
dynamic changes in injury, 421
Sprouting
induced by injury, 473
Submucosal neurons, 36
Substance P, 95,123,217,237,347
and CP 96,345, 240
and hyperexcitability, 353,430
and motoneurons, 255
and nitric oxide, 244
mechanism of action, 244
Tachykinin receptors (see also
neurokinins),217
and pain, 224,338,383
antagonists, 219
heterogeneity, 221
in motoneurons, 259
in the dorsal horn, 389
modulating NMDA receptors,
379,430
Tachykinin release
and synaptic activation, 231
Tetraethylammonium (TEA), 74
Tetrodotoxin (TTX), 4,28,187,259,277
resistant Na-channel, 4
Thermal stimulation, 450
Transient transfection Assay, 318
TRH
and motoneurons, 255
Trigeminal neurons, 104

UV-irradiation, 284

VIP, 38
    and hyperalgesia, 353
WDR neurons, 201
    and NMDA, 209, 389
Windup, 13,196,229,379,388,421

Printing: Druckhaus Beltz, Hemsbach
Binding: Buchbinderei Schäffer, Grünstadt

NATO ASI Series H

Vol. 1: Biology and Molecular Biology of Plant-Pathogen Interactions.
Edited by J.A. Bailey. 415 pages. 1986.

Vol. 2: Glial-Neuronal Communication in Development and Regeneration.
Edited by H.H. Althaus and W. Seifert. 865 pages. 1987.

Vol. 3: Nicotinic Acetylcholine Receptor: Structure and Function.
Edited by A. Maelicke. 489 pages. 1986.

Vol. 4: Recognition in Microbe-Plant Symbiotic and Pathogenic Interactions.
Edited by B. Lugtenberg. 449 pages. 1986.

Vol. 5: Mesenchymal-Epithelial Interactions in Neural Development.
Edited by J. R. Wolff, J. Sievers, and M. Berry. 428 pages. 1987.

Vol. 6: Molecular Mechanisms of Desensitization to Signal Molecules.
Edited by T M. Konijn, P J. M. Van Haastert, H. Van der Starre,
H. Van der Wel, and M.D. Houslay. 336 pages. 1987.

Vol. 7: Gangliosides and Modulation of Neuronal Functions.
Edited by H. Rahmann. 647 pages. 1987.

Vol. 8: Molecular and Cellular Aspects of Erythropoietin and Erythropoiesis.
Edited by I.N. Rich. 460 pages. 1987.

Vol. 9: Modification of Cell to Cell Signals During Normal and Pathological Aging.
Edited by S. Govoni and F. Battaini. 297 pages. 1987.

Vol. 10: Plant Hormone Receptors. Edited by D. Klämbt. 319 pages. 1987.

Vol. 11: Host-Parasite Cellular and Molecular Interactions in Protozoal Infections.
Edited by K.-P. Chang and D. Snary. 425 pages. 1987.

Vol. 12: The Cell Surface in Signal Transduction.
Edited by E. Wagner, H. Greppin, and B. Millet. 243 pages. 1987.

Vol. 13: Toxicology of Pesticides: Experimental, Clinical and Regulatory
Perspectives. Edited by L.G. Costa, C.L. Galli, and S.D. Murphy.
320 pages. 1987.

Vol. 14: Genetics of Translation. New Approaches.
Edited by M.F. Tuite, M. Picard, and M. Bolotin-Fukuhara. 524 pages. 1988.

Vol. 15: Photosensitisation. Molecular, Cellular and Medical Aspects.
Edited by G. Moreno, R. H. Pottier, and T. G. Truscott. 521 pages. 1988.

Vol. 16: Membrane Biogenesis. Edited by J.A.F Op den Kamp. 477 pages. 1988.

Vol. 17: Cell to Cell Signals in Plant, Animal and Microbial Symbiosis.
Edited by S. Scannerini, D. Smith, P. Bonfante-Fasolo, and V. Gianinazzi-
Pearson. 414 pages. 1988.

Vol. 18: Plant Cell Biotechnology.
Edited by M.S.S. Pais, F. Mavituna, and J. M. Novais. 500 pages. 1988.

Vol. 19: Modulation of Synaptic Transmission and Plasticity in Nervous Systems.
Edited by G. Hertting and H.-C. Spatz. 457 pages. 1988.

Vol. 20: Amino Acid Availability and Brain Function in Health and Disease.
Edited by G. Huether. 487 pages. 1988.

NATO ASI Series H

Vol. 21: Cellular and Molecular Basis of Synaptic Transmission.
Edited by H. Zimmermann. 547 pages. 1988.

Vol. 22: Neural Development and Regeneration. Cellular and Molecular Aspects.
Edited by A. Gorio, J. R. Perez-Polo, J. de Vellis, and B. Haber. 711 pages.
1988.

Vol. 23: The Semiotics of Cellular Communication in the Immune System.
Edited by E.E. Sercarz, F. Celada, N.A. Mitchison, and T. Tada. 326 pages.
1988.

Vol. 24: Bacteria, Complement and the Phagocytic Cell.
Edited by F. C. Cabello und C. Pruzzo. 372 pages. 1988.

Vol. 25: Nicotinic Acetylcholine Receptors in the Nervous System.
Edited by F. Clementi, C. Gotti, and E. Sher. 424 pages. 1988.

Vol. 26: Cell to Cell Signals in Mammalian Development.
Edited by S.W. de Laat, J.G. Bluemink, and C.L. Mummery. 322 pages.
1989.

Vol. 27: Phytotoxins and Plant Pathogenesis.
Edited by A. Graniti, R. D. Durbin, and A. Ballio. 508 pages. 1989.

Vol. 28: Vascular Wilt Diseases of Plants. Basic Studies and Control.
Edited by E. C. Tjamos and C. H. Beckman. 590 pages. 1989.

Vol. 29: Receptors, Membrane Transport and Signal Transduction.
Edited by A. E. Evangelopoulos, J. P. Changeux, L. Packer, T. G.
Sotiroudis, and K.W.A. Wirtz. 387 pages. 1989.

Vol. 30: Effects of Mineral Dusts on Cells.
Edited by B.T. Mossman and R.O. Begin. 470 pages. 1989.

Vol. 31: Neurobiology of the Inner Retina.
Edited by R. Weiler and N.N. Osborne. 529 pages. 1989.

Vol. 32: Molecular Biology of Neuroreceptors and Ion Channels.
Edited by A. Maelicke. 675 pages. 1989.

Vol. 33: Regulatory Mechanisms of Neuron to Vessel Communication in Brain.
Edited by F. Battaini, S. Govoni, M.S. Magnoni, and M. Trabucchi.
416 pages. 1989.

Vol. 34: Vectors asTools for the Study of Normal and Abnormal Growth and
Differentiation.
Edited by H. Lother, R. Dernick, and W. Ostertag. 477 pages. 1989.

Vol. 35: Cell Separation in Plants: Physiology, Biochemistry and Molecular
Biology. Edited by D. J. Osborne and M. B. Jackson. 449 pages. 1989.

Vol. 36: Signal Molecules in Plants and Plant-Microbe Interactions.
Edited by B.J.J. Lugtenberg. 425 pages. 1989.

Vol. 37: Tin-Based Antitumour Drugs. Edited by M. Gielen. 226 pages. 1990.

Vol. 38: The Molecular Biology of Autoimmune Disease.
Edited by A.G. Demaine, J-P. Banga, and A.M. McGregor. 404 pages.
1990.

NATO ASI Series H

Vol. 39: Chemosensory Information Processing.
Edited by D. Schild. 403 pages. 1990.

Vol. 40: Dynamics and Biogenesis of Membranes.
Edited by J. A. F. Op den Kamp. 367 pages. 1990.

Vol. 41: Recognition and Response in Plant-Virus Interactions.
Edited by R. S. S. Fraser. 467 pages. 1990.

Vol. 42: Biomechanics of Active Movement and Deformation of Cells.
Edited by N. Akkas. 524 pages. 1990.

Vol. 43: Cellular and Molecular Biology of Myelination.
Edited by G. Jeserich, H. H. Althaus, and T. V. Waehneldt. 565 pages.
1990.

Vol. 44: Activation and Desensitization of Transducing Pathways.
Edited by T. M. Konijn, M. D. Houslay, and P. J. M. Van Haastert.
336 pages. 1990.

Vol. 45: Mechanism of Fertilization: Plants to Humans.
Edited by B. Dale. 710 pages. 1990.

Vol .46: Parallels in Cell to Cell Junctions in Plants and Animals.
Edited by A. W Robards, W. J . Lucas, J . D. Pitts, H . J . Jongsma,
and D. C. Spray. 296 pages. 1990.

Vol. 47: Signal Perception and Transduction in Higher Plants.
Edited by R. Ranjeva and A. M. Boudet. 357 pages. 1990.

Vol. 48: Calcium Transport and Intracellular Calcium Homeostasis.
Edited by D. Pansu and F. Bronner. 456 pages. 1990.

Vol. 49: Post-Transcriptional Control of Gene Expression.
Edited by J. E. G. McCarthy and M. F. Tuite. 671 pages. 1990.

Vol. 50: Phytochrome Properties and Biological Action.
Edited by B. Thomas and C. B. Johnson. 337 pages. 1991.

Vol. 51: Cell to Cell Signals in Plants and Animals.
Edited by V. Neuhoff and J. Friend. 404 pages. 1991.

Vol. 52: Biological Signal Transduction.
Edited by E. M . Ross and K . W. A. Wirtz. 560 pages. 1991.

Vol. 53: Fungal Cell Wall and Immune Response.
Edited by J. P. Latge and D. Boucias. 472 pages. 1991.

Vol. 54: The Early Effects of Radiation on DNA.
Edited by E. M. Fielden and P. O'Neill. 448 pages. 1991.

Vol. 55: The Translational Apparatus of Photosynthetic Organelles.
Edited by R. Mache, E. Stutz, and A. R. Subramanian. 260 pages. 1991.

Vol. 56: Cellular Regulation by Protein Phosphorylation.
Edited by L. M. G. Heilmeyer, Jr. 520 pages. 1991.

NATO ASI Series H

Vol. 57: Molecular Techniques in Taxonomy.
Edited by G . M . Hewitt, A. W. B. Johnston, and J. P. W. Young .
420 pages. 1991.

Vol. 58: Neurocytochemical Methods.
Edited by A. Calas and D. Eugene. 352 pages. 1991.

Vol. 59: Molecular Evolution of the Major Histocompatibility Complex.
Edited by J. Klein and D. Klein. 522 pages. 1991.

Vol. 60: Intracellular Regulation of Ion Channels.
Edited by M. Morad and Z. Agus. 261 pages. 1992.

Vol. 61: Prader-Willi Syndrome and Other Chromosome 15q Deletion Disorders.
Edited by S. B. Cassidy. 277 pages. 1992.

Vol. 62: Endocytosis. From Cell Biology to Health, Disease and Therapie.
Edited by P. J. Courtoy. 547 pages. 1992.

Vol. 63: Dynamics of Membrane Assembly.
Edited by J. A. F. Op den Kamp. 402 pages. 1992.

Vol. 64: Mechanics of Swelling. From Clays to Living Cells and Tissues.
Edited by T. K. Karalis. 802 pages. 1992.

Vol. 65: Bacteriocins, Microcins and Lantibiotics.
Edited by R. James, C. Lazdunski, and F. Pattus. 530 pages. 1992.

Vol. 66: Theoretical and Experimental Insights into Immunology.
Edited by A. S. Perelson and G. Weisbuch. 497 pages. 1992.

Vol. 67: Flow Cytometry. New Developments.
Edited by A. Jacquemin-Sablon. 1993.

Vol. 68: Biomarkers. Research and Application in the Assessment of
Environmental Health. Edited by D. B. Peakall and L. R. Shugart.
138 pages. 1993.

Vol. 69: Molecular Biology and its Application to Medical Mycology.
Edited by B. Maresca, G. S. Kobayashi, and H. Yamaguchi. 271 pages.
1993.

Vol. 70: Phospholipids and Signal Transmission.
Edited by R. Massarelli, L. A. Horrocks, J. N. Kanfer, and K. Löffelholz.
448 pages. 1993.

Vol. 71: Protein Synthesis and Targeting in Yeast.
Edited by A. J. P. Brown, M. F. Tuite, and J. E. G. McCarthy. 425 pages.
1993.

Vol. 72: Chromosome Segregation and Aneuploidy.
Edited by B. K. Vig. 425 pages. 1993.

Vol. 73: Human Apolipoprotein Mutants III. In Diagnosis and Treatment.
Edited by C. R. Sirtori, G. Franceschini, B. H. Brewer Jr. 302 pages. 1993.

NATO ASI Series H

Vol. 74: Molecular Mechanisms of Membrane Traffic.
Edited by D. J. Morré, K. E. Howell, and J. J. M. Bergeron. 429 pages.
1993.

Vol. 75: Cancer Therapy. Differentiation, Immunomodulation and Angiogenesis.
Edited by N. D'Alessandro, E. Mihich, L. Rausa, H. Tapiero, and T. R.Tritton.
299 pages. 1993.

Vol. 76: Tyrosine Phosphorylation/Dephosphorylation and Downstream Signalling.
Edited by L. M. G. Heilmeyer Jr. 388 pages. 1993.

Vol. 77: Ataxia-Telangiectasia. Edited by R. A. Gatti, R. B. Painter. 306 pages. 1993.

Vol. 78: Toxoplasmosis. Edited by J. E. Smith. 272 pages. 1993.

Vol. 79: Cellular Mechanisms of Sensory Processing. The Somatosensory System.
Edited by L. Urban. 514 pages. 1994.

Vol. 80: Autoimmunity: Experimental Aspects.
Edited by M. Zouali. 318 pages. 1994.

Springer-Verlag
and the Environment

We at Springer-Verlag firmly believe that an international science publisher has a special obligation to the environment, and our corporate policies consistently reflect this conviction.

We also expect our business partners – paper mills, printers, packaging manufacturers, etc. – to commit themselves to using environmentally friendly materials and production processes.

The paper in this book is made from low- or no-chlorine pulp and is acid free, in conformance with international standards for paper permanency.